MW00685420

Atlas of Minimally Invasive Surgery

Editor-in-Chief
Daniel B. Jones, M.D.

Chief of Minimally Invasive Surgical Services, Beth Israel Deaconess Medical Center
Associate Professor of Surgery, Harvard Medical School

Associate Editor
Shishir K. Maithel, M.D.

Minimally Invasive Surgical Services, Beth Israel Deaconess Medical Center
Clinical Fellow in Surgery, Harvard Medical School

Associate Editor
Benjamin E. Schneider, M.D.

Minimally Invasive Surgical Services, Beth Israel Deaconess Medical Center
Instructor in Surgery, Harvard Medical School

Illustrations by Brooks Hart, C.M.I.

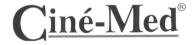

Published by: Cine-Med, Inc.
                  127 Main Street North
                  Woodbury, CT 06798
                  203-263-0006

Copyright © 2006

All rights reserved. No part of this publication may be reproduced, stored in a retrieval system, or transmitted in any form or by any means electronic, mechanical, photocopied, recorded, or otherwise, without prior written permission of the publisher.

ISBN: 0-9749358-7-5

Publisher   Kevin McGovern

Project Manager   Mary Panagrosso

Book and Cover Design   Cara McArdle Forbes

Notice: Our knowledge in clinical sciences is constantly changing. As new information becomes available, changes in treatment and in the use of drugs or medical devices become necessary. The authors and the publisher of this volume have taken care to make certain that the doses of drugs, uses of medical devices, and schedules of treatment are correct and compatible with the standards generally accepted at the time of publication. The reader is advised to consult carefully the instruction and information material included in the package insert of each drug or therapeutic agent before administration. This advice is especially important when using new or infrequently used drugs. One must be thoroughly conversant with any drugs used in order to advise the patient about signs and symptoms of potential adverse reactions and incompatibilities.

Printed in Canada

About the Editors

DANIEL B. JONES is Chief of Minimally Invasive Surgical Services, Beth Israel Deaconess Medical Center, Boston, Massachusetts, and Associate Professor of Surgery, Harvard Medical School. He is the founder of the Southwestern Center for Minimally Invasive Surgery in Dallas and is co-director of the Center for Minimally Invasive Surgery at the Harvard teaching hospitals. An internationally recognized leader in the field, he is the author of more than 150 professional publications. Dr. Jones is the recipient of the James IV Association Travel Award (2005) and the SAGES Gold Laparoscope Award (2001). He serves on the Society of American Gastrointestinal and Endoscopic Surgeons Board of Governors, and he is an active member of the American College of Surgeons, Society for Surgery of the Alimentary Tract Foundation, the Association of Surgical Education, and the American Society for Bariatric Surgery. He received his M.D. from Cornell University Medical College and Masters in Medical Management from the University of Texas at Dallas.

SHISHIR K. MAITHEL is a Clinical Fellow in Surgery at Beth Israel Deaconess Medical Center. He has completed a combined research fellowship in minimally invasive surgery at Beth Israel Deaconess Medical Center and Massachusetts General Hospital. He is also the author of *Critical Care: Physiology and Management*, and is active in the American College of Surgeons, Society of American Gastrointestinal and Endoscopic Surgeons, Society for Surgery of the Alimentary Tract, and American Hepato-Pancreato-Biliary Association. He received his M.D. from the University of Chicago, Pritzker School of Medicine, Chicago, Illinois.

BENJAMIN E. SCHNEIDER is a Surgical Faculty in Minimally Invasive Surgical Services, Beth Israel Deaconess Medical Center and Instructor in Surgery, Harvard Medical School. He completed postgraduate MIS Fellowship training at UT Southwestern and Beth Israel Deaconess Medical Center. He is a member of the American College of Surgeons, Society of American Gastrointestinal and Endoscopic Surgeons, Society for Surgery of the Alimentary Tract, and American Society for Bariatric Surgery. He received his M.D. from the University of Colorado, Denver.

Dedication

The editors wish to thank the numerous teachers who donated their valuable time and expertise to our education, in particular our department chairs: Samuel A. Wells, Jr., G. Tom Shires, C. James Carrico, Carol Scott-Conner, and Josef E. Fischer. This text represents on our part a humble attempt at pedagogical atonement. We believe that surgeons in practice will find this atlas to be a useful reference in their adoption of new techniques.

We wish to dedicate this text to those who have suffered from our absence on late nights and weekends. In particular, we thank our spouses, Stephanie, Sheetal, and Janie, and children, Ryan, Cara, Leah, Karina, Benjamin, and William.

Additionally, we thank our contributors and Ciné-Med, without whom this text could not have possibly been completed, let alone on schedule.

Daniel B. Jones, M.D.

Shishir K. Maithel, M.D.

Benjamin E. Schneider, M.D.

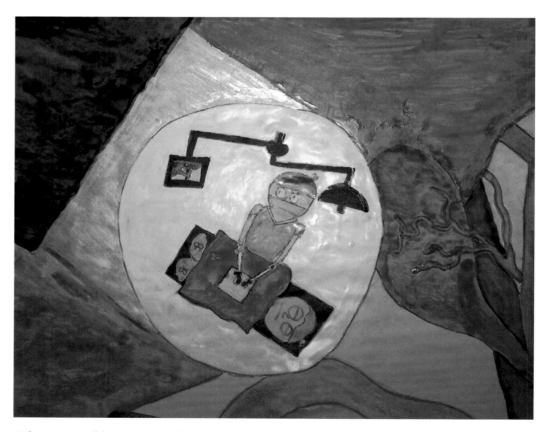

This is a self-portrait of Ryan M. Jones, age 10, titled "When I grow up," based on observations from Beth Israel Deaconess Skills and Simulation Lab and anatomical illustrations scattered throughout his home in preparation of the Atlas of Minimally Invasive Surgery.

Atlas of Minimally Invasive Surgery
Table of Contents

Dedication IV

Foreword 3

Contributors 6

Operating Endosuite 11

Biliary Surgery

Cholecystectomy 12

Common Bile Duct Exploration 40

Cholecystojejunostomy 72

Foregut Surgery

Nissen Fundoplication 98

Paraesophageal Hernia 128

Heller Myotomy 144

Partial Gastrectomy 166

Management of Peptic Ulcer Disease 196

Gastrojejunostomy 226

Enteral Access

Gastrostomy (T-Fasteners Technique) 244

Janeway Permanent Gastrostomy 262

Jejunostomy 276

Obesity Surgery

Roux-en-Y Gastric Bypass 298

Adjustable Gastric Banding 332

Solid Organ

Hepatic Resection 356

Adrenalectomy 382

Distal Pancreatectomy 406

Splenectomy 430

Nephrectomy 460

Thoracic

Pulmonary Wedge Resection 484

Esophagectomy 496

Hernia

Inguinal 524

Transabdominal Preperitoneal Repair (TAPP) 526

Totally Extraperitoneal Repair (TEP) 536

Ventral 550

Colorectal

Colectomy 570

Right Colectomy 572

Left Colectomy 594

Low Anterior Resection (LAR) 602

Abdominoperineal Resection (APR) 610

Appendectomy 626

Foreword

Josef E. Fischer, M.D.

Twenty years ago, a leader of American surgery declared general surgery dead. The corollary of that statement was that people should stop worrying about general surgery, abandon it, and let general surgery evolve into a series of subspecialties without the mother church, as it were, to survive.

Three individuals, George Block, Ward Griffen, and Alexander Walt, stepped into the breach and kept general surgery alive. Two cardiac surgeons, W. Gerald Austin, then Chair at the Massachusetts General Hospital, and Frank Spencer, Chair at New York University Medical Center, also helped keep general surgery alive socioeconomically by reviving the role that the American College of Surgeons had representing general surgery. And while perhaps things socioeconomically have not turned out as well as they might have, this appears to be more the desire of CMS or its antecedent, Medicare, to do things like devalue "overvalued procedures," most of which were general surgery procedures such as cholecystectomies, colectomies, and hernias. My comment on that was, "Who said they were overvalued, on what basis did they say they were overvalued, and why in fact were they considered overvalued?" This devaluation poses not only a perpetual detriment to the field of general surgery, but presumably also poses future difficulties for patients' access to care.

But I wander. The fact is that minimally invasive surgery saved general surgery. It rekindled the interest, it made young people aware of the fact that general surgery was doing something that was novel, which was forward-looking, which was forthright, and which benefited patients by performing procedures in a less traumatic fashion.

Initially, minimally invasive surgery started in the private sector and academic medical centers were woefully slow in teaching other surgeons how to do minimally invasive procedures or integrating it into their own residency programs. Indeed, although progress has been made in the latter area as far as integrating it into general surgical training, the number of post-general surgery fellowships in minimally invasive surgery speaks volumes to the fact that most people who finish general surgery training programs do not feel adequately trained in minimally invasive surgery.

Minimally invasive surgery, although extraordinarily popular and forward-looking, remains a technique. I consider that extremely unfortunate and would have hoped that by now there would be a science surrounding minimally invasive surgery. There would be a science concerning the metabolic changes or lack of metabolic changes, the advantages, the immunologic changes as compared to open general surgery, but alas, none of these have been forthcoming. Thus, minimally invasive surgery will remain a technique, at least for the foreseeable future, only to be replaced when another, better, technique takes its place.

In an effort to improve the training of general surgeons in minimally invasive surgery, the American College of Surgeons has established a system of accreditation of surgical skills laboratories, which will become standardized throughout the country. There will be two model laboratories, there will be approximately 30 comprehensive surgical skills laboratories, and the rest will be basic surgical skills laboratories. The Residency Review Committee has committed itself to having each residency program have at least a basic surgical skills laboratory by the year 2008 as defined by the American College of Surgeons, and additionally, has tied the 10% educational work hours exemption to surgical skills labs and minimally invasive teaching in surgical residencies.

It is highly unlikely that a surgical resident or indeed, a surgical staff or faculty member, can learn everything they need to know by going to a surgical skills lab alone, and that is the reason for this atlas. There is an immense need for an inexpensive, clearly illustrated book as to how to do the common, both basic and advanced, minimally invasive procedures. This volume accomplishes that goal admirably. The drawings are to the point and clearly illustrate the critical steps in carrying out various minimally invasive procedures. They are not tremendously lifelike but close enough so that the surgeon should be able to learn how to do the procedure. It is clear that this atlas assumes some knowledge of minimally invasive surgery on the part of the reader who will be doing the procedure.

One additional device that the authors have, I suspect, borrowed from *Mastery of Surgery*, of which Dr. Jones is an assistant editor, is the commentary by 70 experts. In an effort to be direct and to the point, the text is somewhat directed and terse, and the experience, as well as the writing of the surgical minimally invasive gurus, many of whom are represented in this book, will help to explain the nuances of the various procedures.

I am enthusiastic about this volume. It meets a real need, and as far as I'm aware, does not have any peers or competitors in the area. It is very well done by Dr. Jones, a leader in the field and the Chief of our Minimally Invasive Laboratory and Section, who has taken the minimally invasive laboratory, which he built from scratch in this institution, to the leadership of surgical skills centers in the United States. The quality of the commentaries also is superb and adds a great deal to the value of the book. True, some of the commentaries are slightly terse and are almost in code, but given some experience, the reader will well understand what the commentators, first-class all, are getting at.

As for the co-authors, Dr. Schneider, an extremely promising and excellent clinical surgeon who is devoted to the residents and the residents to him, and Dr. Maithel, a resident, who has spent a profitable 2 years in the laboratory, have put this book together. Hurray for them!

Josef E. Fischer, M.D.
Chairman, Department of Surgery
Surgeon-in-Chief
Beth Israel Deaconess Medical Center
McDermott Professor of Surgery
Harvard Medical School
Boston, Massachusetts

Contributors

Jeff W. Allen, M.D.
Associate Professor of Surgery
University of Louisville
Louisville, Kentucky

Horacio J. Asbun, M.D.
Director
Minimal Access and Robotic Surgery
John Muir Health
Walnut Creek, California

Stanley W. Ashley, M.D.
Brigham and Women's Hospital
Frank Sawyer Professor and Vice Chairman
Harvard Medical School
Boston, Massachusetts

Robert Bailey, M.D.
Director – Miami Laparoscopic Center
University of Miami
Miami, Florida

George L. Blackburn, M.D., Ph.D.
Beth Israel Deaconess Medical Center
S. Daniel Abraham Associate Professor of Nutrition
Harvard Medical School
Boston, Massachusetts

Fred Brody, M.D., M.B.A
Associate Professor of Surgery
The George Washington University Medical Center
Washington, District of Columbia

David C. Brooks, M.D.
Director of Minimally Invasive Surgery
Brigham & Women's Hospital
Associate Professor
Harvard Medical School
Boston, Massachusetts

L. Michael Brunt, M.D.
Barnes-Jewish Hospital
Associate Professor of Surgery
Washington University School of Medicine
St. Louis, Missouri

Jo Buyske, M.D.
Chief of Surgery
Penn Presbyterian Medical Center
University of Pennsylvania
Philadelphia, Pennsylvania

Jeffrey A. Cadeddu, M.D.
Parkland Hospital
Associate Professor of Urology
University of Texas Southwestern Medical Center
Dallas, Texas

Mark P. Callery, M.D.
Chief, Division of General Surgery
Beth Israel Deaconess Medical Center
Associate Professor of Surgery
Harvard Medical School
Boston, Massachusetts

Craig G. Chang, M.D.
General Surgeon
Citizens Medical Center
Victoria, Texas

Kevin C. Conlon, M.D., M.B.A.
The Adelaide & Meath Hospital
Professor of Surgery
The University of Dublin
Trinity College Dublin
Dublin, Ireland

Jonathan F. Critchlow, M.D.
Beth Israel Deaconess Medical Center
Assistant Professor of Surgery
Harvard Medical School
Boston, Massachusetts

Malcolm DeCamp, Jr., M.D.
Chief, Thoracic Surgery
Beth Israel Deaconess Medical Center
Visiting Associate Professor of Surgery
Harvard Medical School
Boston, Massachusetts

Eric J. DeMaria, M.D.
Chief of Endosurgery
Duke University Medical Center
Durham, North Carolina

Daniel J. Deziel, M.D.
Professor of Surgery
Rush University Medical Center
Chicago, Illinois

J. Michael DiMaio, M.D.
Associate Professor
Department of Cardiovascular & Thoracic Surgery
University of Texas Southwestern Medical Center
Dallas, Texas

David W. Easter, M.D.
Professor of Clinical Surgery
University of California at San Diego
San Diego, California

Michael A. Edwards, M.D.
Beth Israel Deaconess Medical Center
Minimally Invasive Surgery Fellow
Harvard Medical School
Boston, Massachusetts

James Ellsmere, M.D.
Beth Israel Deaconess Medical Center
Minimally Invasive Surgery Fellow
Harvard Medical School
Boston, Massachusetts

Josef E. Fischer, M.D.
Surgeon-in-Chief
Chief of Surgery, Beth Israel Deaconess Medical Center
Chairman, Department of Surgery
McDermott Professor of Surgery
Harvard Medical School
Boston, Massachusetts

James W. Fleshman, M.D.
Barnes-Jewish Hospital
Professor of Surgery
Washington University School of Medicine
St. Louis, Missouri

David R. Flum, M.D., M.P.H.
Associate Professor of Surgery
University of Washington Medical Center
Seattle, Washington

Morris E. Franklin, Jr., M.D.
Director
Texas Endosurgery Institute
San Antonio, Texas

Michel Gagner, M.D.
Chief, Division of Laparoscopic and Bariatric Surgery
New York-Presbyterian Hospital
Professor of Surgery
Weill College of Medicine of Cornell University
New York, New York

Antonio Garcia-Ruiz, M.D.
Section Head
Minimally Invasive Surgery
Hospital Central Militar
Mexico City, Mexico

Ronit Grinbaum, M.D.
Beth Israel Deaconess Medical Center
Minimally Invasive Surgery Fellow
Harvard Medical School
Boston, Massachusetts

Elizabeth C. Hamilton, M.D.
Parkland Hospital
Assistant Professor of Surgery
University of Texas Southwestern Medical Center
Dallas, Texas

Michael D. Holzman, M.D., M.P.H.
Assistant Professor of Surgery
Vanderbilt University Hospital
Nashville, Tennessee

Matthew M. Hutter, M.D., M.P.H.
Director, Center of Clinical Effectiveness in Surgery
Massachusetts General Hospital
Instructor in Surgery
Harvard Medical School
Boston, Massachusetts

Scott R. Johnson, M.D.
Director, Renal Transplantation
Beth Israel Deaconess Medical Center
Assistant Professor
Harvard Medical School
Boston, Massachusetts

Stephanie B. Jones, M.D.
Beth Israel Deaconess Medical Center
Assistant Professor of Anesthesia
Harvard Medical School
Boston, Massachusetts

Namir Katkhouda, M.D.
USC Chief of Minimally Invasive Surgery
Professor of Surgery
University of Southern California
Los Angeles, California

Khalid Khwaja, M.D.
Director of Pancreatic Transplantation
Beth Israel Deaconess Medical Center
Harvard Medical School
Boston, Massachusetts

James D. Luketich, M.D.
Professor and Chief
Heart, Lung and Esophageal Surgery Institute
University of Pittsburgh Medical Center
Pittsburgh, Pennsylvania

Jeffrey Marks, M.D.
Associate Professor of Surgery
University Hospitals of Cleveland
Case Western Reserve University
Cleveland, Ohio

W. Scott Melvin, M.D.
Professor of Surgery
Chief, Division of General Surgery
The Ohio State University
Columbus, Ohio

Kenric M. Murayama, M.D.
Vice-Chair, Clinical & Hospital Affairs
University of Hawaii
Professor
John A. Burns School of Medicine
Honolulu, Hawaii

Ninh T. Nguyen, M.D.
Associate Professor of Surgery
Chief, Division of Gastrointestinal Surgery
University of California, Irvine Medical Center
Orange, California

Michael S. Nussbaum, M.D.
Vice-Chairman, Clinical Affairs
Chief of Staff, The University Hospital
Associate Professor of Surgery
University of Cincinnati
Cincinnati, Ohio

Paul E. O'Brien, M.D.
Director – Centre for Obesity Research and Education
  (CORE)
The Alfred Hospital
Emeritus Professor of Surgery
Monash University
Melbourne, Australia

Adrian E. Park, M.D.
Campbell and Jeanette Plugge Professor of Surgery
Chief, Division of General Surgery
University of Maryland Medical Center
Baltimore, Maryland

Arjun Pennathur, M.D.
Heart, Lung and Esophageal Surgery Institute
Assistant Professor of Surgery
University of Pittsburgh Medical Center
Pittsburgh, Pennsylvania

Jeffrey L. Ponsky, M.D.
Oliver H. Payne Professor and Chairman
Department of Surgery
Case School of Medicine and
  University Hospitals of Cleveland
Cleveland, Ohio

David A. Provost, M.D.
Director, Clinical Center for the
  Surgical Management of Obesity
Associate Professor of Surgery
University of Texas Southwestern Medical Center
Dallas, Texas

David W. Rattner, M.D.
Chief, Division of General & Gastrointestinal Surgery
Massachusetts General Hospital
Professor of Surgery
Harvard Medical School
Boston, Massachusetts

Robert V. Rege, M.D.
Professor and Chairman, Surgery
University of Texas Southwestern Medical Center
Dallas, Texas

Christine Ren, M.D.
Assistant Professor of Surgery
New York University School of Medicine
New York, New York

Steven M. Rudich, M.D., Ph.D.
Director, Liver Transplant Services
Associate Professor of Surgery
University of Cincinnati College of Medicine
Cincinnati, Ohio

Vivian M. Sanchez, M.D.
Beth Israel Deaconess Medical Center
Instructor in Surgery
Harvard Medical School
Boston, Massachusetts

Philip R. Schauer, M.D.
Director
Advanced Laparoscopic & Bariatric Surgery
Cleveland Clinic Foundation
Cleveland, Ohio

Bruce David Schirmer, M.D.
Stephen H. Watts Professor of Surgery
University of Virginia
Charlottesville, Virginia

Steven D. Schwaitzberg, M.D.
Cambridge Hospital
Associate Professor of Surgery
Harvard Medical School
Boston, Massachusetts

Daniel J. Scott, M.D.
Director, Tulane Center for Minimally Invasive Surgery
Charity Hospital
Associate Professor and William Henderson Chair
Tulane University School of Medicine
New Orleans, Louisiana

C. Daniel Smith, M.D.
W. Dean Warren Professor of Surgery
Emory University School of Medicine
Atlanta, Georgia

Nathaniel J. Soper, M.D.
Chief, Division of GI/Endocrine Surgery
Director, Minimally Invasive Surgery
Northwestern Memorial Hospital
Professor of Surgery
Northwestern University
Chicago, Illinois

Steven C. Stain, M.D.
Professor & Chairman
Department of Surgery
Albany Medical College
Albany, New York

Lee L. Swanstrom, M.D.
Director, Division of Minimally Invasive Surgery
Legacy Health System
Clinical Professor of Surgery
Oregon Health Sciences University
Portland, Oregon

John F. Sweeney, M.D.
Chief, Division of General Surgery
Chief, Minimally Invasive Surgery
Associate Professor of Surgery
Baylor College of Medicine
Houston, Texas

Alastair M. Thompson, M.D.
Ninewells Hospital and Medical School
Professor of Surgical Oncology
University of Dundee
Dundee, Scotland

Ashley Haralson Vernon, M.D.
Brigham & Women's Hospital
Instructor in Surgery
Harvard Medical School
Boston, Massachusetts

Leonardo Villegas, M.D.
Beth Israel Deaconess Medical Center
Clinical Fellow in Surgery
Harvard Medical School
Boston, Massachusetts

Charles M. Vollmer, Jr., M.D.
Beth Israel Deaconess Medical Center
Assistant Professor of Surgery
Harvard Medical School
Boston, Massachusetts

Mark J. Watson, M.D.
Parkland Hospital
Assistant Professor of Surgery
University of Texas Southwestern Medical Center
Dallas, Texas

Steven D. Wexner, M.D.
Professor and Chair, Colorectal Surgery
Cleveland Clinic Foundation Health Sciences Center of
 the Ohio State University
University of South Florida
Weston, Florida

Justin S. Wu, M.D.
Kaiser Permanente Medical Center
Assistant Clinical Professor of Surgery
University of California, San Diego
San Diego, California

Operating Endosuite

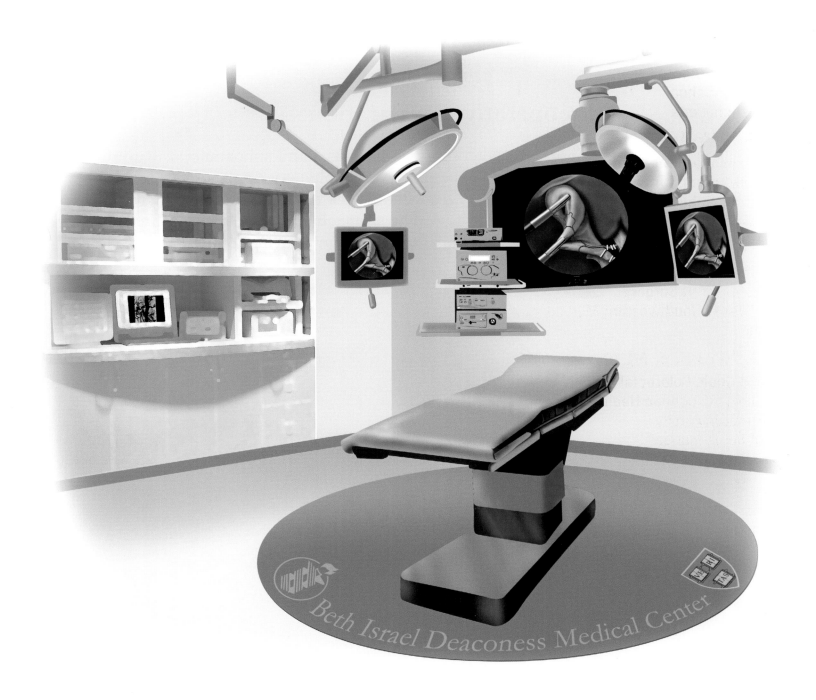

Monitors and equipment float from booms hanging from the ceiling. Voice recognition controls key systems. Integrated communication links radiology, pathology, and/or doctors' offices to the operating room.

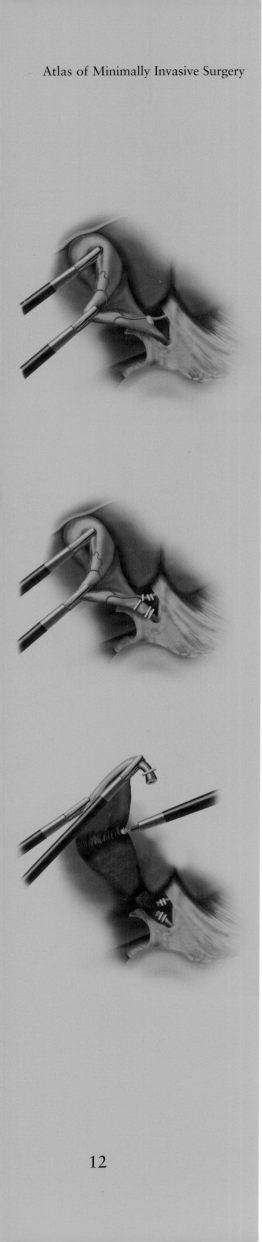

Laparoscopic Cholecystectomy

Laparoscopic cholecystectomy is the standard of care for symptomatic gallbladder disease, of which most are performed for symptomatic cholelithiasis. Other indications include acute cholecystitis, chronic cholecystitis, biliary dyskinesia, and gallstone pancreatitis

Preoperative Preparation

1. Sequential compression devices and subcutaneously administered heparin may be used for prophylaxis against deep venous thrombosis. We administer a first-generation cephalosporin prophylactically. The stomach is routinely decompressed with an orogastric tube after induction of general anesthesia.

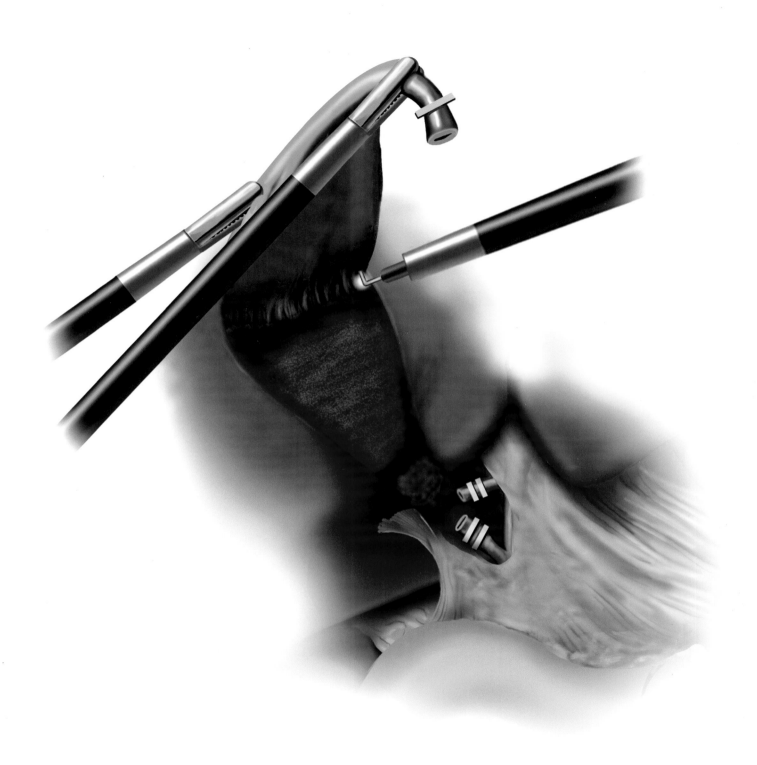

Operating Room Setup

2. The patient is placed supine on the operating table. The surgeon stands to the patient's left, while the first assistant stands to the right. A second assistant may be used on the surgeon's side to hold the laparoscopic camera.

3. Alternatively, the surgeon may choose to hold the camera with the left hand, or may choose to operate with a two-handed technique, in which the first assistant or scrub nurse may operate the camera.

4. The video monitors are arranged at the head of the operating room table as shown.

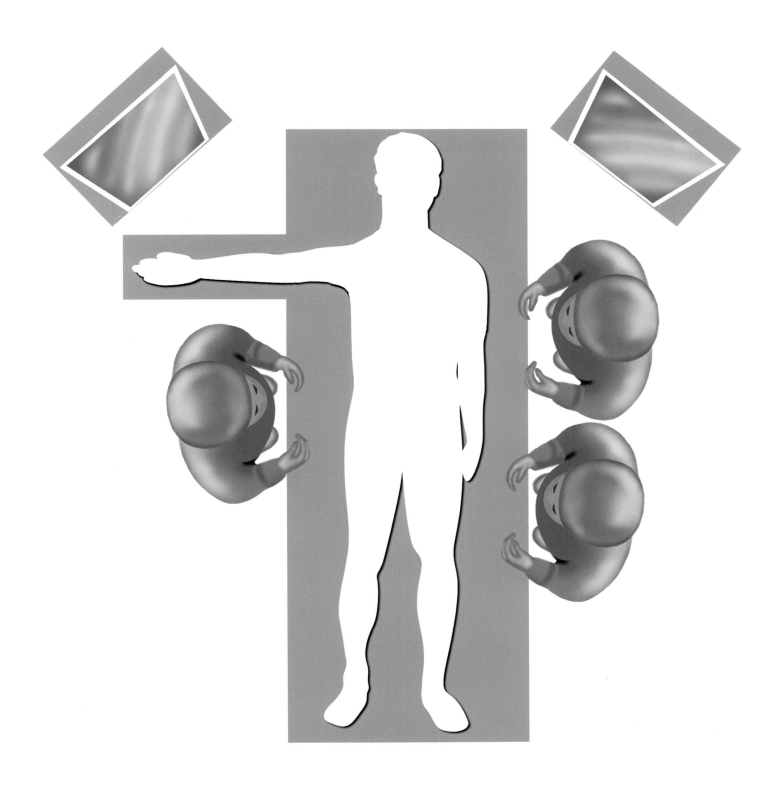

Access and Port Placement

5. After an infraumbilical incision is made, the open technique is used to gain access to the peritoneal cavity and a 11 mm Hasson port is secured to the fascia with a 0 Vicryl suture. Pneumoperitoneum is set to a pressure of 15 mm Hg.

6. Either a straight or 30° angled laparoscope can be used, although the angled scope is preferred as it facilitates obtaining crucial images during the operation if a skilled camera holder is available. A careful exploration of the abdomen is performed to ensure that no injury occurred during port insertion and that no other surface structure abnormalities are present.

7. With the patient in reverse Trendelenburg position, planned port sites are marked and the skin and peritoneum are injected with local anesthetic. A radially expanding 11 mm trocar is placed through an oblique incision in the midline of the epigastrium below the xiphoid process and is angled right of the falciform ligament aiming toward the gallbladder.

8. Two 5 mm ports are placed in the right upper quadrant under direct laparoscopic visualization. The first port is placed in the anterior axillary line between the twelfth rib and the iliac crest, two finger breadths below the costal margin. A second 5 mm port is inserted in roughly the midclavicular line, allowing for adequate spacing between ports (10 cm). Care should be taken to orient the three ports to facilitate making an open subcostal incision should conversion to an open approach become necessary.

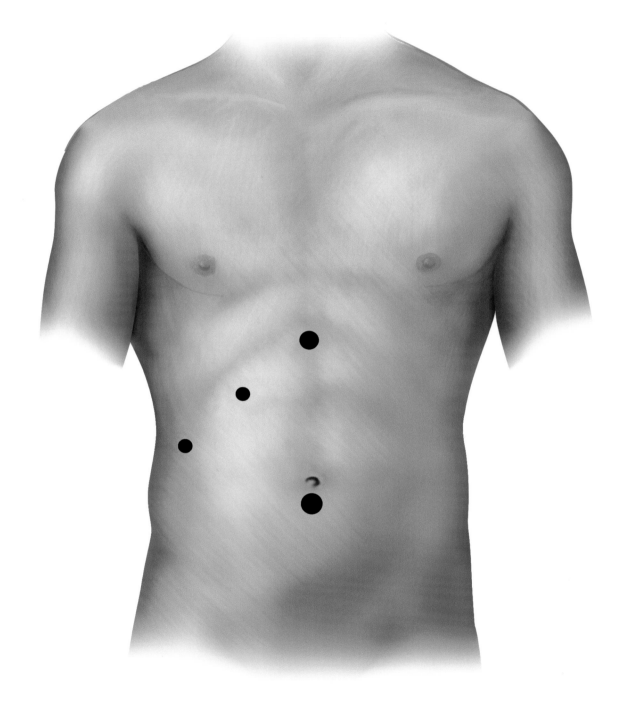

FIGURE C

Exposing Calot's Triangle

9. Grasping forceps, passed through the 5 mm ports by the assistant, are used to lock and retract the fundus of the gallbladder in a lateral and cephalad direction (toward the right shoulder of the patient) so that the entire right lobe of the liver is retracted as well. If excessive distension of the gallbladder prohibits grasping the fundus, the gallbladder can be aspirated and drained with a large needle to restore flaccidity to the wall.

10. A second 5 mm grasping forcep is used to distract the infundibulum laterally away from the CBD and common hepatic bile duct. This maneuver is performed by either the surgeon or assistant, depending on whether a two-handed or one-handed operative technique is utilized.

11. The surgeon, using a blunt dissector placed through the epigastric port, then peels away any adhesions between the gallbladder and omentum, hepatic flexure, stomach, and duodenum, being careful to grasp adhesions close to the gallbladder, pulling them "away" bluntly. Vascular adhesions may be divided with hook cautery. Calot's lymph node overlying the cystic artery is swept away, sometimes requiring brief cautery to obtain hemostasis. This initial dissection exposes Calot's, or the hepatocystic, triangle which is bounded by the cystic duct, common hepatic duct, and liver edge.

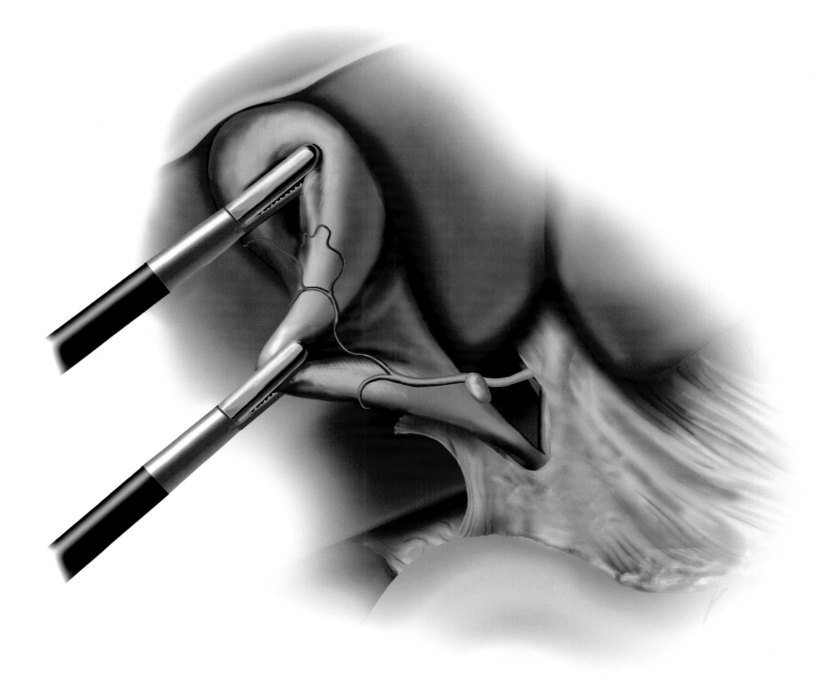

Exposing the Reverse Triangle

12. The reverse side of the hepatocystic triangle, bordered by the cystic duct, inferior lateral border of the gallbladder, and right lobe of the liver, is exposed by placing the infundibulum on stretch in a superior and medial direction and the fundus in a superior and lateral direction. Alternating between this view and the anterior view of the hepatocystic triangle, precise indentification of the junction of the infundibulum and the cystic duct is possible.

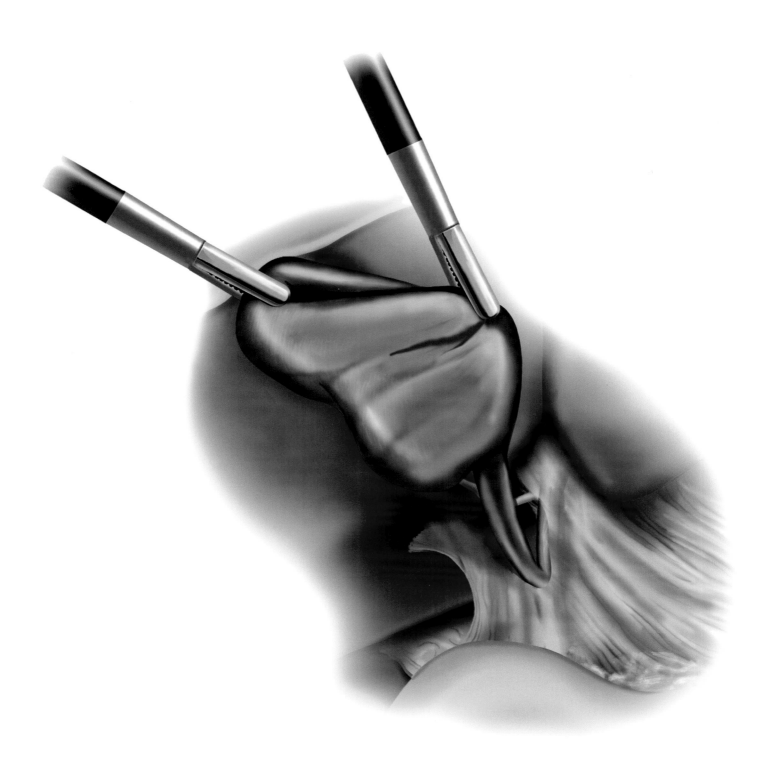

Obtaining the "Critical View"

13. No structure should be divided until this "critical view" is attained. The critical view clearly identifies the cystic duct at its origin from the infundibulum. Curved dissecting forceps are used to create a "window" around the posterior aspect of the duct, thus creating a circumferential plane around the cystic duct to enable safe transection. The cystic artery may be dissected free from surrounding tissue using a similar technique.

14. After the cystic duct is clearly exposed, static or fluoroscopic cholangiography may be performed on a routine or selective basis. The cholangiogram should be scrutinized for the following: 1) size of the common bile duct (CBD), 2) location of the cystic duct and CBD confluence, 3) presence of intraluminal filling defects, 4) free flow of contrast into the duodenum, 5) anatomy of the proximal biliary tree with both the left and right systems filling, and 6) presence of aberrant biliary radicals entering the gallbladder directly.

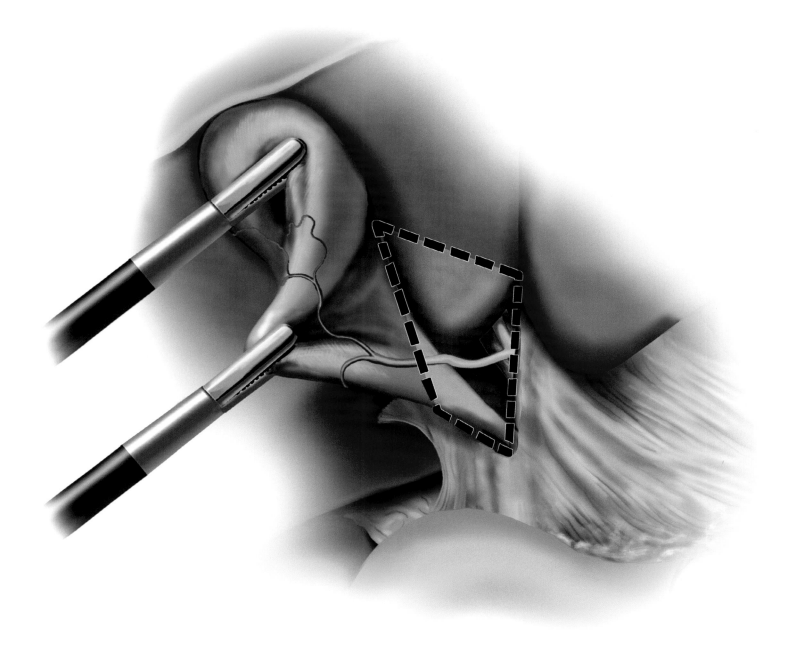

Dividing the Cystic Duct and Artery

15. Whether or not a cholangiogram is performed, the cystic duct is doubly clipped distally, and a single clip is placed near its origin from the gallbladder, before the cystic duct is divided using scissors. The posterior jaw of the clip applier must be visualized before applying each clip. A particularly large or friable cystic duct can be further secured with a preformed loop ligature or suture.

16. Attention is then directed toward the cystic artery, being careful not to mistake the right hepatic artery for the cystic artery. The artery is dissected, doubly clipped, and divided in a similar manner. Care must be taken not to miss a posterior branch of the cystic artery. The ligated stumps of both the cystic duct and artery are examined.

17. A suction-irrigation catheter can be used to remove any debris or blood that has accumulated from the dissection, although suction should not be directly applied to the clip sites as this may risk dislodgement.

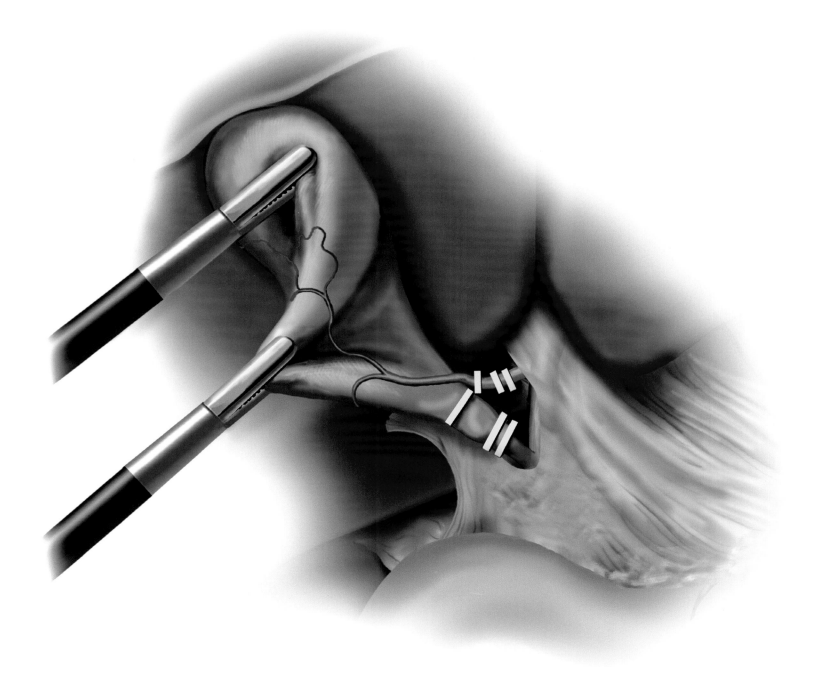

Dissecting the Gallbladder From the Liver

18. Separation of the gallbladder from its bed is performed with electrocautery. The infundibulum is retracted superiorly and laterally and is distracted anteriorly away from its hepatic bed. With the tissue connecting the gallbladder to its fossa placed under tension, the surgeon uses an electrocautery hook or spatula in a gentle sweeping motion with low-power wattage (25-30 W) to coagulate and divide this connective tissue (Figure G-a).

19. The gallbladder retraction is alternated between a lateral and medial direction to provide maximal countertraction and continuously expose tissue under tension in the appropriate plane that may be easily divided (Figure G-b). Any bleeding from the liver during this dissection can usually be controlled with direct pressure, further cauterization, or application of a topical hemostatic agent.

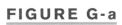

FIGURE G-a

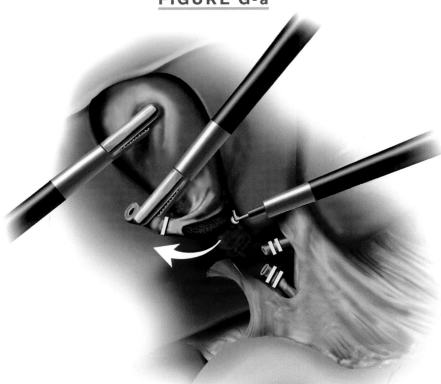

FIGURE G-b

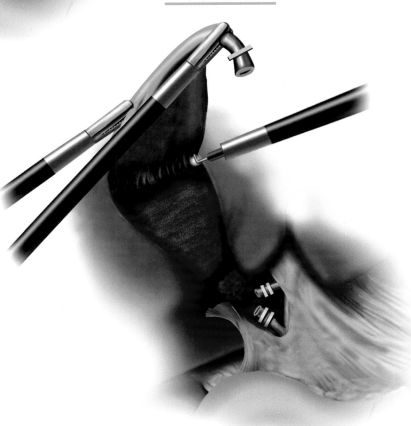

Preparing for Extraction

20. Using the gallbladder for traction, the liver bed and cystic duct and artery stumps are carefully inspected for hemostasis and bile leakage, making sure the clips are secure. Any bleeding points from the liver bed can usually be controlled with cauterization. The final attachments to the gallbladder are then divided.

21. If inadvertent rupture of the gallbladder occurs, loose stones can be retrieved with a spoon grasper (Figure H-a). For removal of the gallbladder from the abdominal cavity, the laparoscope is switched to the epigastric port and the gallbladder is removed through the umbilical incision. Either large grasping forceps or an entrapment sack is used for extraction (Figure H-b). A sack is recommended, especially if the gallbladder is purulent, fragmented, or perforated.

FIGURE H-a

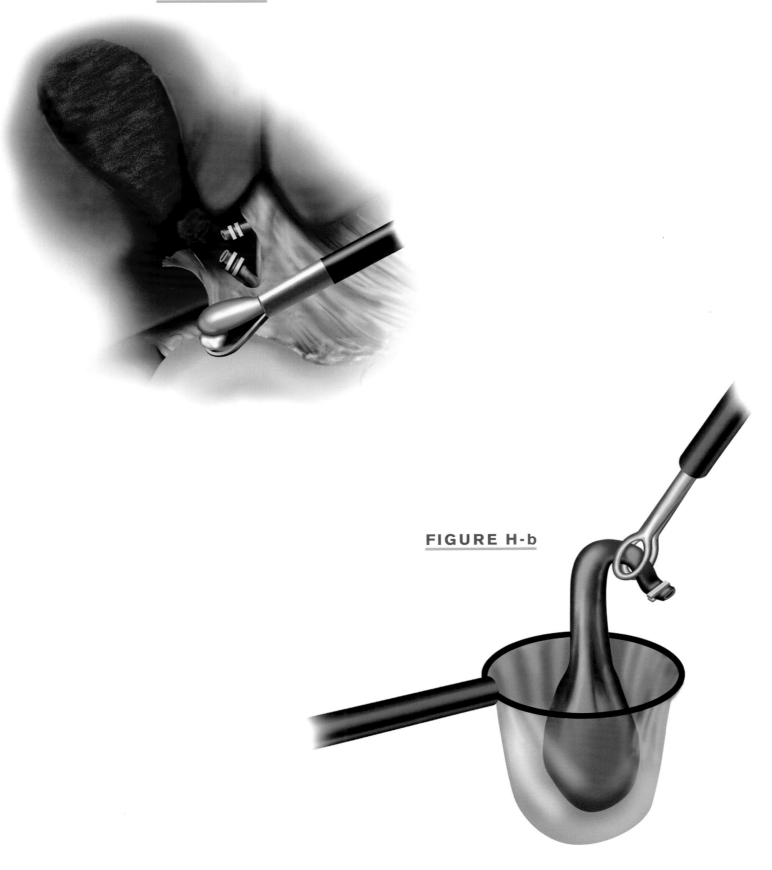

FIGURE H-b

FIGURE I

Extracting the Gallbladder

22. The grasping forceps or entrapment sack, umbilical port, and gallbladder neck are retracted as a unit through the umbilical incision. The neck of the gallbladder is thus exposed on the anterior abdominal wall, with the distended fundus remaining within the abdominal cavity. If bile or large stones prevent removing the gallbladder with gentle traction, the bile can be aspirated and the stones can be crushed or extracted with stone forceps. Alternatively, the fascial incision may be dilated or extended to deliver large stones.

23. Once the gallbladder is extracted from the abdominal cavity, the laparoscope is returned to the umbilical site. The right upper quadrant is again inspected for hemostasis and the ports are removed under direct laparoscopic visualization to ensure hemostasis at each of the three ports sites as well. Each incision is irrigated with saline solution. The fascia at the umbilical incision is closed with a 0 absorbable suture. The skin incision at each port site is closed with a 4-0 subcuticular absorbable suture.

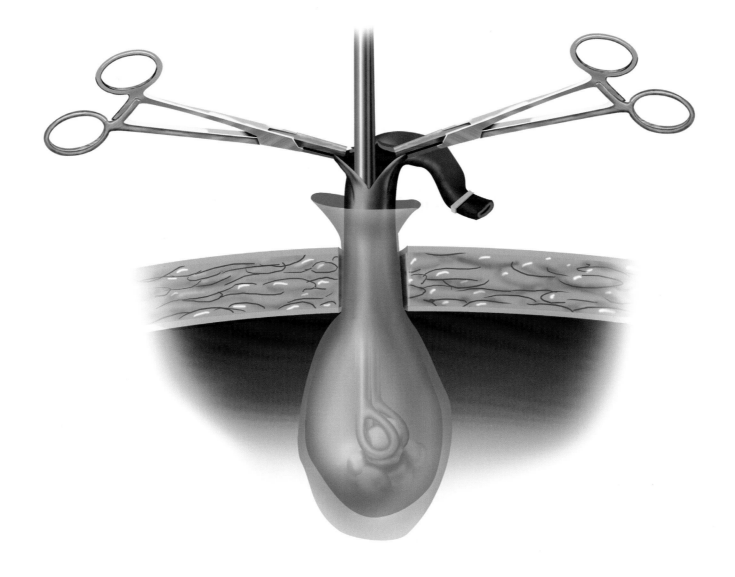

Postoperative Care

Pneumatic compression devices and/or subcutaneous heparin may be continued postoperatively. Continued use of antibiotics is at the discretion of the surgeon, although it is usually not necessary. Patients are usually able to tolerate liquids and solid food within 24 hours after the operation. The majority of uncomplicated cases are performed as outpatient surgery with patients being discharged home the same day.

Suggested Readings

1. National Institutes of Health Consensus Development Conference Statement on Gallstones and Laparoscopic Cholecystectomy. *Am J Surg.* 1993; 165:390-398.

2. Soper NJ. Laparoscopic cholecystectomy. *Curr Probl Surg.* 1991; 28:585-655.

3. Strasberg SM, Hertl M, Soper NJ. An analysis of the problem of biliary injury during laparoscopic choleystectomy. *J Am Coll Surg.* 1995; 180:101-125.

4. Strasberg SM. Biliary injury in laparoscopic surgery: part 1. Processes used in determination of standard of care in misidentification injuries. *J Am Coll Surg.* 2005; 201:598-603.

5. Strasberg SM. Biliary injury in laparoscopic surgery: part 2. Changing the culture of cholecystectomy. *J Am Coll Surg.* 2005; 201:604-611.

Commentary

David Brooks, M.D., Brigham and Women's Hospital
Harvard Medical School

Laparoscopic cholecystectomy is the progenitor of all laparoscopic procedures performed by general surgeons. It was the first and remains the best. Indeed, it could easily be termed a "perfect operation." It provides complete symptom relief in nearly 100% of patients, has a low complication rate, is remarkably well accepted by patients, and is an enjoyable operation to perform. That notwithstanding, it has taken more than 15 years and millions of operations for us to refine the techniques to enhance safety and facilitate the performance of the procedure.

The description provided in this atlas is excellent, and I have only minor disagreements with the author's technique. I, too, favor an open access technique, although I typically make a vertical incision in a supraumbilical location. This can be easily extended for a large gallbladder or stone and is almost imperceptible after healing. Likewise, I agree with the port placement positions, although I place the lateral, 5 mm port first, reflect the gallbladder and liver, and then place the midclavicular port and the subxyphoid port. This allows me to position the subxyphoid port in a direct line to the infundibulum so that there will be no torque on the instruments when dissecting in the triangle.

The area in which I have the most major departure from the author's description is in the exposure of Calot's triangle. I reverse the order in which the right and left sides of the triangle are dissected. Over the years I have found that the safest, least bloody, and most expeditious way to expose the infundibular-cystic duct junction is to start on the lateral or right side of the gallbladder. Using a two-handed technique, I reflect the infundibulum to the patient's left and gently strip the peritoneal attachments from the lateral aspect of the gallbladder. As the authors point out, it is important to strip the attachments close to the gallbladder. This minimizes bleeding. Moving from patient's right to patient's left and using almost no electrocautery, I quickly come to the anterior aspect of the cystic duct and clear this so that the duct is easily seen.

Once this has been visualized, I retract the infundibulum back to the patient's right and anteriorly to begin exposure of the triangle. By dissecting the peritoneum over the triangle and stripping it toward the liver (rather than down to the portal structures), the entire triangle opens. Using a Kittner or other blunt instrument, the loose areolar tissue in this area can be gently pushed toward the liver, further opening the space and exposing the cystic artery. This also ensures that there is no other structure (i.e., common hepatic duct) in this space. I don't use the recently popular term "critical view," but the concept of opening this window fully is extremely important to ensure that no vital structures in the porta are disturbed.

Once the duct and the artery have been visualized, clipped, and tied, the gallbladder is removed from the liver bed using electrocautery as the authors have described. I prefer to use a spatula rather than a hook because it allows me to perform blunt dissection, but the technique is essentially the same.

Several other points are worth reiterating. First, the operating surgeon should be encouraged to use a two-handed technique with the left hand manipulating the grasper on the infundibulum rather than holding the camera. For neophyte laparoscopists, this starts the process of becoming comfortable with a bimanual surgery, a skill that will be critical in advanced procedures. Second, always be on the lookout for a posterior branch of the cystic artery. It has caused me untold grief. Lastly, dropped stones are more than a nuisance. They can and will lead to significant late postoperative morbidity from abscess or granuloma. Make every effort to prevent spillage and when it occurs, retrieve all the stones.

Antonio Garcia-Ruiz, M.D., Hospital Central Militar

I have three priorities during a laparoscopic cholecystectomy: 1) safety—prevent bile duct injury, 2) efficiency—keep the procedure as simple as possible, and 3) least invasive surgery—maintain trocars to the smallest diameter. The previous description is excellent; I have few additional comments:

I make the umbilical incision right at the bottom of the umbilicus, running down to the edge of the umbilical fossa. For most patients this will be enough. However, if needed (large stone or specimen) I can enlarge the incision up to an inch by cutting through the center of the umbilicus up to the upper edge of the umbilical fossa. The result of this incision is more cosmetically appealing than the subumbilical incision as it will be well hidden inside the umbilicus. To avoid the risk of postoperative herniation, through any 10 mm to 12 mm incision, and improve the cosmetic results, I use a 5 mm trocar in the subxyphoid position. Therefore I have to use 5 mm clip appliers.

Exposing and dissecting the cholecystohepatic triangle is of outmost importance. To avoid any bile duct injury, I perform five "high-security maneuvers" before attempting to clip or cut any structure within the triangle. First maneuver—my assistant elevates the gallbladder fundus to the center of the right clavicle, to avoid lacerating the liver by excessive traction on the round or falciform ligament insertion as this may cause unnecessary bleeding that will obscure my view. Second maneuver—with my left-hand instrument, I grasp the gallbladder infundibulum and pull it laterally toward the left lower corner of my monitor. This will increase the angle between the common bile duct and the cystic duct, making it easier to correctly identify the safe spot to start the dissection. Third maneuver—starting at the Hartmann's pouch, by clearing the peritoneum at the lower border of the cholecystohepatic triangle, I dissect what seems to be the cystic duct. Fourth maneuver—with blunt dissection, I dissect the central portion of the triangle, identifying what seems to be the cystic artery. Sometimes using the aspiration cannula as a blunt dissecting instrument while making small aspirations will nicely do the job of keeping the optical view as clean as possible. Fifth maneuver—to complete my safe dissection, I always try to start the dissection of the liver bed bluntly with a Maryland dissector, in order to make sure that there is not any ductal structure coming back from the gallbladder infundibulum to the porta hepatis. I like to call this my "highest security maneuver," as it gives me the critical view mentioned in this chapter.

Dissecting the gallbladder from the liver is much simpler if you keep the dissection preferably from medial to lateral using an "L-shaped" electrosurgical hook. Usually, I start with the infundubulum and medial portion, achieving exposure by contertraction with my left-hand instrument. Then I take down the fundus and, finally, the lateral peritoneum. Routinely, I extract the gallbladder through the umbilical incision and I prefer to prevent wound infection by introducing the specimen in a latex bag (sterile condom) prior to extraction. This is extremely useful and considerably diminishes our operating room costs. Finally, instead of opening the gallbladder to crush large calculi (which increases the risk of bag rupture and potential wound infection), I prefer to enlarge the incision just enough to retrieve the specimen.

Daniel J. Deziel, M.D.
Rush University Medical Center

The authors describe the standard retrograde technique for laparoscopic cholecystectomy. Alternatively, an antegrade ("fundus first" or "top-down") method can be accomplished laparoscopically, although it is more difficult. This approach may be useful for cases in which the anatomy of the cystic duct—gallbladder junction is less clear.

Like the authors, I prefer open placement of a blunt Hasson cannula at the initial access site. Use of a Veress needle to establish the pneumoperitoneum with subsequent blind placement of the initial umbilical trocar is also acceptable providing that proper techniques are followed. A visible periumbilical scar can be avoided by use of a vertical incision placed directly through the middle of the umbilicus. While 15 mm Hg intraperitoneal pressure is routinely described, most cases can be performed at a slightly lower pressure of 10 mm Hg to 12 mm Hg. The precise cephalad-caudal position of the anterior axillary line trocar will vary according to the patients' body habitus and the location of the gallbladder fundus. It may be just below the costal margin, as illustrated or commonly lower, even down to the level of the umbilicus.

During initial dissection, I suggest avoiding direct manipulation of the cystic duct node, if possible, as this typically will cause bleeding. The node is usually a good landmark for the location of the cystic artery, which lies just behind or dorsal to the node. The cystic artery can also be identified by tracing the vessel back from the surface of the body of the gallbladder where it is usually apparent. Anatomic purists will note that Calot originally described an anatomic area bounded by the cystic duct, the common hepatic duct, and the cystic artery. The authors' description of Calot's triangle, identifying the liver edge as the superior border, has become the commonly accepted working definition.

The concept of careful dissection until the "critical view of safety" is obtained is crucial for proper identification of the cystic duct. This involves dissection of all tissues between the presumed cystic duct-gallbladder junction and the liver edge until it is certain that no other duct structures are coursing upward toward the liver. This is facilitated by opening the ventral and dorsal peritoneal reflections to allow the gallbladder neck and body to be further separated from the liver

Operative imaging of the bile ducts can be obtained by cholangiography or by laparoscopic ultrasonography. The techniques are complementary; each can identify common bile duct stones and bile duct anatomy. Cholangiography is better for visualizing the anatomy of the proximal extrahepatic ducts. Proper interpretation of intraoperative cholangiography requires complete visualization of the distal and proximal ducts, including both the right anterior and right posterior segmental ducts.

Division of the cystic artery is accomplished as close to the gallbladder as possible. This is to avoid any compromise of the right hepatic artery. Also, the classic anatomic studies of Michels demonstrated that some individuals have a recurrent artery to the common bile duct that originates from the cystic artery. If present, this could be impaired if the cystic artery is taken proximal to its origin. Beware of multiple cystic artery branches and of multiple cystic arteries. I have divided as many as five separate cystic arteries coming off of a right hepatic artery as it coursed parallel to the body of the gallbladder before finally turning cephalad into the liver.

I prefer to always use a retrieval bag and to remove the gallbladder from the umbilical port site. Extraction of large specimens is best accomplished by midline extension of the fascial incision and skin as necessary. Opening the gallbladder risks contamination. Avoid pulling on the retrieval bag alone and exerting undue tension on the specimen because the bag will rupture. If not done prior to trocar placement, a longer-acting local anesthetic agent can be injected at each port site under direct laparoscopic visualization prior to port removal.

Elizabeth C. Hamilton, M.D., Parkland Hospital
University of Texas Southwestern Medical Center

More than one million cases of symptomatic cholelithiasis and cholecystitis are diagnosed per year in the United States. As such, gallbladder disease is a very common surgical problem and a significant component of the general surgical practice. In the early 1990s, laparoscopic cholecystectomy replaced the open technique as the treatment of choice for appropriate surgical candidates with symptomatic gallstone disease. The technique is considered safe and effective. Open cholecystectomy is reserved, in most cases, to situations in which the anatomy is obscured by severe inflammation or bleeding, there is a suspicion of malignancy, or there is a need to perform an open common bile duct exploration. Most commonly, laparoscopic cholecystectomy is performed on patients who return home on the same day. Recovery is usually quick with the majority of patients being able to return to normal daily activities within 7 to 9 days.

Although many pearls to performing the laparoscopic cholecystectomy safely and effectively are already included in the chapter, I believe some deserve re-emphasis.

Access to the abdominal cavity can be gained using either a closed (Veress needle) or open technique depending on the approach with which the surgeon is most familiar.

The inability to clearly define the anatomy using the laparoscopic approach mandates prompt conversion to the open technique and should not be considered a sign of weakness or a complication.

Lateral and inferior retraction of the gallbladder infundibulum helps enlarge the angle between the cystic duct and common duct, making inadvertent injury to the common bile duct less likely.

Clearly obtaining the "critical view" of the cystic duct and cystic artery directly entering the infundibulum of the gallbladder with the liver visible in the background is mandatory before clipping and dividing any structures.

Transcystic cholangiogram prior to dividing any structures is helpful for defining anatomy in cases where the anatomy is unclear.

Clips should be placed across the cystic duct and artery so that the entire lumen is ligated. Endoloops can be helpful when a cystic duct is inadvertently avulsed or the lumen is too large for a 10 mm clip.

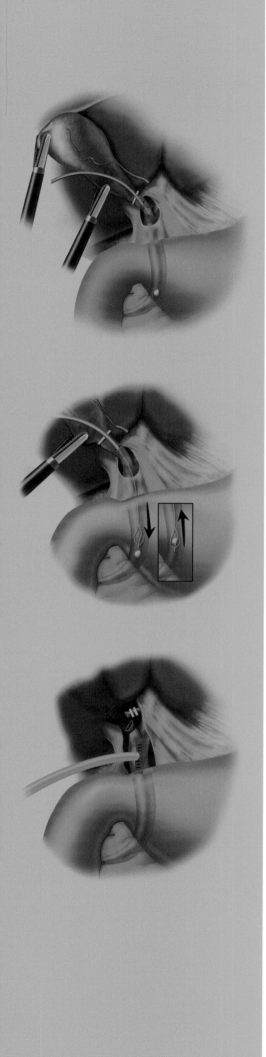

Laparoscopic Common Bile Duct Exploration

Choledocholithiasis may be treated by percutaneous transhepatic, endoscopic, open surgical, and laparoscopic approaches. Now that laparoscopic cholecystectomy has become the standard of care for symptomatic gallstones, proficiency in performing intraoperative cholangiography and laparoscopic common bile duct exploration is a viable alternative to manage common bile duct (CBD) stones in one setting.

Preoperative Preparation

1. Sequential compression devices and subcutaneously administered heparin may be used for prophylaxis against deep venous thrombosis. A first-generation cephalosporin is administered for antibiotic prophylaxis. The stomach is decompressed with an orogastric tube after induction of general anesthesia.

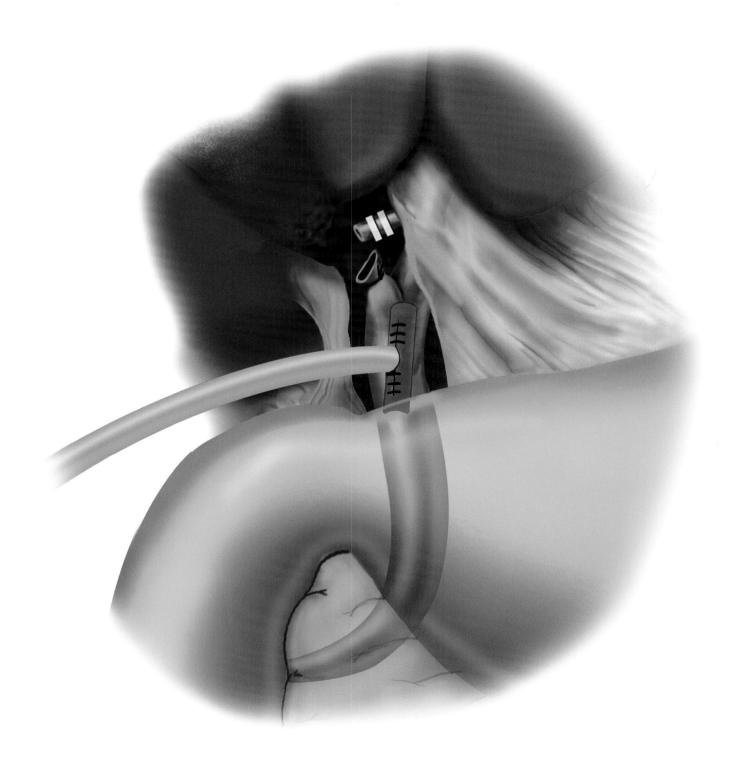

FIGURE A

Operating Room Setup

2. Before starting a laparoscopic common bile duct exploration, it is imperative that the surgeon is familiar with all the equipment necessary to perform the operation and that all equipment is available.

3. The patient is placed in the supine position. It is important to position the patient properly on an appropriate bed such that a fluoroscope may intraoperatively image the right upper quadrant.

4. The surgeon stands to the patient's left, while the first assistant stands to the right. A second assistant may be used on the surgeon's side to hold a 30° laparoscopic camera. Alternatively, the first assistant or scrub nurse may operate the camera.

5. The video monitors are placed at both sides of the patient's head to facilitate viewing from either side of the table.

6. Proper arrangement must be made to have C-arm fluoroscopy in the operating room, as well as a second tower for the choledochoscope, second camera, light source, and monitor.

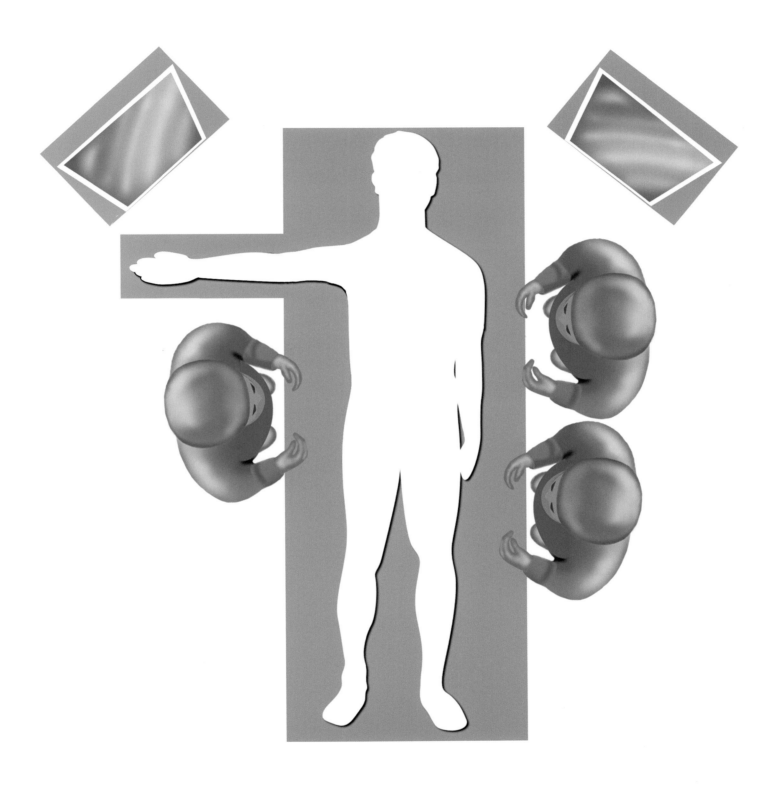

Access and Port Placement

7. An infraumbilical incision is used to establish pneumoperitoneum, setting a maximum pressure limit of 15 mm Hg. This is established with either an open or closed technique. A 10/11 mm port is placed here and the laparoscope is inserted. Either a straight or 30° angled scope can be used, although the angled scope, if available, is preferred as it facilitates obtaining crucial images during the operation. A careful exploration is performed to ensure that no injury occurred during port insertion and that no other abnormalities are present.

8. A 10/11 mm trocar is placed through an oblique incision in the midline of the epigastrium. This is generally placed 2 cm below the xiphoid process and is angled right of the falciform ligament aiming toward the gallbladder.

9. Two 5 mm ports are placed in the right upper quadrant. The first 5 mm port is placed in the anterior axillary line between the twelfth rib and the iliac crest. A second 5 mm port is inserted midway between the axillary and epigastric port. Care should be taken to orient the three ports to facilitate making an open subcostal incision should conversion be necessary.

10. The cholangiogram catheter and choledochoscope can be introduced into the abdomen via one of the lateral ports or via a separate site that is located in between the epigastric and lateral ports.

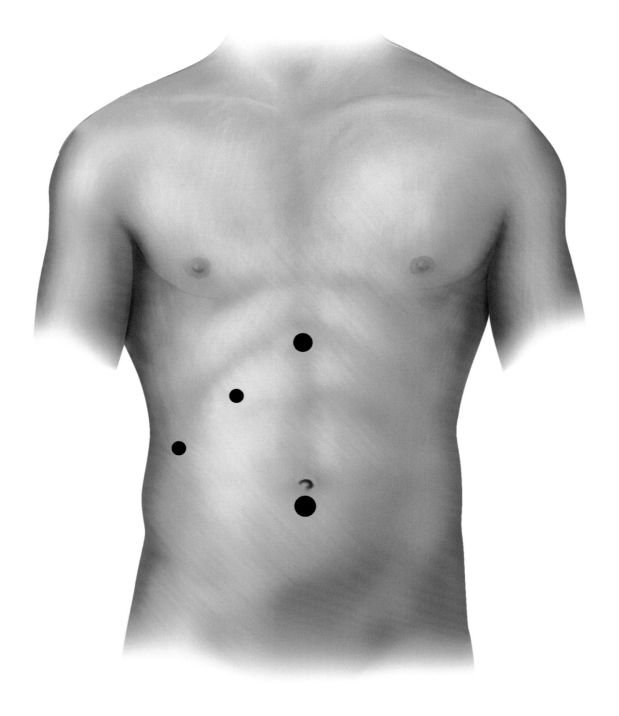

FIGURE C

Performing a Cholangiogram

11. The cystic duct is clearly exposed for a length of 2 cm to 3 cm using the same dissection technique as that described for performing a laparoscopic cholecystectomy, being particularly careful to expose Calot's triangle and obtain the "critical view." A surgical clip is applied across the cystic duct at the level of its insertion into the gallbladder.

12. Next, laparoscopic scissors are used to partially incise the cystic duct below the level of the surgical clip and the cystic duct's lumen is identified. It is often best to incise the cystic duct via the same port through which the cholangiogram catheter will be introduced. This facilitates a simpler introduction as the angle of the incision is optimized.

13. Next, the cholangiogram catheter, which may have an inflatable balloon at its tip, is introduced into the peritoneal cavity and is flushed with saline to remove any air in the system. The catheter is introduced into the cystic duct and is secured in place by inflating the catheter balloon. It is important to ensure that the tip of the catheter remains in the cystic duct so that it does not interfere with the cholangiogram.

14. One-half strength contrast is injected through the catheter under fluoroscopy. If a normal cholangiogram is seen, the catheter is removed, the cystic duct is doubly clipped and divided, and the gallbladder is removed in the usual fashion. However, if a filling defect is noticed in the biliary tree, a diagnosis of choledocholithiasis is confirmed and further manipulation is required.

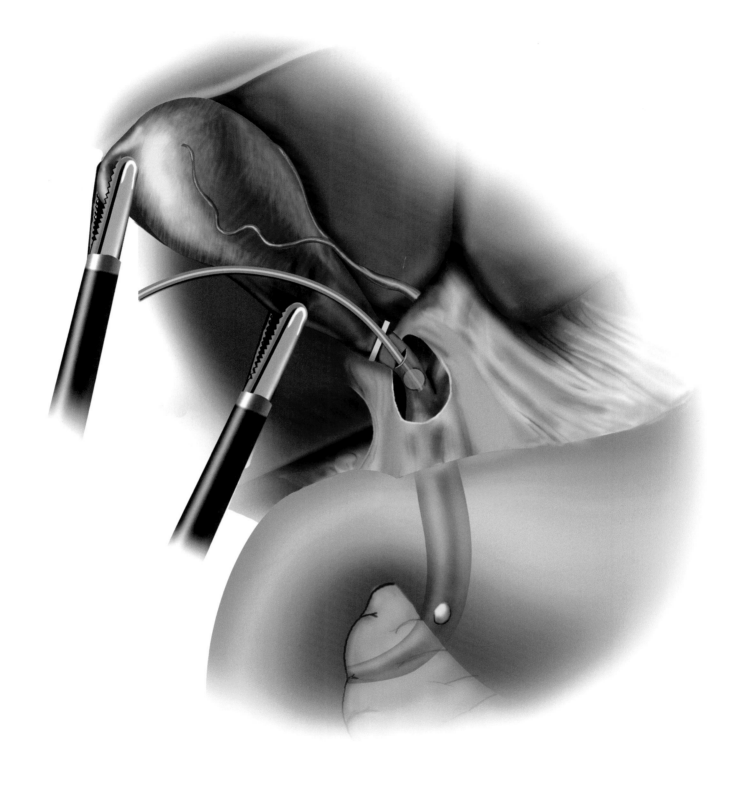

Transcystic Approach

FIGURE D

Flushing the Common Bile Duct

15. The common bile duct is flushed with 20 mL to 30 mL of saline via the cholangiogram catheter. Small stones less than 4 mm in diameter are particularly amenable to this maneuver. Intravenous administration of 1 mg of glucagon can further facilitate stone removal by relaxing the sphincter of Oddi.

16. A repeat cholangiogram is performed. If a normal cholangiogram is observed, the gallbladder can then be removed in the usual fashion.

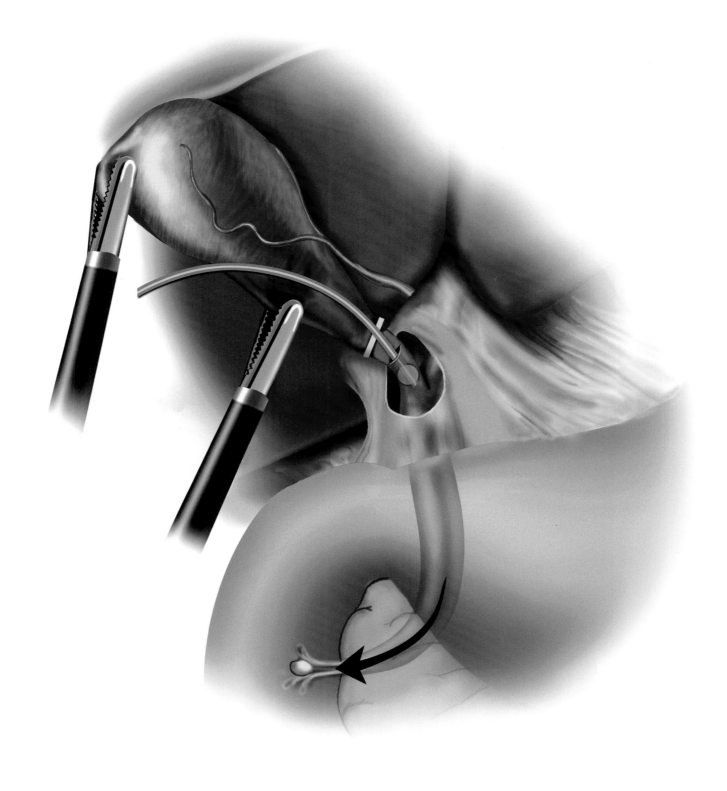

Basket Retrieval of Common Bile Duct Stones

17. Persistent filling defects on the repeat cholangiogram imply that stones remain in the common bile duct. If only small stones (less than 3 mm) are observed and contrast flows freely into the duodenum, expectant management and observation may be considered as the majority of these small stones will spontaneously pass into the duodenum.

18. Alternatively, a stone retrieval basket may be inserted through the cholangiogram catheter into the common bile duct. Under fluoroscopic guidance, the basket is passed beyond the stone. The basket is opened and then closed while being slowly withdrawn. Inability to fully close the basket implies stone capture. The entire unit, including the cholangiogram catheter and the retrieval basket containing a stone, is removed. The process is repeated until a normal cholangiogram is observed.

19. A 4 Fr Fogarty balloon catheter can also be used to withdraw stones from the common bile duct. The catheter is inserted into the common bile duct transcystically and passed beyond the stones. The balloon is inflated and the catheter is withdrawn, pulling the stones into the abdominal cavity while being careful to prevent stones from travelling proximally into the hepatic duct. Stones can be collected in the abdomen and removed later within the same entrapment sac used for gallbladder retrieval. It is important to not leave any stones behind in the peritoneal cavity, as they can be a nidus for subsequent abscess formation.

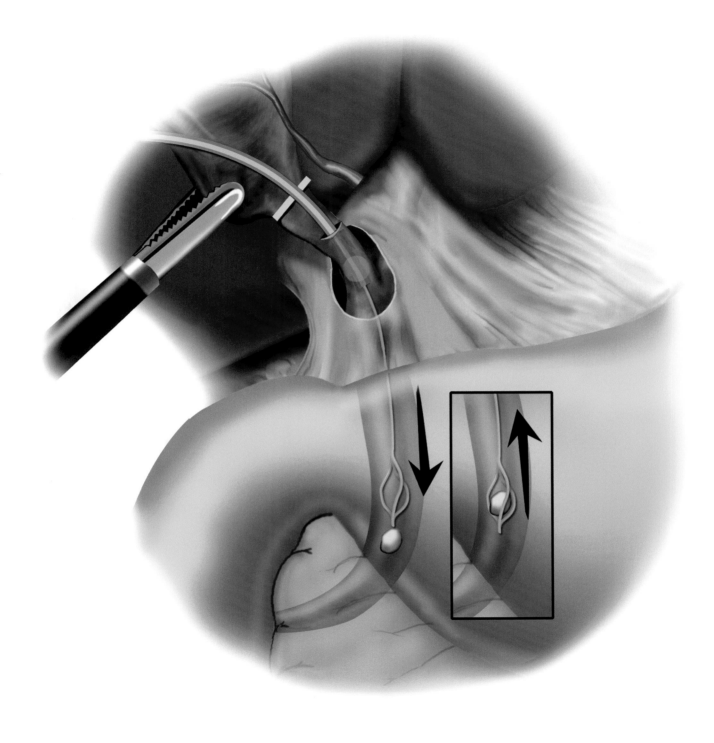

Transcystic Choledochoscopy

FIGURE F

Preparing for Choledochoscopy

20. A 5 Fr catheter is used to perform a trancystic cholangiogram as previously described. This larger catheter enables passage of a 0.035-inch flexible guide wire into the common bile duct and duodenum. The wire's position is confirmed with fluoroscopy. To facilitate passage of the choledochoscope, the cystic duct can be dilated by passing an 8 Fr balloon angioplasty catheter over the guide wire and inflating the balloon to 6 atmospheres of pressure for 5 minutes. The balloon is deflated and the catheter is removed, leaving the wire in place.

21. A 12 Fr diameter plastic sheath is then passed over the wire into the peritoneal cavity, leaving the proximal end of the sheath outside the patient. This will serve as a protective sheath for passage of the choledochoscope. Alternatively, a 3 mm inner cannula, placed in a standard laparoscopic port, can allow for safe passage of the choledochoscope.

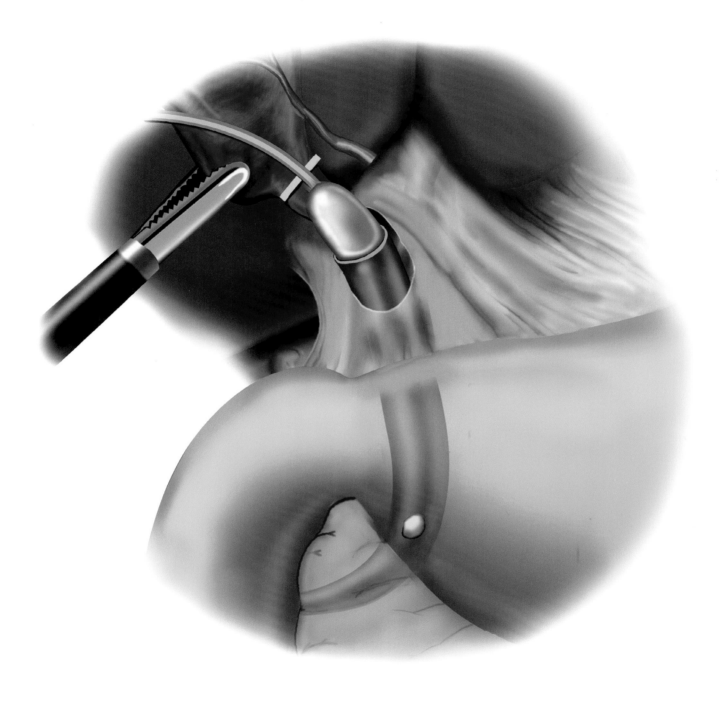

Performing Choledochoscopy

22. A 3 mm choledochoscope is advanced over the guide wire through the protective sheath into the abdomen. Padded graspers are used to facilitate passing the scope into the common bile duct via the cystic duct opening. Pressurized saline is connected to a working side port of the scope to enable adequate visualization inside the biliary system.

23. The guide wire is removed and a stone retrieval basket is inserted through the scope. Stones are removed under direct visualization using the same technique as previously described. The entire unit is removed as each stone is captured in the basket. Attempts at directly reinserting the scope through the cystic duct opening can often take longer than simply repeating the entire sequence of catheter and guide wire insertion. Alternatively, the scope may be used to gently push stones into the duodenum, being careful to not exert excess pressure.

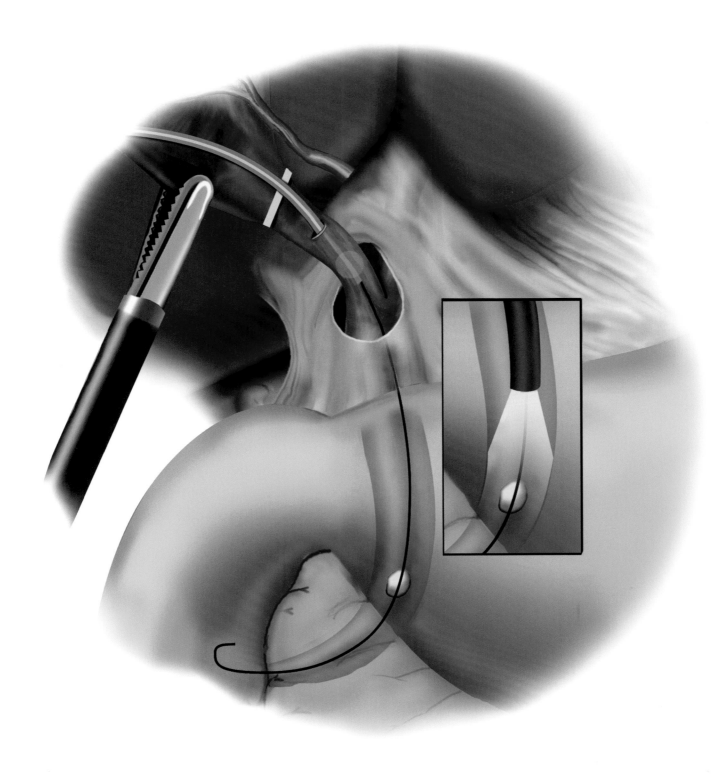

Laparoscopic Choledochotomy

A choledochotomy may be indicated in situations where the cystic duct is extremely short or has a distal insertion into the common bile duct, there are multiple large stones present that cannot be extracted via a transcystic route, and/or there are proximal stones located in the common hepatic duct. However, when the common bile duct is less than 8 mm in diameter and/or surrounded by significant inflammation, the patient may be better served with endoscopic removal of the stones.

FIGURE H

Making a Choledochotomy

24. The cystic and common bile ducts are exposed in the usual manner, using blunt dissection and/or an ultrasonic dissector. The use of electrocautery should be avoided in close proximity to the common bile duct. The cystic duct is clipped at the infundibulum in the usual fashion. For large cystic ducts, an endoscopic ligating loop should be used to secure the duct.

25. A vertical ductomy is made in the common bile duct with small, sharp scissors and is extended to a length of approximately 5 mm to 6 mm, or long enough to allow for removal of stones and placement of a T-tube. The incision is made along the right anterolateral surface of the common bile duct, just distal to the insertion of the cystic duct.

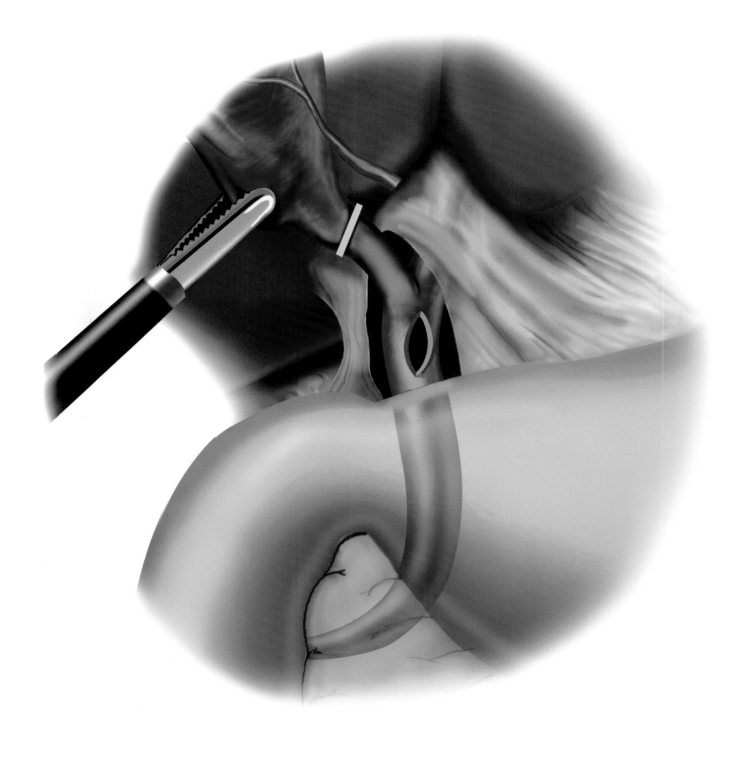

FIGURE I

Extracting the Stones

26. Common bile duct stones are removed using atraumatic graspers or a Fogarty balloon catheter, as previously described. Care should be taken to remove all stones from the peritoneal cavity.

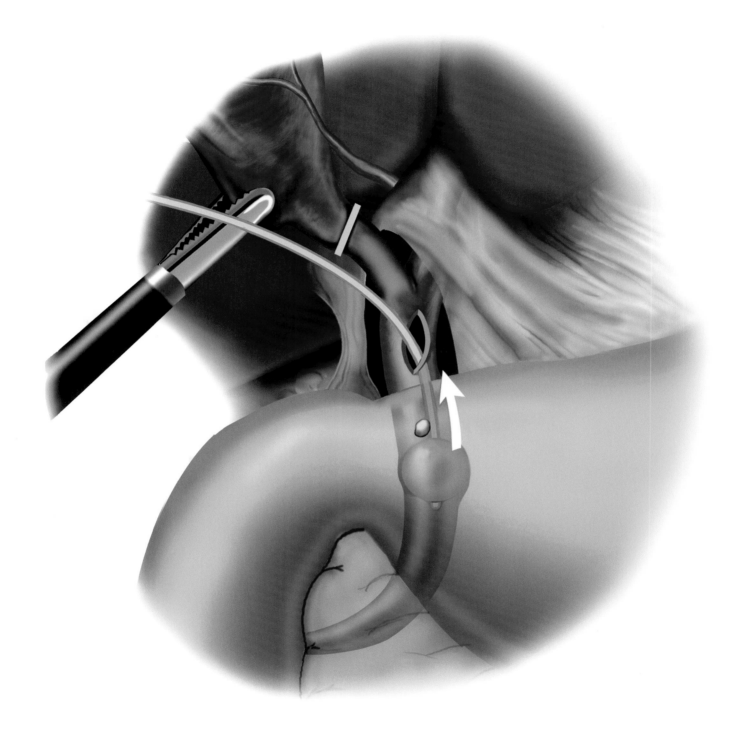

Performing Choledochoscopy and Removing Retained Stones

27. A 3 mm choledochoscope is then inserted into the common bile duct via the choledochotomy, and the proximal common hepatic duct and distal common bile duct are inspected for any retained stones. A stone retrieval basket may be used to extract any remaining stones under direct choledochoscopic visualization.

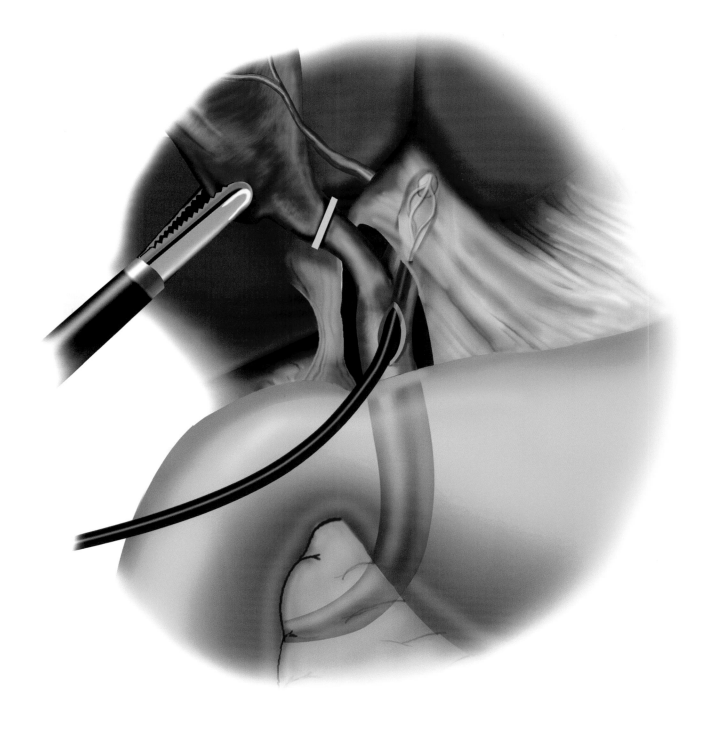

Placing a T-tube

28. Once the bile duct is clear, a 10 to 14 Fr T-tube is fashioned depending on the size of the common bile duct. Atraumatic graspers are used to facilitate placing the tube into the common bile duct. The ductomy is closed around the tube with multiple interrupted 4-0 absorbable sutures. The end of the T-tube is brought out through one of the lateral ports and is sutured to the skin. (Alternatively, primary closure without T-tube is reported.)

29. A completion cholangiogram is performed through the T-tube. The gallbladder is then removed in the usual manner, being careful not to dislodge the T-tube.

30. The right upper quadrant is observed for adequate hemostasis and/or any evidence of a bile leak. A closed suction drain is left in place through one of the lateral port sites. The trocars are removed under direct vision and the fascia and skin incisions are closed in the usual manner.

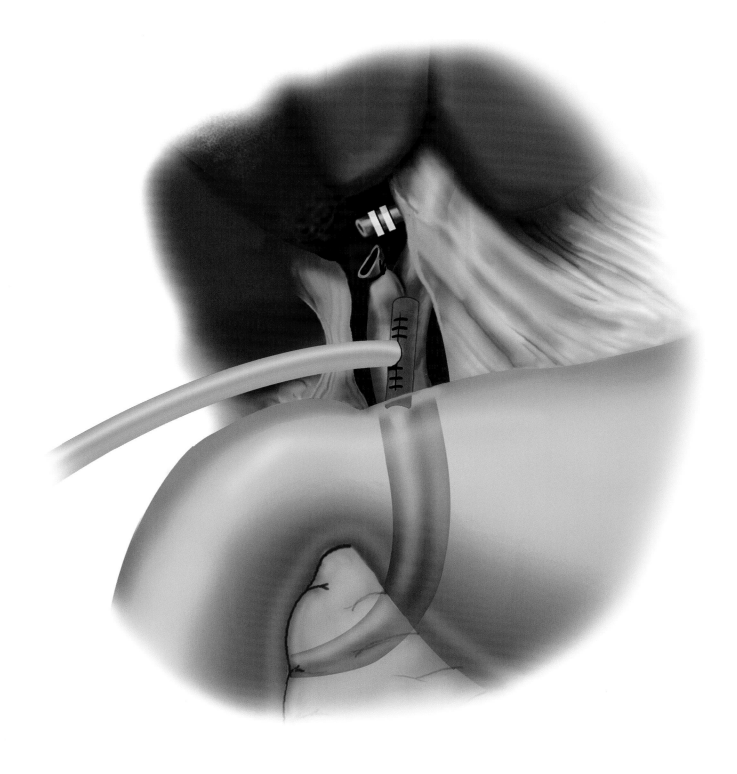

Postoperative Care

Pneumatic compression devices and/or subcutaneous heparin are continued postoperatively. Antibiotics are usually continued for 24 hours postoperatively. Patients are usually able to tolerate liquids and solid food within 24 hours after the operation. The drain is removed if there is no evidence of a bile leak. If a transcystic approach was used, no further treatment is required. If a choledochotomy was performed, the T-tube should be left in place for at least 4 weeks to allow maturation of the tract. However, the tube can be clamped to allow for normal anatomic internal drainage of bile into the duodenum. After 2 weeks, a repeat cholangiogram is taken to confirm a clear ductal system. Residual stones can be removed through the T-tube. If the duct is clear, the tube can be removed at the appropriate time.

Suggested Readings

1. Crawford DL, Phillips EH. Laparoscopic common bile duct exploration. *World J Surg.* 1999;23:343-349.

2. Dorman JP, Franklin ME, Glass JL. Laparoscopic common bile duct exploration by choledochotomy. *Surg Endosc.* 1998;12:926-928.

3. Jones DB, Dunnegan DL, Soper NJ. Results of a change to routine fluorocholangiograhy during laparoscopic cholecystectomy. *Surgery.* 1995;118:693-702.

4. Watson M, Hamilton EC, Jones DB. Laparoscopic common bile duct exploration. In: VanHeerden JA, Farley DR, eds. *Operative Techniques in General Surgery.* 2005;7(1):23-38.

Commentary

Mark J. Watson, M.D., Parkland Hospital
University of Texas Southwestern Medical Center

Clinically relevant bile duct stones are discovered during routine laparoscopic cholecystectomy. Competence in the laparoscopic removal of these stones should be within the grasp of most surgeons and these techniques are beautifully illustrated in this chapter.

Currently, the endoscopist via endoscopic retrograde cholangiopancreatography (ERCP), manages the majority of bile duct stones. There are several reasons why the surgeon should be interested in the techniques described in this chapter. Though endoscopic bile duct stone extraction is a proven procedure with good results, it requires an additional procedure with its inherent risks, costs, and additional anesthesia for the patient. In most cases, endoscopic stone extraction requires sphincterotomy or balloon dilation of the sphincter of Oddi. There is mounting evidence that in the long term, this may be associated with future cholangitis and stenosis of the sphincter. Management of bile duct stones leaving the sphincter intact is preferable.

Competence with intraoperative cholangiography is essential to manage bile duct stones laparoscopically. Debate continues over the indications for performing an intraoperative cholangiogram during a laparoscopic cholecystectomy. The arguments against its routine use typically focus on the additional operative time and expense of this study. In reality, the routine application of intraoperative cholangiography allows the surgeon and operating room staff to become so facile in its performance that it adds little to the operative time of the total procedure. The combined cost of normal, routine cholangiograms is likely offset by the cost of potentially missed, clinically relevant bile duct stones and rare common bile duct injuries that could be avoided or minimized. Cholangiography is one of the three key skills that are necessary to perform the transcystic approach illustrated in this chapter. The other two skills are the Seldinger technique utilizing guide wires and the use of the endoscope. These are skill possessed by most surgeons performing laparoscopic cholecystectomies, and this chapter nicely organizes their use.

In beginning a cholecystectomy, using a 5 mm umbilical port and laparoscope carries certain advantages to the 10 mm equipment. The port site does not require closure at the end of the procedure and the chance of future hernia formation is all but eliminated. With newer laparoscopic equipment, there is little compromise in picture quality. The gallbladder and stones may then be easily removed via the 10 mm subxiphoid port without moving the position of the laparoscope.

If a 5 Fr cholangiogram catheter is used at the outset, the initial step in the transcystic procedure is already completed if bile duct stones are identified during cholangiography. Smaller French catheters will not allow passage of guide wires or baskets. This larger diameter catheter allows better flushing of the common bile duct following administration of glucagon, a procedure that carries a very high success rate for smaller stones (< 4 mm).

Once the guide wire is in place for a transcystic exploration, the remainder of the procedure is more easily accomplished if the surgeon moves to the patient's right side. An additional assistant (tech) can be helpful to manage the end of the guide wires and other equipment. As the choledochoscope is advanced over the guide wire into the abdomen, the assistant must commonly provide caudal motion of the scope into the duct. It is critical that the choledochoscope not be grasped on its flexible tip (several centimeters proximal to the end), even with padded graspers. This will damage the optic fibers of the delicate scope and is expensive to repair.

Laparoscopic choledochotomy is especially helpful in cases of multiple large stones (> 1 cm) in the bile duct. Such stones are difficult to drag through the sphincter of Oddi during ERCP even after sphincterotomy. On the other hand, for smaller bile ducts (< 8 cm) and stones, ERCP avoids opening a bile duct that could potentially lead to stricture formation after closure following surgery. Laparoscopic suturing and intracorporeal tying are additional skills, which are required for treatment by choledochotomy.

Using the illustration provided in this chapter, many surgeons can organize their current skills to perform these procedures. Treating cholelithiasis and bile duct stones at the same procedure can provide improved and more efficient care of these conditions.

Steven C. Stain, M.D.
Albany Medical College

This chapter is well illustrated and includes many technical tips to direct the reader toward efficient completion of the operation. It is timely, as fewer surgeons are choosing laparoscopic common bile duct explorations compared to endoscopic therapy for choledocholithiasis. There are many technical pearls within the chapter, such as using half-strength contrast for the cholangiogram to increase the detection of CBD stones; and the techniques for flushing small stones through the common bile duct after the administration of glucagon.

The author describes a basket retrieval of the common bile duct stones under fluoroscopic guidance. While I believe this description is important for completeness sake, choledochoscopy is often required to accurately place the basket around the common bile duct stone. Trancystic choledochoscopy achieves direct visualization of the common bile duct stone during removal.

The author describes the method of laparoscopic choledochotomy for stone retrieval. Although there are several large series describing the safety of laparoscopic choledochotomy in expert hands, this technique is less frequently utilized than trancystic duct exploration. It may be appropriate for those with excellent laparoscopic suturing skills who can reliably close the common bile duct without it narrowing the common bile duct over a T-tube. Although the laparoscopic choledochotomy stone retrieval offers all of the potential advantages of an open common bile duct exploration, the application of this technique must be weighed against the alternative of endoscopic sphincterotomy for CBD stone removal.

Ashley H. Vernon, M.D., Brigham & Women's Hospital Harvard Medical School

The need for surgical clearance of bile duct stones has diminished as endoscopic procedures have taken on a greater role. Some surgeons may be glad about this since laparoscopic common bile duct exploration is difficult, requiring the most advanced skills. Other surgeons may find themselves in an environment where performance of this procedure is of great benefit to their patients. An example of this is in patients who develop choledocholithiasis after having a bariatric procedure with Roux-en-Y reconstruction in which the biliary tree is difficult to access by endoscopy.

As with the open procedure, laparoscopic common bile duct exploration should not be undertaken without a plan of action and familiarity with the necessary instruments. There are many pieces of equipment available to facilitate successful completion of the procedure; however, they may not be easily obtained without careful planning. The first thing you must do is review the steps of the procedure, anticipate the equipment that will be used during each step and then put all of the equipment in an order that you will be able to find it. This can be accomplished by dedicating a cart in the operating room for this procedure—top drawer for tools used in routine cholangiography, next drawer for instruments used to insert the choledochoscope, and bottom drawer for instruments such as baskets and balloons passed through the working channel of the choledochoscope.

Once stones are detected in the common bile duct during cholangiography, I administer glucagon, 1 mg given twice, and flush the ductal system with saline. This is concurrent with instructing the operating room of the impending workload. Then I repeat the cholangiogram. Generally, manipulations to remove stones with instruments through the cholangiocatheter under fluoroscopic guidance (as in steps 16 and 17) are unsuccessful. A Fogarty balloon leads to stones being pulled up into the proximal ductal system and usually does not get the job done. If the stones are still present, I prepare for a common bile duct exploration.

A guide wire is passed into the common bile duct (0.035-inch coated guide wire with soft tips on both ends) through the cholangiocatheter. The guide wire directs the placement of a dilator (balloon dilators, graduated dilators, pneumatic dilator) into the cystic duct. I use the balloon dilator and inflate it for 5 minutes while I set up the equipment for the rest of the procedure. I take this time to gather the introducer sheath through which the choledochoscope will be passed through the abdominal wall, padded laparoscopic instruments for manipulating the choledochocope, and the balloons and baskets. The choledochoscope should be set up with constant irrigation. The next step is to introduce the sheath through the abdominal wall and pass the choledochoscope into the peritoneal cavity and into the cystic duct. The choledochoscope is 2.8 mm OD with a 1.2 mm working channel and requires a cystic duct at least that size.

The best approach for common bile duct exploration is through the cystic duct. By avoiding opening the common duct, the procedure does not require advanced skills for T-tube placement and does not obligate the patient to prolonged care of a T-tube postoperatively. Even though it is the preferred method, anatomic limitations may make it impossible as when the cystic duct enters the common duct posteriorly or at an acute angle or is very small and cannot be dilated to a large enough size for stone removal. Additionally, it is impossible to extract stones via the cystic duct when the stones are very large (> 6 mm) or when they are located in the hepatic ducts. In those cases, a choledochotomy in the common bile duct must be made. This makes the procedure much more difficult because it involves suturing the common bile duct over a T-tube using laparoscopic instruments and intracorporeal knot tying. Many general surgeons opt to convert to an open procedure at this point.

Leonardo Villegas, M.D., Beth Israel Deaconess Medical Center Harvard Medical School

Surgeons performing intraoperative cholangiogram during laparoscopic cholecystectomy will encounter CBD stones in approximately one third of the patients and must be able to manage them effectively. The most convenient approach is by laparoscopic common bile duct exploration (LCBDE) at the time of laparoscopic cholecystectomy.

The LCBDE approach is preferable because it avoids a two-step procedure (second anesthesia) required by pre- or postoperative ERCP. LCBDE is associated with lower overall cost than postoperative ERCP. The latter is associated with a 5% incidence of morbidity and 1% of mortality, and increasing stenosis complications after sphincterotomy.

Laparoscopic choledocholithotomy represents an exciting option in the armamentarium of laparoscopic surgeons for the management of common bile duct stones. As one can see, a learning curve exists. The literature suggests that this technique is not only feasible, but also safe and effective. There are two ways to approach laparoscopic common bile duct exploration—via the cystic duct (transcystic) or the direct ductal approach (transductal or choledochotomy). Both are highly effective, with the transcystic approach representing the more minimally invasive technique, with low morbidity and mortality, and the postoperative care is identical to a regular laparoscopic cholecystectomy. This approach does not necessitate advanced laparoscopic skills, just basic knowledge of instrumentation and, Seldinger technique. The transcystic approach avoids the need for repair of the common bile duct or placement of a T-tube. Clearing of the common duct of stones can be achieved using the "flushing" technique under fluoroscopic guidance alone or before attempting a transcystic or transductal approach.

Surgeons should consider the laparoscopic management of common bile duct stones as a cost effective, minimally invasive, safe alternative to ERCP and open common bile duct exploration. With experience, laparoscopic common bile duct exploration is successful at clearing the common bile duct approximately 85% to 95%. However certain clinical challenges arise that may necessitate alternative action by the surgeon (see Table 1).

Below is a list of dilemmas commonly encountered during LCBDE, as well as suggestions to aid in management of CBD stones.

Table 1. Clinical Scenarios and Therapeutic Options

Scenario	Management options (in order of attempt)
Small diameter (< 6 mm) CBD	Transcystic approach, using basket, balloon, choledocoscope, try to avoid choledochotomy.
Obstructed cystic duct	Milk stones back toward gallbladder, repeat cystic ductotomy closer to CBD junction, pass hydrophilic guide wire through cholangiogram catheter, or directly through cystic ductotomy over the obstructing stone.
Impacted stone in CBD	Irrigation (distending the wall allows to work with a basket, Fogarty catheter, graspers or lithotripsy; conversion to open CBD exploration.
Stone in proximal biliary tree	Postural positioning, or suction-irrigation, IV glucagon, complete cystic duct dissection (to break the angle limitation of the scope), direct transductal approach.
Big (> 6 mm) CBD stone	Choledochotomy with scope instrumentation, balloon or basket, placement of T-tube or primary closure.
Multiple stones in CBD	Biliary bypass with choledocho-duodenostomy or hepaticojejunostomy
Bleeding from CBD	Irrigation with cold saline or tamponade with balloon angioplasty catheter.
Retained CBD stone	Perform biliary drainage (transcystic or T-tube) and access for postoperative ERCP; consider laparoscopic CBD stent placement and/or laparoscopic anterograde sphincterotomy, if malignancy is ruled out.
Cystic duct injury	Ligation of cystic duct with endoloop or intracorporeal suturing.
Visual impairment	Flush with saline through working port on scope.

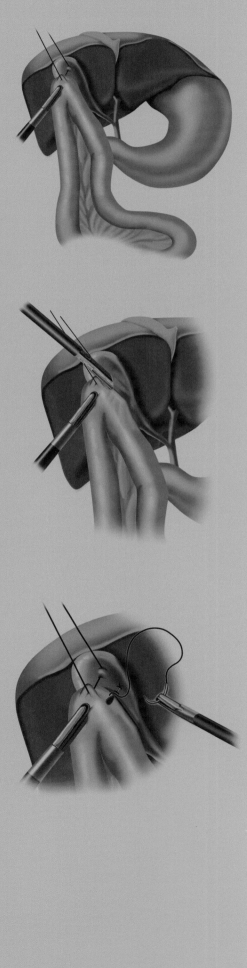

Laparoscopic Cholecystojejunostomy

Periampullary tumors are often unresectable at the time of diagnosis due to local invasion and/or metastatic spread. Palliative surgical therapy of this situation often requires choledochojejunostomy or a cholecystojejunostomy, of which the latter is described here. Each procedure can be performed with either a Roux-en-Y jejunal limb or a jejunal loop reconstruction.

Preoperative Preparation

1. Sequential compression stockings and subcutaneous heparin may be used for prophylaxis against deep venous thrombosis. Intravenous antibiotics, usually a second-generation cephalosporin, is administered prophylactically to cover biliary pathogens. After induction of general anesthesia, the bladder is emptied with a urinary catheter and the stomach is decompressed with a nasogastric tube.

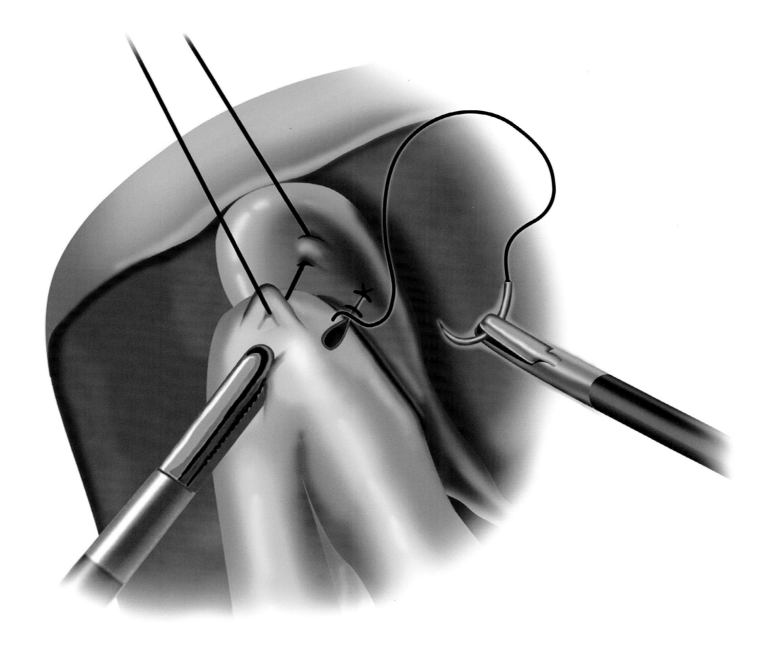

Operating Room Setup

2. The patient is placed in the supine position. All pressure points must be adequately padded.

3. The surgeon stands to the patient's right, while the assistant stands to the left.

4. A video monitor is stationed at each side of the patient's head to provide adequate viewing from both sides of the table.

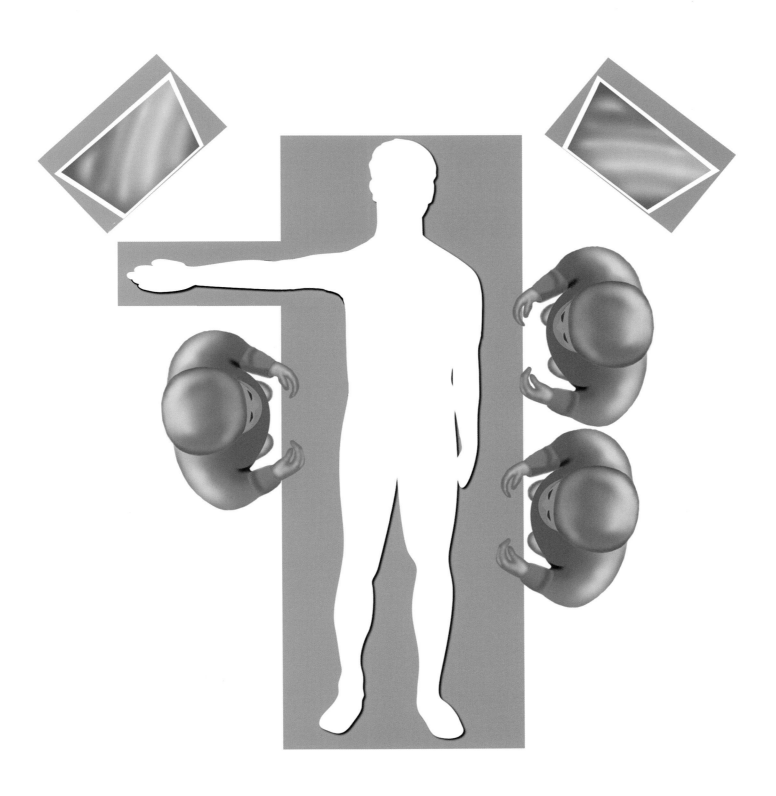

Access and Port Placement

5. An infraumbilical incision is used to establish pneumoperitoneum, setting a pressure limit of 15 mm Hg. This is established either with an open or closed technique. A 10/11 mm port is placed here and the laparoscope is inserted. A 30° angled scope facilitates visualization during the operation. A careful exploration is performed to ensure that no injury occurred during port insertion and that no other abnormalities are present.

6. A 5 mm trocar is placed under direct vision below the right costal margin in the midclavicular line. A second 5 mm port is placed in the left midclavicular line below the costal margin. Finally, a 12 mm port is placed above the right iliac crest.

7. The patient is positioned in 15° of reverse Trendelenburg position to facilitate exposure of the gallbladder and ligament of Treitz.

8. Cholangiography may be performed to determine the position of the cystic duct/common bile duct junction with tumor.

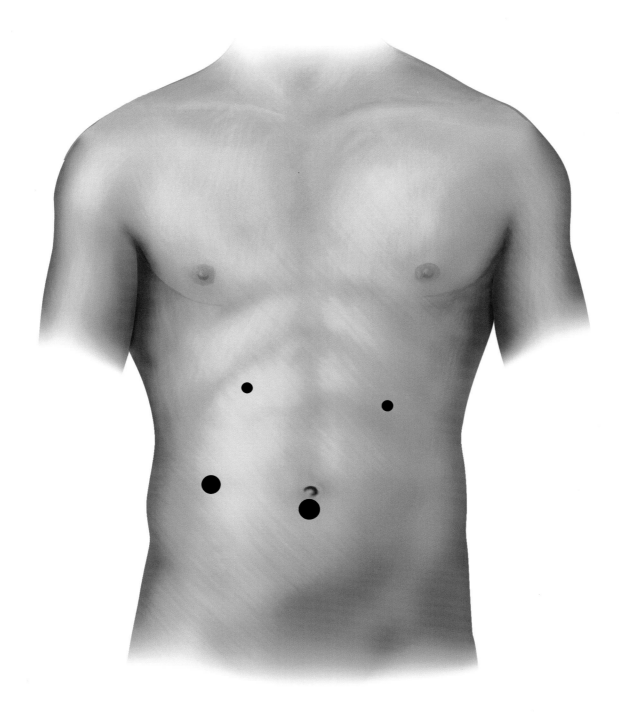

Stapled Anastomosis

FIGURE C

Approximating the Jejunum to Gallbladder

1. A section of jejunum approximately 40 cm to 50 cm distal to the ligament of Treitz is grasped and gently mobilized toward the gallbladder in an antecolic fashion. This distance is usually sufficient to avoid any tension on the anastomosis. Alternatively, a 40 cm Roux limb can be constructed using the same technique as detailed in the section on performing a Roux-en-Y gastric bypass.

2. The loop of jejunum and dilated gallbladder are anchored together using a 3-0 silk suture and an extracorporeal technique. The suture is placed on slight traction, thus promoting apposition of the jejunum to the gallbladder. Alternatively, two stay sutures can be placed at either end of the intended anastomotic site.

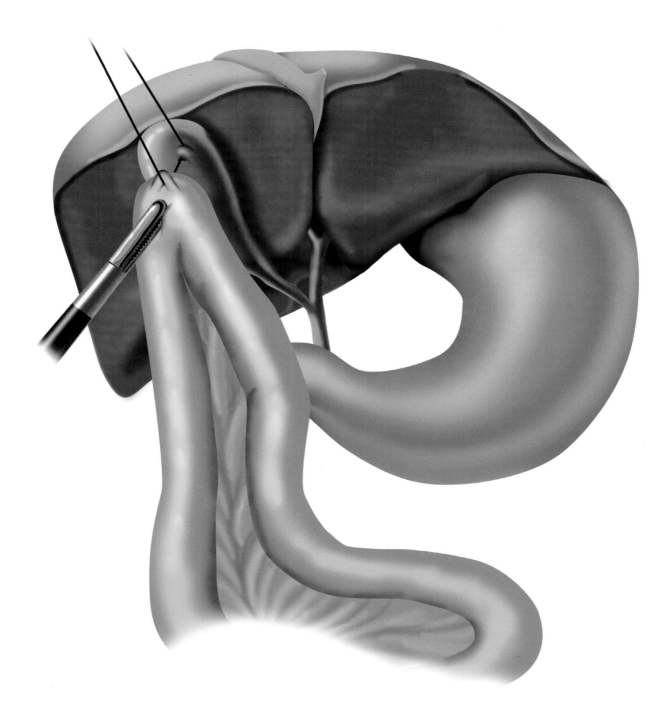

Preparing to Create the Anastomosis

3. The distended gallbladder is decompressed by aspirating its contents using a laparoscopic large-bore needle attached to a 60 cc syringe. This maneuver minimizes the extent of bile spillage in the peritoneal cavity and facilitates handling the gallbladder.

4. Next, a 1 cm long cholecystotomy and enterotomy are created using electrocautery scissors. The enterotomy is created on the antimesenteric side of the jejunum. Hemostasis is obtained with minimal use of electrocautery.

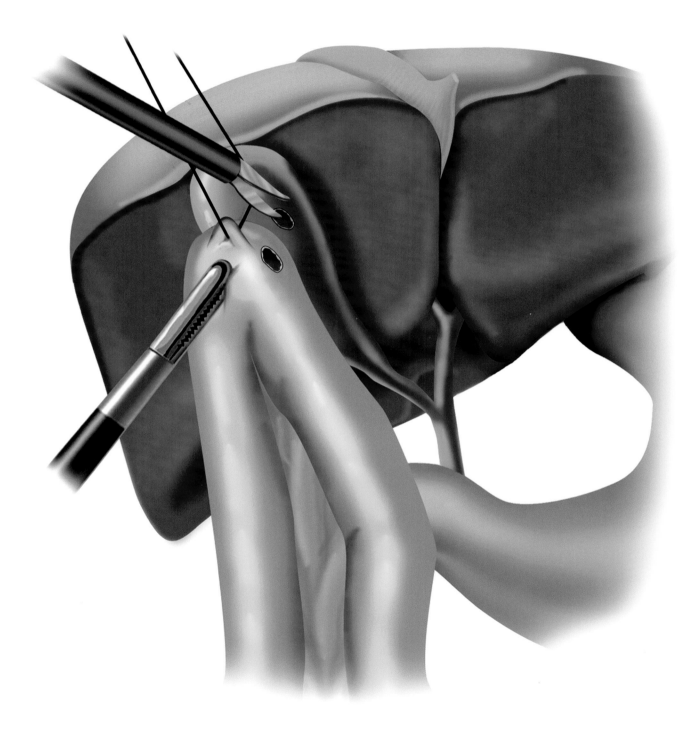

Creating a Stapled Cholecystojejunostomy

5. An endoscopic linear stapler, loaded with 3.5 mm staples, is introduced through the 12 mm port in the right iliac fossa. The stapler should be in line with the long axis of the gallbladder and loop of jejunum. One jaw of the device is inserted into each of the openings (Figure E-a). The stapling device is closed (Figure E-b) and fired to form the anterior and posterior walls of the stapled anastomosis (Figure E-c). An angled stapler can be easier to navigate, particularly in the smaller patient.

FIGURE E-a

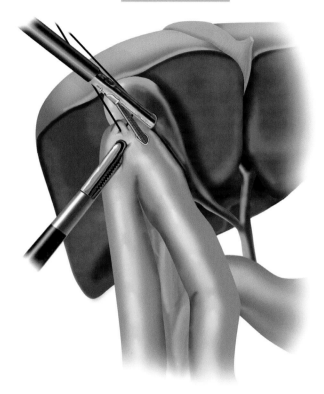

FIGURE E-b

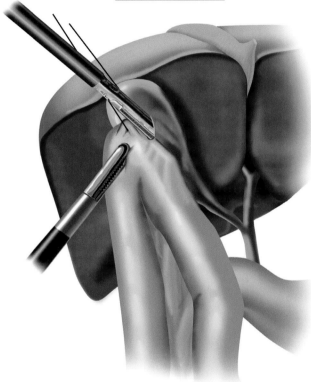

FIGURE E-c

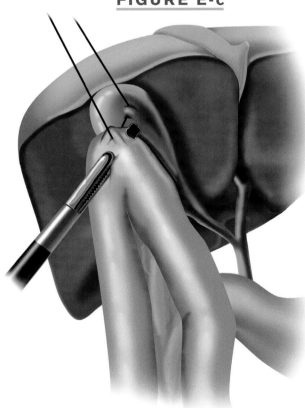

Closing the Enterotomy and Cholecystotomy

6. An intracorporeal 3-0 running, or interrupted, suture is used to close the remaining enterotomy and cholecystotomy. If a running stitch is used, intracorporeal knot tying is utilized. Either knot-tying techniques can be used for an interrupted closure. Full-thickness bites of the gallbladder and seromuscular bites of the jejunum are used to close the defect. This completes the anastomosis.

7. Alternatively, a second firing of the stapler in a transverse fashion can be used to close the enterotomy. If a stapled closure is utilized, care must be taken not to narrow the anastomosis.

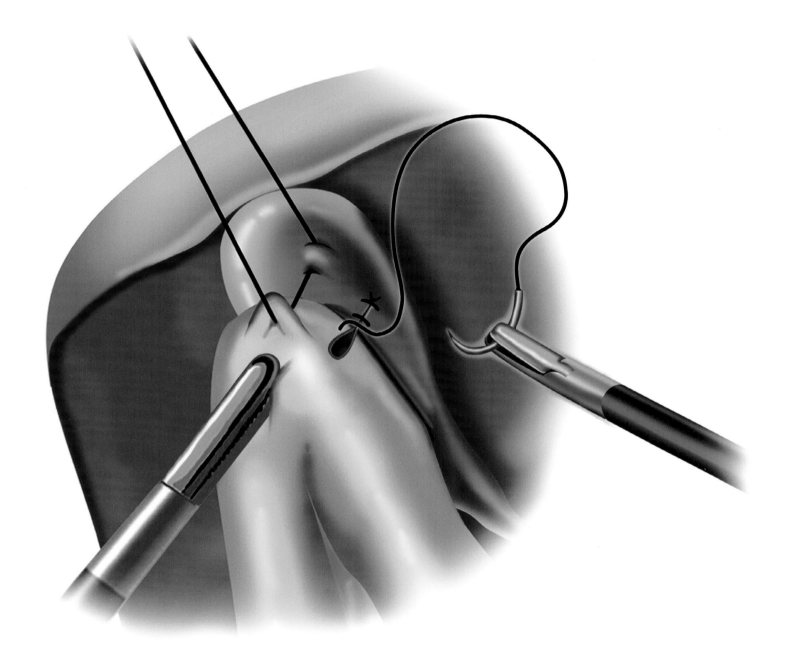

Sutured Anastomosis

Alternatively, a completely hand-sewn anastomosis may be performed.

FIGURE G

Creating the Posterior Layer

1. The loop of jejunum and gallbladder are anchored together as described above. The intended site for anastomosis is selected.

2. The serosa of the gallbladder and antimesenteric border of jejunum are scored with electrocautery to mark the site of the anastomosis, which should be 25 mm to 30 mm in length.

3. A 3-0 nonabsorbable suture is used to approximate the posterior walls of the anastomosis by taking full-thickness bites of the gallbladder and seromuscular bites of the jejunum. If a running stitch is utilized, the suture should be prepared extracorporeally by forming a jamming loop knot at the tail of the suture. After the first pass of tissue is taken from each side, the needle is passed through the loop, which is closed by pulling on the body of the suture. The assistant should maintain slight tension on the suture with an atraumatic grasping forceps as each stitch is placed.

4. Once the posterior layer is complete, an intracorporeal knot is tied at the end to secure the running stitch. Alternatively, interrupted sutures can be placed and secured with either intracorporeal or extracorporeal knot-tying techniques.

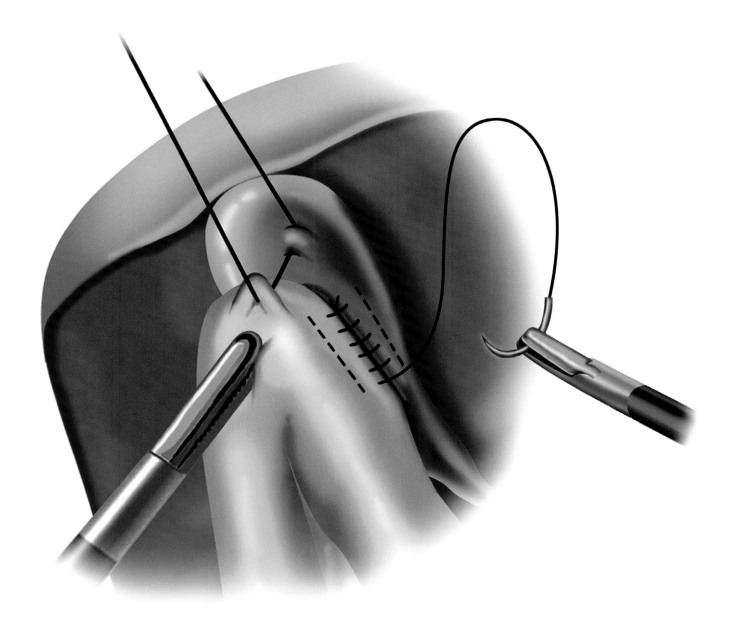

Opening the Gallbladder and Jejunum

5. The distended gallbladder is decompressed by aspirating its contents as previously described. Cauterized hook (Figure H-a) and/or scissors (Figure H-b) are used to open the gallbladder and jejunum along the previously marked line. Care should be taken to minimize bile spillage. Hemostasis is obtained with electrocautery.

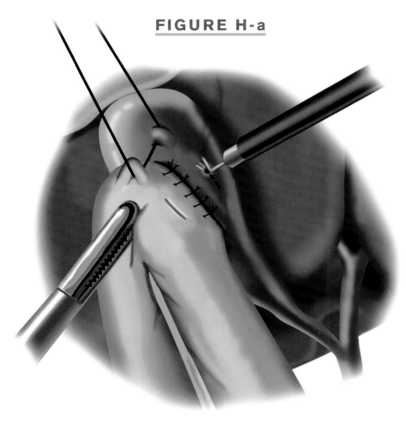

FIGURE H-a

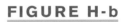

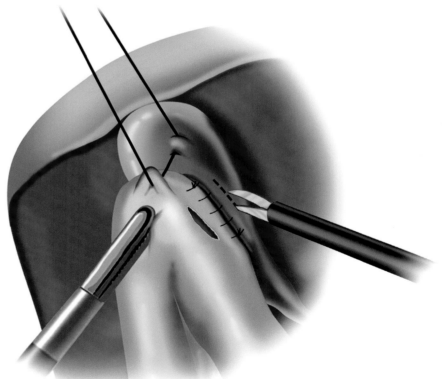

FIGURE H-b

FIGURE I

Closing the Anterior Layer and Completing the Anastomosis

6. The same technique as described for the posterior layer is used to close the anterior layer of the anastomosis. A running, or interrupted, suture is placed along the anterior edge and is secured at the end with an intracorporeal knot.

7. The operative field is again inspected for hemostasis and the ports are removed under laparoscopic visualization to ensure hemostasis at each of the port sites as well. Each incision is infiltrated with a solution of 0.5% bupivacaine and irrigated with saline solution. The fascia of each incision greater than 10 mm is closed with an absorbable suture. The skin incision at each port site is closed with a subcuticular absorbable suture.

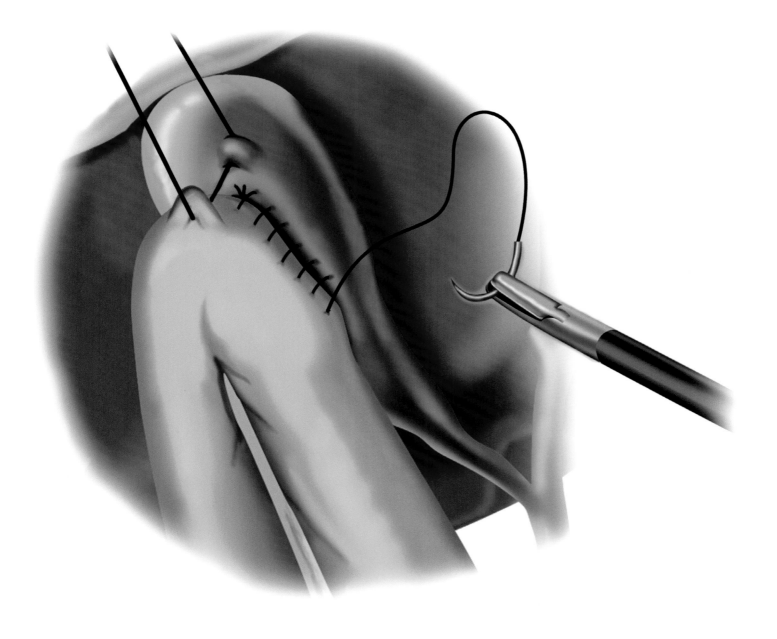

Postoperative Care

Pneumatic compression devices and/or subcutaneous heparin are continued postoperatively. Antibiotics are usually continued for 24 hours after the operation at the discretion of the surgeon. The nasogastric tube is removed after return of bowel function. Oral intake is initiated with clear liquids and advanced as tolerated. Patients are usually discharged within 3 to 4 days after the operation.

Suggested Readings

1. Chekan EG, Clark L, Wu J, Pappas TN, Eubanks S. Laparoscopic biliary and enteric bypass. *Semin Surg Oncol.* 1999;16:313-320.

2. Cuscheri A, Berci G. Laparoscopic management of pancreatic cancer. In: *Laparoscopic Biliary Surgery.* Oxford: Blackwell Scientific Publications. 1992;170-182.

3. O'Rourke N, Nathanson L. Laparoscopic biliary-enteric bypass. In: Paterson-Brown S, Garden J, eds. *Principles and Practice of Surgical Laparoscopy.* London: WB Saunders. 1994;179-189.

4. Urbach DR, Bell CM, Swantstrom CC, Hansen PD. Cohort study of surgical bypass to the gallbladder or bile duct for palliation of jaundice due to pancreatic cancer. *Ann Surg.* 2003;237:86-93.

Commentary

Justin S. Wu, M.D., Kaiser Permanente Medical Center
University of California, San Diego

The incidence of periampullary carcinoma has significantly increased during the past 5 decades, and, unfortunately, the majority of these patients will have unresectable disease. Biliary decompression has improved with the metallic stents as opposed to plastic stents, but nevertheless, they are still a source of infection or obstruction. Surgical biliary bypasses have been shown in multiple studies to have longer patency rate, less infection, and shorter hospitalization. The authors of this chapter have clearly shown the best surgical techniques in providing biliary bypasses, i.e., laparoscopic cholecystojejunostomy, utilizing both the stapling and the hand-sewn technique.

The first laparoscopic cholecystojejunostomy was reported in 1992 and most reports subsequently have involved only small numbers of patients. Early data have been promising, with patients discharged between 10 and 17 days postoperatively. The largest experience reported has been from Duke University Medical Center, revealing similar lengths of operative time and postoperative hospital stay, comparable rates of perioperative morbidity and mortality, and good long-term palliative results following both open and laparoscopic cholecystojejunostomy.

The most important aspect to laparoscopic biliary bypass procedures is the port placement. If the trocars are placed adequately to provide the correct angle of the laparoscopic instruments (needle holders, aspirators, staplers), then half of the operation is already completed. Another key to setting up the gallbladder and jejunum for the anastomosis is extracorporeal stay sutures, which provide important traction and angulation.

Kevin C. Conlon, M.D., M.B.A., The Adelaide and Meath Hospital University of Dublin

Pancreatic cancer remains a lethal disease. Approximately 30,000 new cases of pancreatic adenocarcinoma are reported each year in the United States. Unfortunately, most of these patients initially present with advanced stages of the disease. As such, pancreatic cancer continues to be the gastrointestinal malignancy with the least favorable prognosis with the incidence of new cases correlating closely to the death rate on an annual basis. At the time of diagnosis, approximately, 10% to 15% of patients have disease confined to the pancreas, while 30% exhibit local spread and > 50% demonstrate distant disease.

Since the majority of patients with pancreatic cancer have unresectable disease at the time of presentation, palliation to minimize symptoms and maximize quality of life is a major aim of any treatment plan. Palliation most commonly is required for one of three problems: biliary obstruction, gastric outlet obstruction, and relief of pain.

Obstructive jaundice may occur in up to two thirds of patients at presentation. Historically, relief of biliary obstruction was accomplished at the time of exploratory laparotomy. Currently, improvements in radiological diagnostic and nonoperative staging modalities, as well as the development of nonoperative biliary decompression via transhepatic or endoscopic means, has led to the majority of jaundiced patients being managed non-operatively. However, in selected patients, an operative biliary bypass may be considered preferable. In these patients, it is our preference to perform a laparoscopic procedure if possible.

While both cholecystoenteric and choledochoenteric bypasses have been performed laparoscopically, the latter is much more difficult technically, requiring a high level of laparoscopic skills. A sufficient length of common duct needs to be exposed and a difficult intracorporeal anastomosis between the small bowel and the common duct performed. Cholecystojejunostomy as illustrated in this chapter is the more commonly performed laparoscopic procedure. While a certain degree of controversy exists as to the efficacy of this technique, it is our opinion that it is equally effective when compared to choledochal bypass in selected patients. The anatomical position of the tumor in relation to the cystic duct is critical for selection as tumor impingement within 1 cm of the duct is a predictor of early technical failure. This can occur when either the primary tumor infiltrates the common bile duct above the pancreas, extensive peripancreatic adenopathy is present, or where a low insertion of the cystic duct into the common bile duct occurs. Preoperative imaging studies may provide the necessary information; alternatively, intraoperative cholangiography via the gallbladder or laparoscopic ultrasonography may be used to determine the position of the cystic duct.

As illustrated, the anastomosis can be performed with either a stapled or hand-sewn technique. In general, we favor the former method. We place the 10 mm to 12 mm port midway between the costal margin and the anterior iliac spine as this appears to give the best working angle for placement of the stapler. A single firing of the stapler will create an adequate anastomosis. The resultant enterotomy is closed as described. The operative bed is irrigated to remove any enteric spillage. Postopertaive drainage is not required.

Our experience suggests that successful resolution of jaundice occurs in 90% of patients. We have had no perioperative mortality, and morbidity is minimal with this technique.

Charles M. Vollmer, Jr., M.D., Beth Israel Deaconess Medical Center Harvard Medical School

The optimal approach for relief of biliary obstruction from malignancy remains a hotly debated subject today. Numerous options are available and in a mature hepatobiliary surgical practice there are probably individual circumstances where each is ideal, so having skills in all approaches maximizes versatility and outcomes. Laparoscopic palliation is generally performed by those surgeons who espouse the concept of laparoscopic staging for periampullary malignancy, yet distrust the long-term durability of endoscopic biliary diversion. As such, it is usually employed by either skilled laparoscopists, or hepatobiliary surgical specialists proficient in advanced laparoscopy, who judge this to be the most appropriate procedure for the patient at hand.

This chapter nicely illustrates the procedural layout for laparoscopic cholecystojejunostomy as a minimally invasive option for the relief of obstructive jaundice. It should be emphasized that this procedure falls under the realm of advanced laparoscopy and it would be a mistake to advocate its use by surgeons who do not possess the extra skill-set required to perform intracorporeal knot-tying. Technically, the procedure follows form for any side-to-side stapled anastomosis—either laparoscopic or open. Most often this is performed in the setting of periampullary malignancy with its attendant biliary obstruction and as a result, the gallbladder is frequently dilated, distended, and inflamed (the so-called Courvoisier's gallbladder). This subacute effect provides just enough tissue integrity to allow for a single-layered enterostomy. With a normal, supple gallbladder, this becomes technically more challenging and less reliable. The illustrated technique is essentially the same as that used for laparoscopic enteroenterostomy— frequently performed in conjunction with the biliary bypass for such patients and illustrated elsewhere in this atlas.

In general, I do not advocate cholecystoenterostomy on any occasion unless other approaches are technically impossible, or speed is of the essence. There is always concern about the durability of this approach with the culprit being eventual obstruction of the cystic duct by tumor encroachment or nodal encasement from the periampullary region. The preferred technique is either a choledocho- or hepaticojejunostomy, but currently even few minimally invasive surgeons have the skills to perform these laparoscopically. For now, their application poses more of an academic than practical interest. Perhaps robotics technology will enable promotion of this approach in the future. In addition, I believe that cholecysto- or choledocho-enterostomy via a "lazy loop" of jejunum alone, although quicker and technically simpler, is an inferior operation to that of bypass via a Roux-en-Y loop. In order to prevent recurrent cholangitis or inspissation of enteric contents, it is preferable to provide a disconnected and defunctional conduit from the biliary system.

These points of emphasis are substantiated by a nice analysis spanning 1991-1996, where national patterns of operative biliary bypass for malignant obstruction were compared for their efficacy. It should be noted that these were overwhelmingly open procedures, as this predated the advanced laparoscopic era, but the technical considerations should translate to the current era. Interestingly, cholecystoenterostomy was employed equally as often as was choledochoenterostomy (51-49%). Not surprisingly, however, rates of failure and need for further interventions were both higher at 1, 2, and 5 years for cholecystoenterostomy. Patients who have bypass via the gallbladder are four times as likely to need further biliary surgery, and three times as likely to need any further biliary intervention. Median survival is lower.

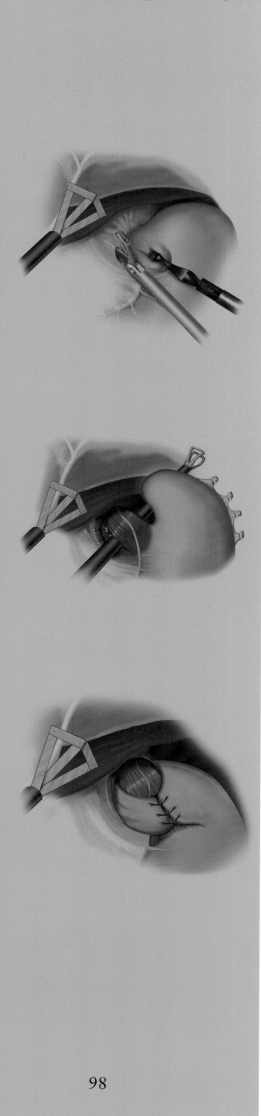

Laparoscopic Nissen Fundoplication

Gastroesophageal reflux disease (GERD) may cause heartburn, regurgitation, esophageal stricture, and Barrett's dysplasia, which can lead to the development of esophageal adenocarcinoma. Preoperative diagnostic tests can include 24-hour pH monitoring, esophageal manometry, upper endoscopy, and/or contrast studies. The three main components of the Nissen fundoplication that contribute to its therapeutic effect are: 1) closing the hiatal defect, 2) creating a short, loose wrap around the gastroesophageal (GE) junction, and 3) returning the GE junction to the abdominal cavity, which is possibly the most important step.

Preoperative Preparation

1. Sequential compression stockings and subcutaneous heparin may be used for prophylaxis against deep venous thrombosis. Intravenous antibiotics, usually a first-generation cephalosporin, are administered prophylactically. After induction of general anesthesia, the bladder is emptied with a urinary catheter and the stomach is decompressed with an orogastric tube.

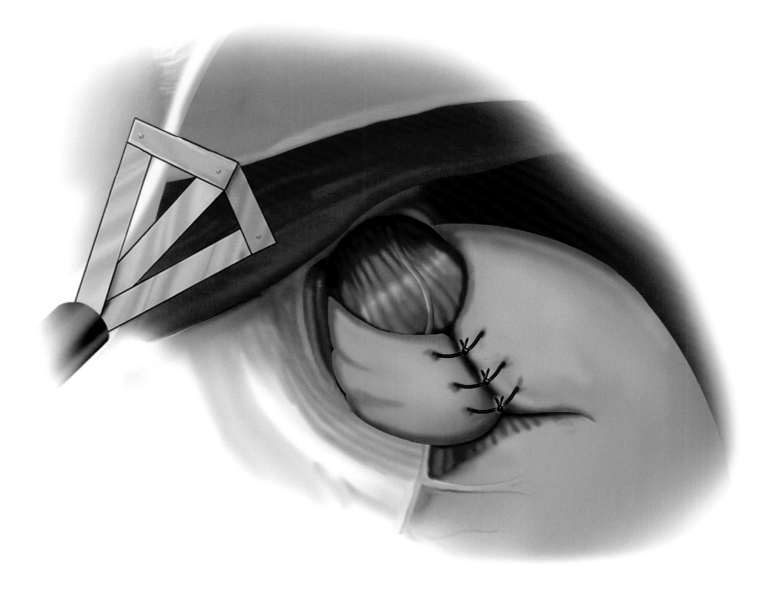

Operating Room Setup

2. The patient is placed on a cushioned bean bag and spreader bars with the surgeon standing between the legs. All pressure points must be adequately padded and the bean-bag device is used to secure the patient's position when rotating the table to facilitate exposure and viewing during the procedure.

3. The assistant is situated to the patient's right, while the camera operator stands on the patient's left side.

4. Alternatively, the patient can be placed supine with the surgeon standing to the patient's right, and the assistant on the left.

5. The video monitors are stationed at both sides of the patient's head to facilitate adequate viewing from either side of the table.

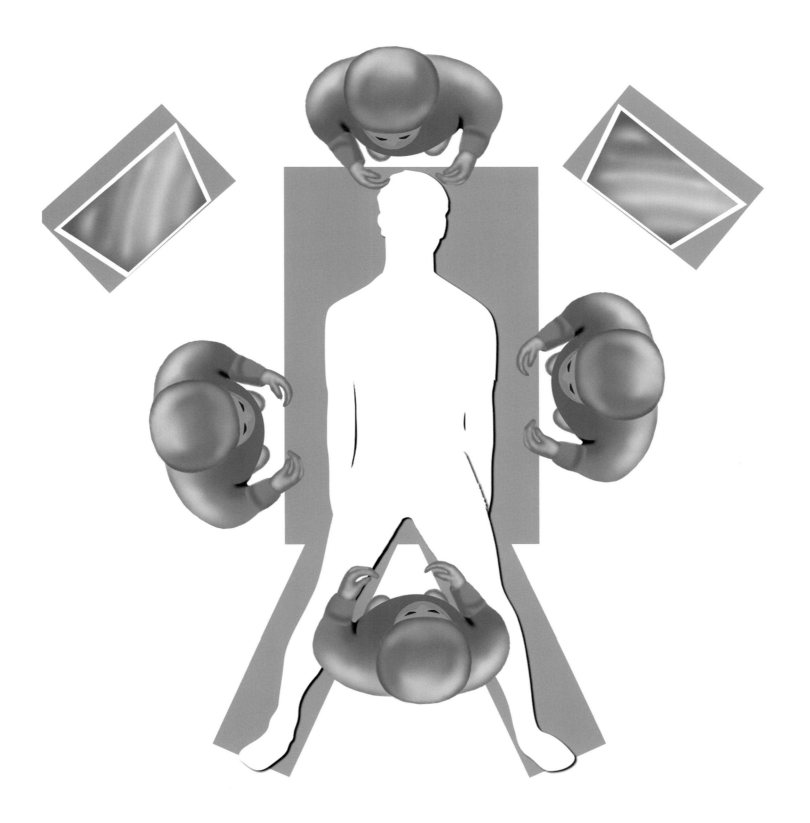

Access and Port Placement

6. Pneumoperitoneum is obtained through a left upper subcostal incision with a closed technique using a Veress needle. An optical trocar is used for initial port placement 15 cm beneath the xiphoid process, slightly left of the umbilicus. The 0° scope is switched for a 30° angled laparoscope, and the abdomen is inspected for adhesions or injuries.

7. Next, four radially expanding 11 mm ports are placed under direct vision in the configuration as shown (alternatively three 5 mm ports and one 11 mm port in the left subcostal area can be used).

8. In general, the most inferior port should be placed no more than 15 cm below the xiphoid process in order to facilitate maximal manipulation and range of motion of the instruments.

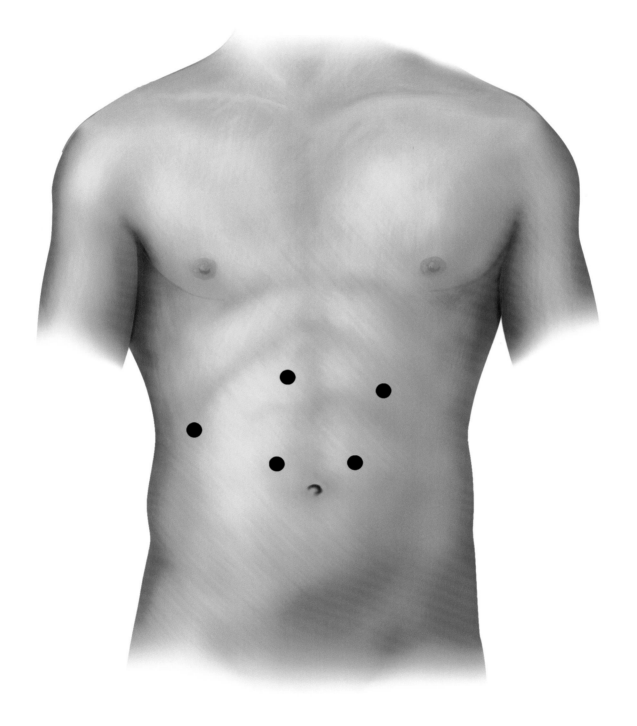

FIGURE C

Exposing the Esophageal Hiatus

9. The patient is placed in the reverse Trendelenburg position to provide gravity retraction. A self-retaining liver retractor is used to displace the left lateral lobe of the liver anteriorly and laterally. The gastroesophageal fat pad is grasped with a Babcock grasper and distracted inferiorly to the patient's left while the gastrohepatic ligament is divided with ultrasonic shears, starting superior to the hepatic branch of the vagus nerve. Care is taken to identify and preserve an aberrant left hepatic artery. The gastrohepatic ligament is opened to the level of the right crus of the diaphragm, after which the phrenoesophageal ligament is divided.

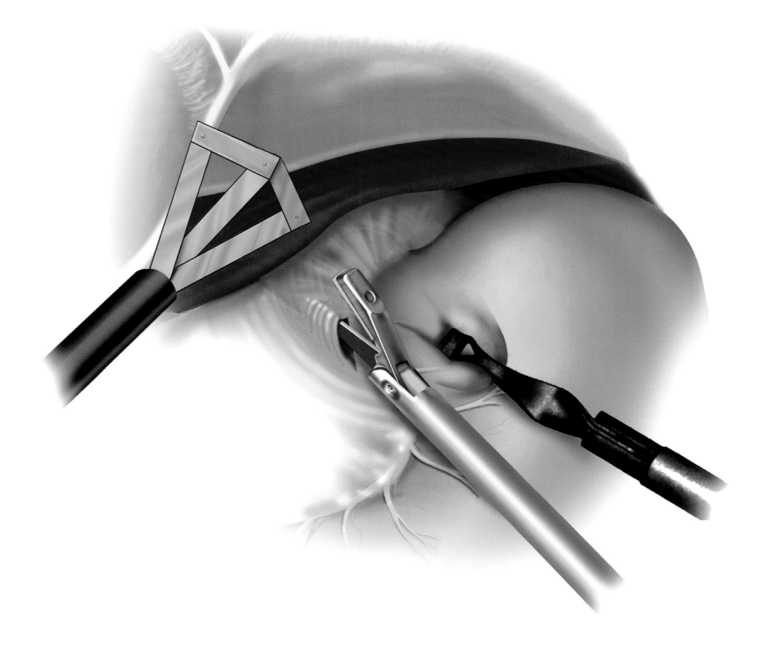

Exposing the Esophageal Hiatus, Part II

10. Once the phrenoesophageal ligament is adequately opened, both crura of the diaphragm and the anterior vagus nerve must be identified. The right crus is retracted laterally to expose and identify the posterior vagus nerve. If a hiatal hernia is present, it is gently reduced into the abdominal cavity by dividing any surrounding adhesions.

11. A plane is bluntly developed between the crura and posterior esophageal wall. Appropriate use of the angled laparoscope greatly facilitates this step. The esophagus overlying this posterior window may be retracted anteriorly with a Babcock grasper or a Penrose drain passed through this window.

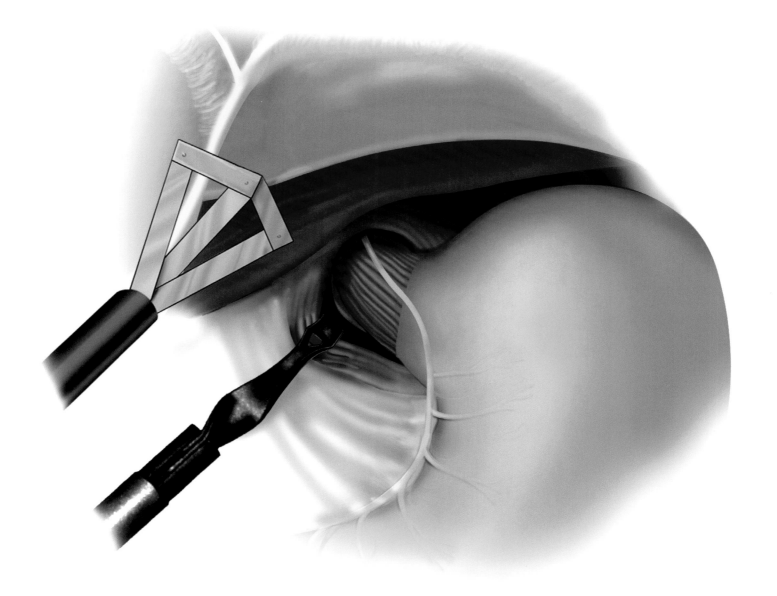

Mobilizing the Gastric Fundus

12. The gastrosplenic ligament and the short gastric vessels contained within are divided with an ultrasonic coagulator from a point on the greater curve 8 cm to 10 cm distal to the esophageal junction to the level of the diaphragm to fully mobilize the gastric fundus. Alternatively, the ligament can be divided with a ligasure device or with surgical clips. Regardless of the technique used, adequate hemostasis must be obtained when dividing the short gastric vessels. Any posterior retroperitoneal adhesions to the fundus must also be divided.

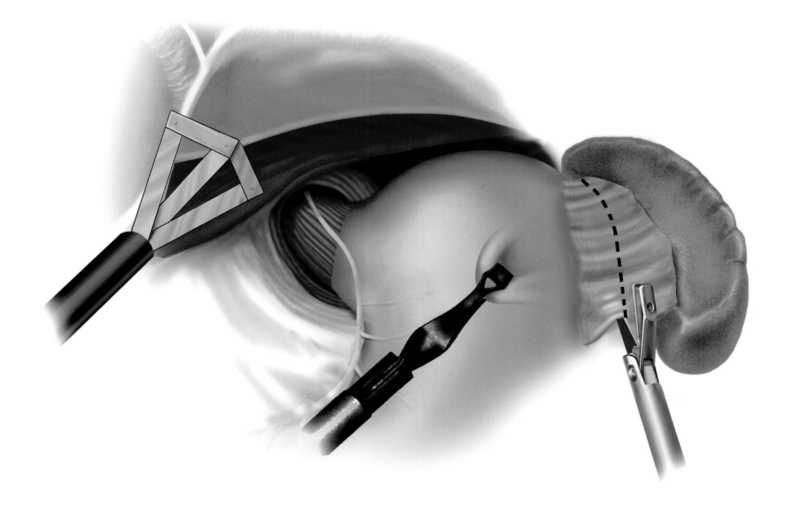

Closing the Hiatal Defect

13. The right and left crura are reapproximated posterior to the esophagus using 0 braided nonabsorbable polyester sutures. Pledgets may be used, especially if the crura are attenuated. Performing this step posterior to the esophagus is important because it enables keeping the GE junction in the abdominal cavity. Retracting the esophagus anterolaterally with a previously placed Penrose drain may facilitate this step. Intracorporeal or extracorporeal knot-tying techniques can be used.

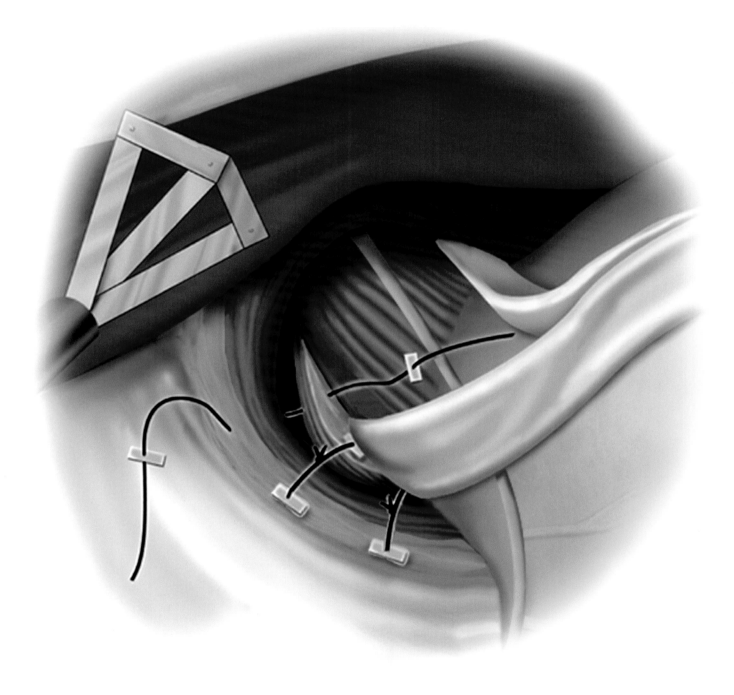

Creating the Fundoplication

14. Once the fundus is completely mobilized, a Babcock grasper is passed from right to left through the previously developed window between the crura and the posterior esophageal wall. Keeping the esophagus on gentle anterior retraction using a previously placed Penrose drain may facilitate this step.

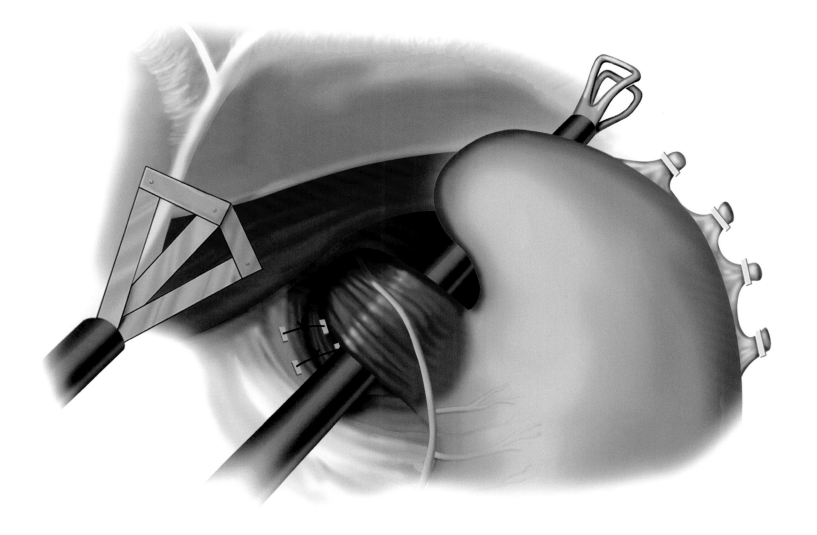

Creating the Fundoplication, Part II

15. The Babcock clamp grasps the lateral edge of the fundus and pulls it left to right through the posterior esophageal window (Figure H-a). The fundus should stay in place once the Babcock clamp is released (Spring sign). If it retracts behind the esophagus, further mobilization of the short gastric vessels is necessary because otherwise the wrap will be too tight.

16. Care should also be taken not to inadvertently twist the wrap (Figure H-b). Pulling on the right and left sides of the wrap (Shoeshine maneuver) helps to ensure proper orientation.

FIGURE H-a

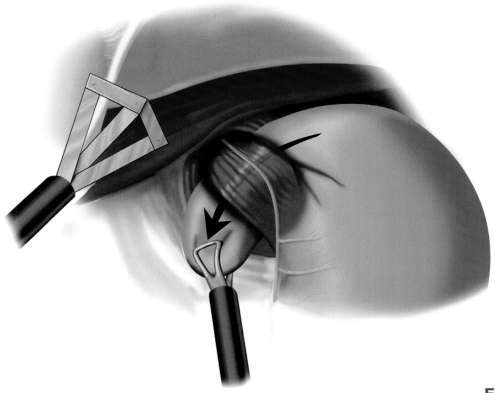

FIGURE H-b

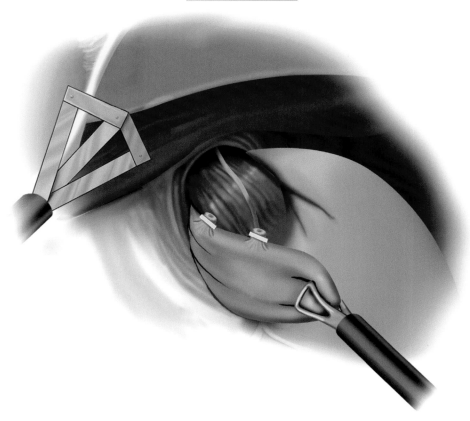

FIGURE I

Securing the Fundoplication

17. The orogastric tube is removed, and a 50-60 Fr Maloney dilator is gently introduced into the esophagus, around which the wrap will be calibrated. This step must be performed cautiously as long-standing reflux may have caused an esophageal stricture or severe inflammation.

18. Seromuscular bites of the fundus on both sides of the esophagus are taken to approximate the two areas of the stomach around the esophagus, thus creating a 360° fundoplication. Usually, three interrupted sutures are adequate to create an ideal wrap of 2 cm to 3 cm in length. Either intracorporeal or extracorporeal knot-tying techniques can be used. It is recommended to include the anterior esophageal wall (away from the anterior vagus nerve) in at least one of the sutures in order to prevent slippage of the wrap.

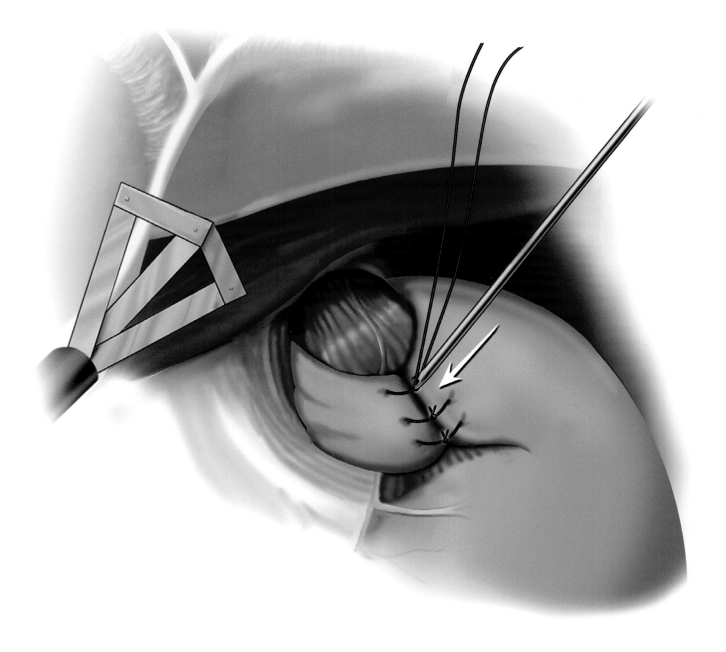

Completion and Closure

19. The dilator is removed by the anesthesiologist and the Nissen fundoplication is complete. A 10 mm instrument should be able to slide easily under an appropriately constructed wrap.

20. The operative field is inspected for adequate hemostasis and any evidence of leak. The fascial and skin incisions are closed in the usual manner.

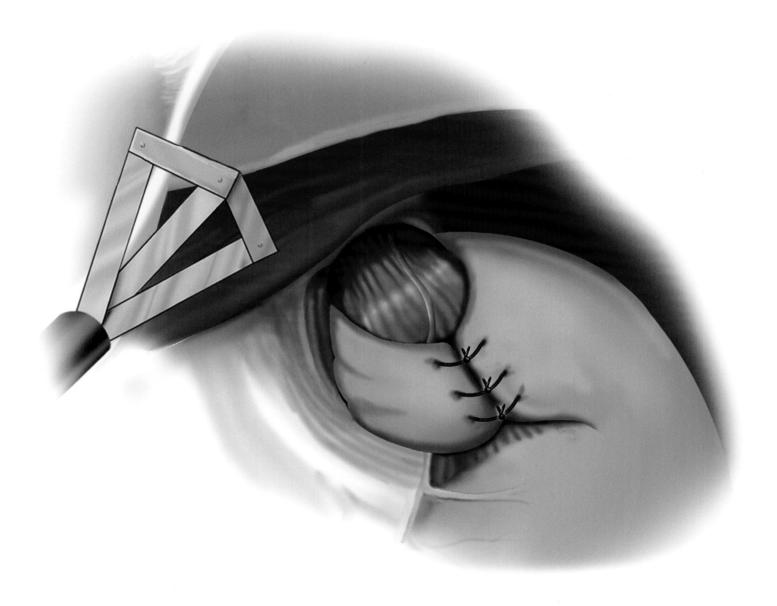

Postoperative Care

Sequential compression devices and/or subcutaneous heparin are continued postoperatively. Postoperative antibiotics are usually not necessary, but may be continued for 24 hours at the surgeon's discretion. Oral intake is initiated with clear liquids on the evening after surgery or on the morning of the first postoperative day. The patient is advanced to a soft mechanical diet as tolerated and maintained for approximately 2 weeks while the postoperative esophageal edema resolves. Patients are usually discharged from the hospital the day after surgery. Antireflux medications may be discontinued.

Suggested Reading

1. Hunter JG, Trus TL, Branum GD, et al. A physiologic approach to laparoscopic fundoplication for gastroesophageal reflux disease. *Ann Surg*. 1996; 223:673-685.

2. Peters JH, DeMeester TR, Crookes P, et al. The treatment of gastroesophageal reflux disease with laparoscopic Nissen fundoplication: prospective evaluation of 100 patients with "typical" symptoms. *Ann Surg*. 1998;228:40-50.

3. Desai KM, Soper NJ, Jones DB. Nissen fundoplication. In: Jones DB, Wu JS, Soper NJ, eds. *Laparoscopic Surgery: Principles and Procedures*, 2nd ed. New York: Marcel Dekker. 2004;259-272.

Commentary

Nathaniel J. Soper, M.D., Northwestern Memorial Hospital Northwestern University

The preoperative evaluation is perhaps one of the most important steps in the appropriate performance of this procedure. One must prove that gastroesophageal reflux is occurring with at least two pieces of evidence. If a patient has typical symptoms of reflux (heartburn and/or regurgitation), as well as endoscopic evidence of esophagitis, a 24-hour pH test is probably not necessary. However, documentation of abnormal reflux on a 24-hour pH test is one of the most sensitive indicators of a good response to surgery, so this test should be applied liberally. For those patients with atypical manifestations of reflux (such as nausea, dental erosions, respiratory symptoms, etc), the 24-hour pH test is mandatory. If a sizeable hiatal hernia is present, a barium swallow is of value to assess the type of hiatal hernia and to get some idea of where the GE junction is in relation to the diaphragm itself.

There are very few absolute contraindications to laparoscopic Nissen fundoplication. Certain characteristics, however, render the operation more difficult and may require additional intraoperative maneuvers beyond what is required in the routine case. These include individuals with paraesophageal hernias, Barrett's esophagus or strictures, and those who are markedly obese. One particularly problematic group of patients is those who have undergone a prior operation at the esophageal hiatus who require a reoperative procedure. In these patients, adhesions between the gastroesophageal junction and the surrounding tissue, particularly involving the left lateral section of the liver, can require an extensive and tedious adhesiolysis. The entire upper stomach and esophagus must be fully mobilized, including taking down the prior fundoplication before reconstructing the anatomy.

In regard to preoperative preparation, the appropriate instrumentation and personnel must be available. The key pieces of equipment are an adequate self-retaining liver retractor, atraumatic grasping instruments, and a good needle holder. We no longer routinely place a Foley catheter, but ask that the patient void immediately preoperatively. The patient's positioning is important, and he or she must be fixed securely to the operating table, as the table is placed in a steep reverse Trendelenburg position throughout the operation. The surgeon stands between the patient's abducted legs. The camera operator must be facile at using an angled laparoscope, generally a 30° laparoscope. The port positions outlined by Dr. Jones et al are similar to those that we have used.

During the performance of the operation, we attempt to preserve the hepatic branch of the vagus nerve. However, not infrequently this structure may render the dissection much more difficult, and may be sacrificed if needed. The phrenoesophageal ligament is divided and the esophagus dissected bluntly from the mediastinum. Great care is taken to identify the anterior and posterior vagus nerves, and these are preserved and kept alongside the esophagus and will ultimately be positioned within the encircling fundoplication. If one is to perform the "short floppy" fundoplication, the gastric fundus needs to be fully mobilized. The harmonic shears ultrasonic device facilitates this process. All connections between the fundus and the lateral and posterior structures must be divided. If this process is skipped, it may be necessary to construct the fundoplication according to the Rossetti modification, wrapping the anterior portion of the fundus around the esophagus, rather than the posterior lateral border, as is done with the "short floppy" technique. We generally use large-gauge braided polyester sutures both for the crural repair and for the fundoplication. Pledgets are used selectively, and only when the crura are attenuated. We generally align the fundoplication such that the two approximated edges of fundus line up just to the right of the anterior midline, whereas others advocate that the fundoplication be performed along the right side of the esophagus.

There is debate as to whether a Maloney dilator needs to be placed at the time a fundoplication is constructed. A small prospective randomized trial performed by Lee Swanstrom's group in Portland, Oregon, has shown an increased rate of postoperative dysphagia when a dilator is not used. We generally use a 60 Fr dilator and use three sutures in the fundoplication, each spaced approximately 1 cm apart. One or two of the sutures incorporate the anterior wall of the esophagus. The resulting fundoplication is approximately 2 cm in length. The fundoplication must be constructed around the distal esophagus, rather than being allowed to drift down onto the proximal stomach. Intraoperatively, if one is not positive where the gastroesophageal junction resides, intraoperative endoscopy may be very helpful to clarify the anatomical relationships. Likewise, endoscopy performed after the wrap has been completed may help demonstrate an adequate fundoplication.

Postoperative care is also important. We begin the patient on clear liquids immediately postoperatively. The patients are usually admitted on a "23-hour" basis and are allowed a soft diet the following morning. This soft mechanical diet is maintained for 2 to 4 weeks postoperatively—the worst foods that result in early postoperative dysphagia are bread products and coarse meats. Early postoperatively, many patients complain of dysphagia and may have a host of other symptoms, most of which spontaneously resolve during the first month. Should a patient complain of severe ongoing dysphagia or symptoms of reflux, the first test that we usually perform is a barium swallow study. Rarely will postoperative endoscopy with dilatation be necessary as long as the patient can be counseled and nurtured until the postoperative edema and/or hematoma of the wrap subsides. Using the concepts and technique that Dr. Jones et al have detailed in this chapter, the majority of patients undergoing laparoscopic Nissen fundoplication should enjoy excellent outcomes.

Daniel J. Deziel, M.D.
Rush University Medical Center

Laparoscopic Nissen fundoplication can be performed with the patient in standard supine position or in the leg-spread position described. Location of the trocar sites and trocar sizes will also vary somewhat, depending on the surgeon's preference and the patients' body habitus. The primary optical port is optimally positioned left of the midline for most portions of the procedure. Care is required to avoid the superficial and deep superior epigastric vessels at nonmidline trocar sites. I prefer to use a direct cutdown and Hasson cannula at the initial access site, although the Veress needle technique or use of an optical trocar are appropriate alternatives.

Dissection can be commenced at the gastrohepatic ligament superior to the hepatic branch of the anterior vagus nerve or at the greater curvature of the stomach with division of the short gastric vessels. In either case, the edges of the right and left crura must be identified, the cardia and proximal fundus must be completely freed from the crura and posterior attachments, the anterior phrenoesophageal membrane must be divided and an adequate (3.5 cm) length of esophagus must be freely mobilized below the diaphragm.

The plane between the border of the right crus and the esophagogastric junction is developed bluntly. The surgeon uses two hands to sweep the structures apart in a medial-lateral direction. The esophagus is elevated anteriorly with a blunt-tipped instrument as the posterior window is developed. When working from the right side of the patient's esophagus, the left pleura will be entered if instruments are inadvertently directed dorsal to the left crus and oriented in too cephalad a direction. The posterior medial aspect of the left crus should be visualized from the right side and the dissection should be anterior or ventral to this. The posterior vagus is identified during this dissection; most descriptions leave the nerve with the esophagus and hence within the eventual wrap, but some describe leaving the nerve outside the wrap.

The extent of fundic mobilization necessary to construct a floppy fundoplication is variable. Typically, short gastric vessels are divided beginning about 10 cm from the angle of His. As the authors note, complete division of the dorsal retroperitoneal attachments to the fundus is key to establishing an adequate wide posterior window.

Retraction of the esophagus can be achieved with blunt instruments, with a Penrose drain, or by using the wrapped fundus as a retractor. Approximation of the crura requires substantial bites of tissue on each side. Whether or not pledgets are used, suture bites should incorporate the whitish crural fascia in addition to muscle fibers.

Instead of passing the mobilized fundus using Babcock clamps, one end of a Penrose drain can be sutured to the appropriate spot on the fundus and used to draw it posterior to the esophagus. To achieve proper geometry of the wrap, it is the posterior fundus that is passed behind to the right of the esophagus and sutured to the anterior fundus on the left side. Laxity of the wrap must be ensured. If the fundus is grasped too far distally, the proximal portion can torse and a paraesophageal hernia can result. The esophageal sutures should be placed toward the right side of the anterior wall to avoid the anterior vagal fibers.

Passage of any bougie or nasogastric tube should be done under direct videoscopic vision by both the surgeon and the team member advancing the esophageal tube. The surgeon and/or assistant should hold the gastroesophageal junction in a nonangled position during passage. This usually requires anterior, i.e., ventral, retraction of the proximal stomach.

Treatment with metoclopramide for approximately 1 to 3 weeks postoperatively may minimize any gas or bloating sensations.

Alastair M. Thompson, M.D., Ninewells Hospital and Medical School University of Dundee

Despite the wide range of medications available to treat esophageal reflux and the developing intralumenal endoscopic techniques, anti-reflux surgery plays an important role in symptom control, particularly where medications have failed. Laparoscopic Nissen fundoplication gives excellent long-term symptom control after suitable patient selection, which includes endoscopy and esophageal manometry.

The key components of antireflux surgery (revising the anatomy of the hiatus to give a length of intra-abdominal esophagus, a suitably sized hiatus, and a snug 360° wrap) can be achieved by following the method described here.

Attention to patient and port positioning, exposure of the structures passing through the hiatus, and adequate mobilization of the fundus should be facilitated by firm but gentle tissue handling in an operating field with meticulous hemostasis.

First-time, accurate, seromuscular suture placement and correctly tensioned knots of 2 cm to 3 cm of fundus wrapped around the esophageal dilator are key to the longevity of symptom control. Unless the hiatal repair is sound and the fundus mobilization sufficient, this will not be achieved.

Postoperative recovery is surprisingly rapid, although dietary restraint and modification is initially required. After successful laparoscopic Nissen fundoplication, patients can be extremely grateful.

Jeffrey L. Ponsky, M.D., University Hospitals of Cleveland Case School of Medicine

The Nissen fundoplication is the most widely accepted and practiced operation for the treatment of gastroesophageal reflux disease. Its precision and popularity have markedly increased since the introduction of the laparoscopic approach over a decade ago. The authors correctly define the preoperative assessment and evaluation of the patient. The key to excellent results lies in proper patient selection, as well as good operative technique.

The arrangement of the abdominal trocar sites as depicted by the authors is quite satisfactory, although the exact location of the trocars varies somewhat based on the patient's body habitus and surgeon's preference. Some surgeons choose to place the camera operator on the patient's right and the assistant to the patient's left. While the authors describe use of the Veress needle for abdominal access, many surgeons prefer a direct cutdown (Hasson) technique.

The key to the safe dissection of the esophageal hiatus is the careful identification of the diaphragmatic crura. The phrenoesophageal ligament is opened around the top of the esophagus and the crura exposed. Many surgeons emphasize the complete dissection of the left crus as a first step. The peritoneum over the crus is opened and the crus is dissected inferiorly to its passage under the esophagus. Then, in like fashion, the right crus is dissected. The plane between the crural muscle and esophagus is gently and bluntly spread on each side. As the right crus is followed inferiorly, it will be seen to join the left crus. At this point, the esophagus is bluntly elevated and the retro-esophageal window created. The key point is that the esophagus is surrounded by dissection of the crura, not by dissection of the esophagus.

The authors describe the remainder of the operation as it is performed by most all surgeons. Some use a posterior stitch to fix the back of the wrap to the crural closure. The keys to success of the operation are: 1) careful dissection of the crura, 2) attainment of at least 2 cm of intra-abdominal esophagus, 3) adequate crural closure, and 4) absence of tension on the fundic wrap.

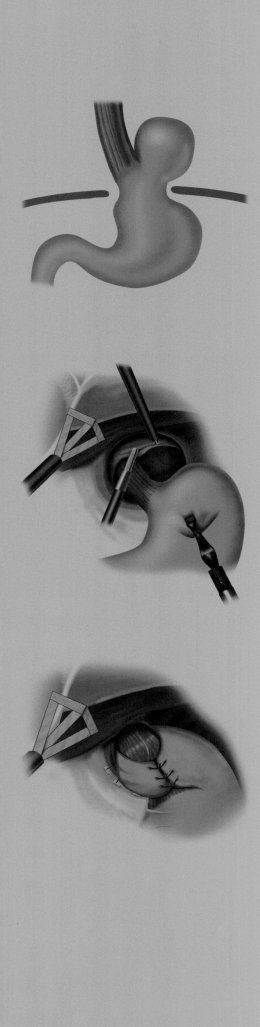

Laparoscopic Paraesophageal Hernia Repair

A hiatal hernia is characterized by the superior migration of the gastroesophageal (GE) junction into the chest and may be diagnosed by upper GI, CT, or endoscopy. The proximal stomach is subjected to the negative intrathoracic pressures of normal respiration, and this condition in part predisposes to the development of gastroesophageal reflux disease (GERD).

FIGURE A-a,b,c,d

Classification of Hiatal Hernias

Hiatal hernias have traditionally been classified into four types, as depicted in Figure A-a,b,c,d. Type I (Figure A-a) represents a sliding hiatal hernia as described above and represents the most common type, comprising approximately 90% of all hiatal hernias. Type II (Figure A-b) hernias are characterized by the herniation of the gastric fundus into the chest while the GE junction remains fixed in its normal position. Type III (Figure A-c) hernias represent a combination of the first two, characterized by herniation of both the fundus and GE junction. Type II and III hernias, as opposed to the Type I variety, contain a true hernia sac and are thus considered "true" paraesophageal hernias. Type III hernias constitute approximately 90% of these sac-containing paraesophageal hernias. When a Type III hernia involves concurrent herniation of other abdominal organs, such as the spleen, it is designated a Type IV (Figure A-d) hernia.

FIGURE A-a

FIGURE A-b

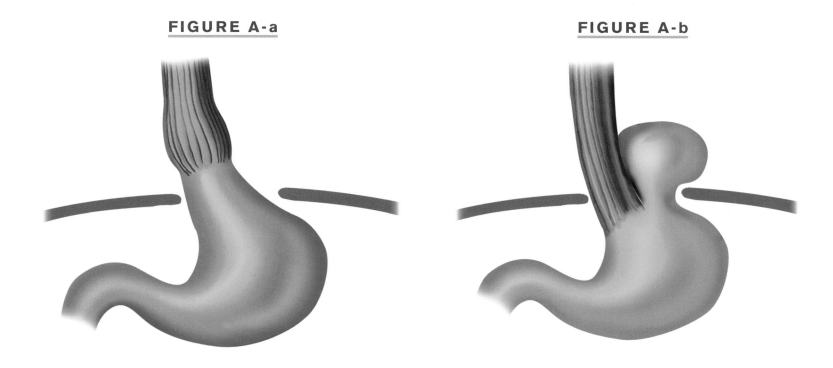

FIGURE A-c

FIGURE A-d

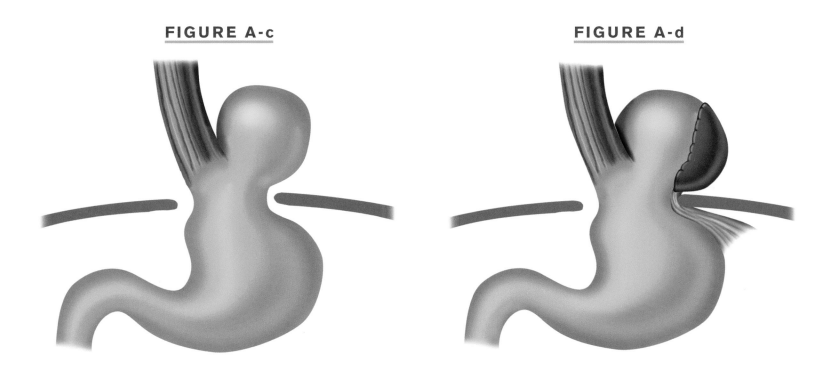

Potential Complications of Paraesophageal Hernias

Gastric volvulus is a potentially devastating complication of paraesophageal hernias. Volvulus can occur around either the organoaxial (Line A, Figure B-b) or mesenteroaxial axis (Line B, Figure B-c), and can result in a closed-loop obstruction of the stomach. GERD is a common complication of paraesophageal hernias as well. Symptomatic reflux is often demonstrated in all three types of hernias, including the Type II variant, thus compelling most surgeons to advocate performing a concurrent antireflux procedure at the time of the hernia repair. Even if reflux is not demonstrated preoperatively, the dissection performed around the GE junction necessary for hernia reduction predisposes to the development of reflux after the operation. Fundoplication anchors the stomach in the abdominal cavity and treats existing or potential reflux.

FIGURE B-a

FIGURE B-b

FIGURE B-c

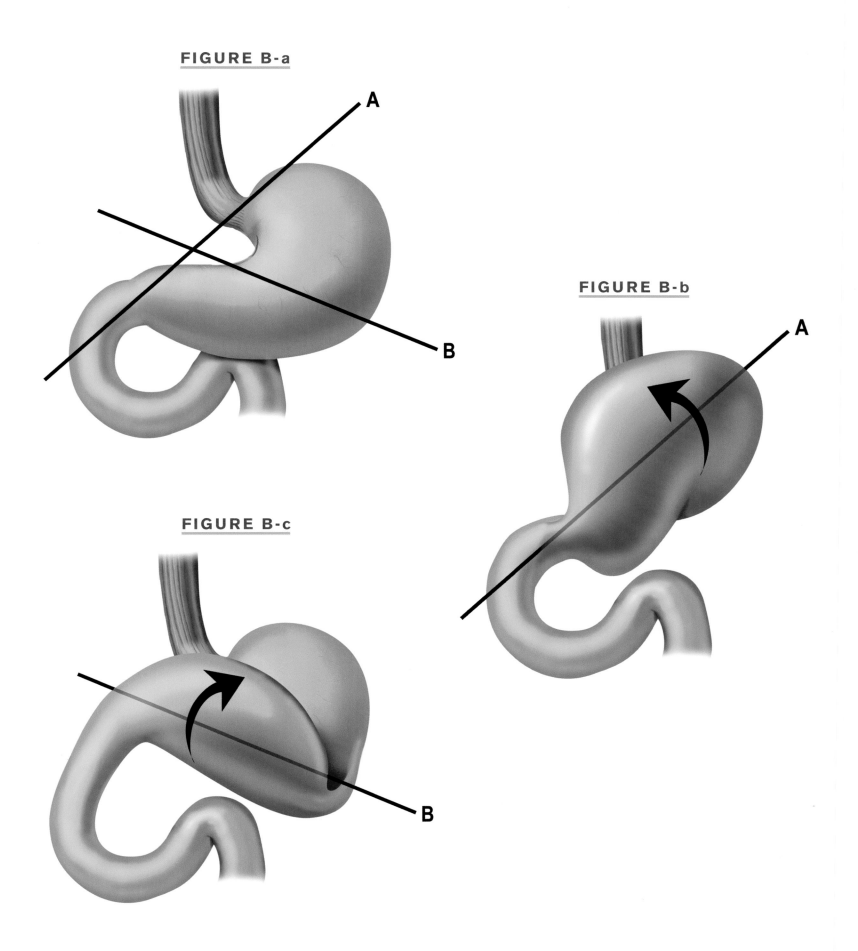

Preoperative Preparation

1. Sequential compression stockings and subcutaneous heparin may be used for prophylaxis against deep venous thrombosis. Intravenous antibiotics, usually a first-generation cephalosporin, are administered prophylactically. After induction of general anesthesia, the bladder is emptied with a urinary catheter and the stomach is decompressed with an orogastric tube.

FIGURE C

Operating Room Setup

2. The patient is placed on a cushioned bean bag and spreader bars with the surgeon standing between the legs. All pressure points must be adequately padded and the bean-bag device is used to secure the patient's position when rotating the table to facilitate exposure and viewing during the procedure.

3. The assistant is situated to the patient's right, while the camera operator stands on the patient's left side.

4. The video monitors are stationed at both sides of the patient's head to facilitate adequate viewing from either side of the table.

FIGURE D-a

FIGURE D-b

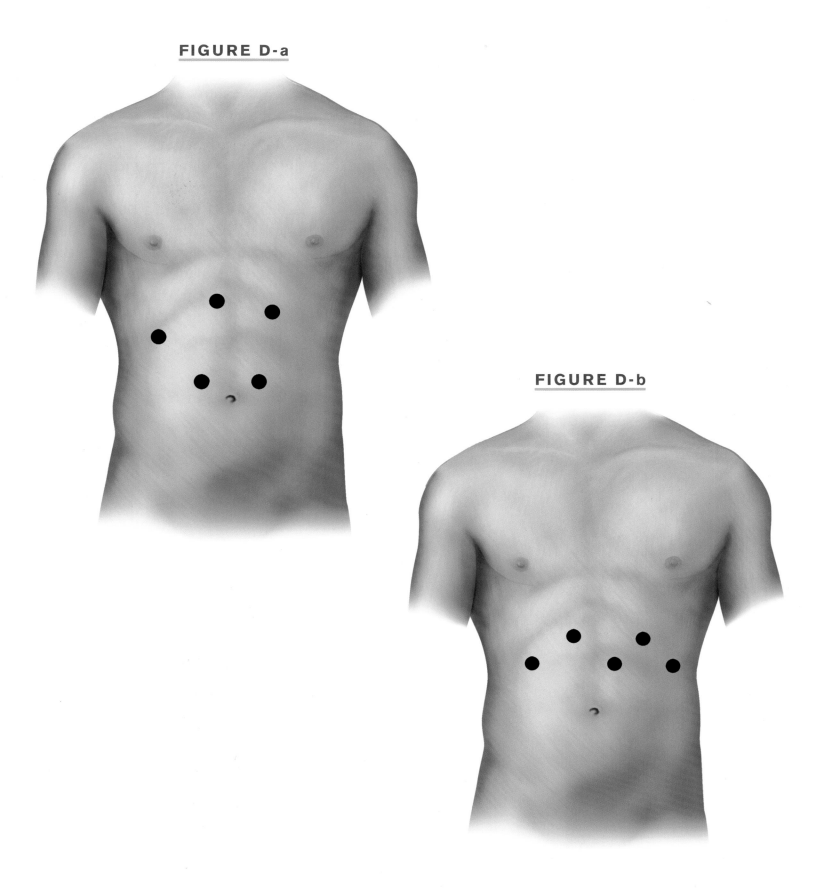

Reducing the Hernia

9. After the liver is retracted anterolaterally, the initial step is to reduce the paraesophageal hernia contents, which often occurs spontaneously after obtaining pneumoperitoneum.

10. The gastrohepatic ligament is opened to better expose the diaphragmatic hiatus. Care is taken to identify and preserve an aberrant left hepatic artery, as well as the vagus nerves. The hernia sac is incised along the hernia orifice and blunt dissection is used to reduce the sac from the mediastinum, which is usually best accomplished in a right to left direction. This maneuver may be complicated by pneumothorax or injury to other mediastinal structures. Pneumothorax can usually be managed by releasing pneumoperitoneum and then reinsufflating to a lower pressure, provided there is no injury to the lung parenchyma.

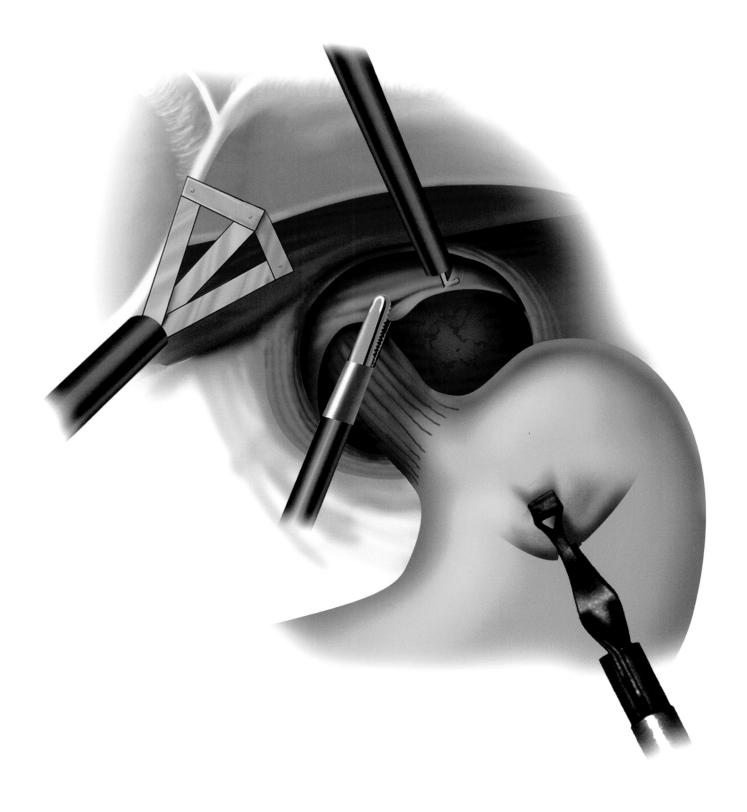

Crural Closure and Fundoplication

11. The rest of the operative repair, including hiatal dissection and exposure, closing the diaphragmatic defect (Figure F), and creating a fundoplication (Figure G) is the same as that described in detail for performing a laparoscopic Nissen fundoplication.

12. Very large crural defects may not be amenable to simple suture approximation. Instead, a mesh repair allows for closure without undo tension. Mesh (xenograft or ePTFE) may be fixed posteriorly but risks erosion.

13. Anterior fixation of the mesh to the abdominal fascia is performed using several horizontal mattress sutures in a manner similar to that employed in laparoscopic ventral hernia repair.

FIGURE F

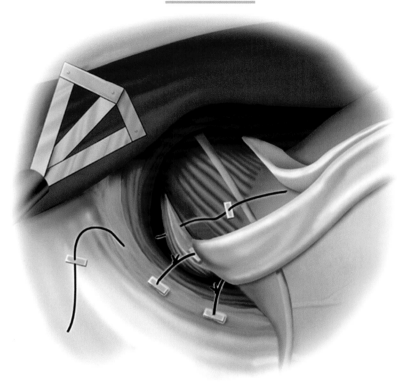

FIGURE G

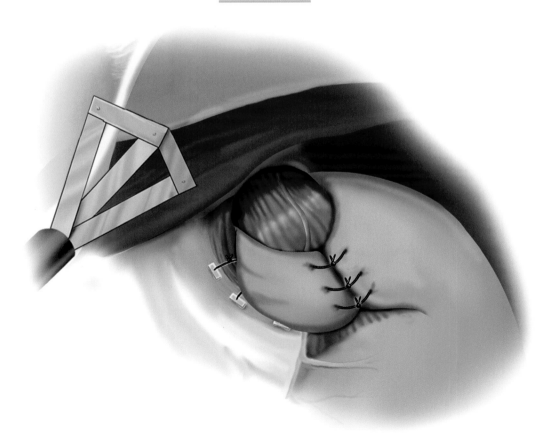

Postoperative Care

Sequential compression devices and/or subcutaneous heparin are continued postoperatively. Postoperative antibiotics are usually not necessary, but may be continued for 24 hours at the surgeon's discretion. After extensive dissection, a gastrograffin swallow may be performed prior to initiating clear liquids on the morning of the first postoperative day. The patient is advanced to a soft mechanical diet as tolerated and maintained on this diet for approximately 2 weeks while the postoperative esophageal edema resolves. Patients are usually discharged from the hospital on postoperative day 1 or 2.

Suggested Reading

1. Schauer PR, Ikramuddin S, McLaughlin RH, et al. Comparison of laparoscopic versus open repair of paraesophageal hernia. *Am J Surg.* 1998;176:659-665.

2. Swanstrom LL, Jobe BA, Kinzie LR, Horvath KD. Esophageal motility and outcomes following laparoscopic paraesophageal hernia repair and fundoplication. *Am J Surg.* 1999;177:359-363.

3. Mattar SG, Bowers SP, Galloway KD, Hunter JG, Smith CD. Long-term outcome of laparoscopic repair of paraesophageal hernia. *Surg Endosc.* 2002;16:745-749.

Commentary

Jo Buyske, M.D., Penn Presbyterian Medical Center
University of Pennsylvania

This chapter presents a crisp summary of the management of paraesophageal hernias. I would emphasize the absolute necessity of upper GI fluoroscopy in the evaluation of paraesophageal hernias. These studies provide a road map for the surgeon, outlining the anatomy of the hernia and allowing it to be visualized in dynamic form. Although endoscopy can suggest or make the diagnosis, it can also be very misleading. The procedure itself might deform the stomach and reduce the hernia, so that the paraesophageal component can be missed. Similarly, CT scanning may not distinguish a sliding hernia from a paraesophageal type, although it helps distinguish between a Type III and IV hernia. I always require a recent (within 12 months, sooner if change in symptoms) upper GI fluoroscopy in these patients.

The diagrams provide a simple schematic to help delineate between these types of hernias. I especially like the diagrams that distinguish between organoaxial and mesenteroaxial volvulus, a difference that can be elusive when described verbally. Regarding complications, in addition to volvulus and reflux, these hernias can cause irritation of the thoracic portion of the stomach with gastritis and either brisk or low-level bleeding resulting in anemia. They can also produce symptoms of esophageal obstruction when they fill with food or with air, so that some patients regurgitate saliva or undigested food, or complain that food sticks in their chest. Others complain of a sensation of chest pressure or shortness of breath during meals, likely related to the space occupying presence of food, gas, and viscera in the chest. Although these last complaints almost always elicit a cardiology evaluation, it is important not to overlook this possibility if it has not already been addressed. More than a few patients will have both paraesophageal hernias and coronary artery disease, and it behooves the good surgeon to establish that prior to operating on the hernia.

Fundoplication can guard against postoperative reflux, as well as recurrence of the hernia. The surgeon must balance this against the incidence of presbyesophagus in these patients, and the risk of inducing debilitating dysphagia with a wrap or an overtightened hiatus. Anterior gastropexy and temporary gastrostomy have both been proposed to help minimize the risk of recurrence of the hernia. Gastrostomy has the additional benefit of offering a "vent" for a stomach that may not empty very well in the early postoperative period. These techniques can all be applied selectively.

The use of mesh is controversial. Although the use of mesh in inguinal and incisional hernias has certainly reduced the incidence of recurrence, that benefit in this area might be outweighed by the risk of erosion of mesh into the esophagus in this highly mobile location. It is my opinion that mesh should be used only when other efforts, including esophageal lengthening, Nissen fundoplication, pledgetted sutures, and gastropexy, appear inadequate to affect durable repair. If mesh is used it must be placed such that it does not come in direct contact with the esophagus.

Laparoscopic paraesophageal hernias are one of the most challenging of the GE junction cases. The anatomy is distorted and sometimes confusing, and the patients are often frail. Careful attention to preoperative evaluation and to operative technique can yield excellent results.

C. Daniel Smith, M.D., Emory University Hospital
Emory University School of Medicine

Hiatal hernia has an increasing prominence in our care of surgical patients. We have seen increasing numbers of patients with hiatal hernias, either as the primary indication for surgical referral or as an exacerbating factor in GERD. This is likely a reflection of both our aging population and the trend toward referring patients only with more complicated GERD. This chapter provides basic details regarding the steps in performing a hiatal hernia repair, and I commend the authors for digesting this into a few illustrative steps. I would like to add to the topics of reducing the hernia, crural closure, and fundoplication.

One of the most common reasons for recurrence after hiatal hernia repair is failure to reduce and excise the hernia sac. When repairing a hiatal hernia, we now initiate the hiatal dissection from the patient's left, first dividing the short gastric vessels to gain exposure of the base of the left crus. The peritoneum as it drapes over the base of the left crus is then incised and a flap of peritoneum elevated off of the undersurface of the left crus and up into the mediastinum. With this, the thin areolar tissue of the retroesophageal plane in the mediastinum is entered and the sac and herniated content easily reduced. This continues ventrally along the left crus, through the crural arch and down to the base of the right crus. With the sac now well mobilized and the retroesophageal window open above the sac, a Penrose drain can be used to encircle the esophagus and complete the dissection and sac excision. Opening the retroesophageal window through, rather than above, the sac will result in leaving sac behind and increase the risk of recurrence.

The primary issue in crural closure is whether to use mesh. While many advocate a "tension-free" repair similar to what is done with abdominal wall hernias, this is not the abdominal wall, but rather, a very mobile and dynamic region where rigid and proinflammatory material near the esophagus has the potential for significant esophageal dysfunction and even ulceration and erosion. Those of us whose daily practice involves caring for these patients have all performed an esophagectomy for a piece of mesh that has eroded into an esophagus, a devastating outcome after hiatal hernia repair. Therefore, we reserve the use of mesh for only those cases where all other measures to get crural closure fail, and when placing mesh, we almost never place it against the esophagus, but rather, create a defect in the diaphragm just medial to the right crus, thereby allowing the right and left crus to approximate directly behind the esophagus and the mesh placement to cover the medial defect. Steps to facilitate avoiding mesh include decreasing pneumoperitoneum during crural closure and varying the depth of crural bites so as to avoid fraying of the crus.

The technique of creating the fundoplication doesn't vary from what is commonly done with GERD surgery; however, correct placement of the fundoplication is critical in hiatal hernia repair. The most common error we see in fundoplication during hiatal hernia repair is placing the wrap on the proximal stomach rather than distal esophagus. This is the result of inadequate esophageal mobilization out of the mediastinum or failure to recognize a short esophagus. To assess esophageal length and ensure correct placement of the fundoplication, we liberally use intraoperative esophagoscopy to localize the Z-line.

Laparoscopic Heller Myotomy

Heller myotomy is performed for the treatment of achalasia, a primary motor disorder of the esophagus characterized by an absence of the myenteric neural plexus. This leads to the loss of normal coordinated peristalsis and failure of the lower esophageal sphincter (LES) to relax. Typical symptoms include dysphagia, heartburn, and chest pain. Prior to surgery, diagnostic tests may include upper endoscopy, esophageal manometry, and an upper gastrointestinal contrast study, which typically reveals a "bird's beak" deformity. Management options include endoscopic pneumatic balloon dilation, botulinum toxin injections, and esophagomyotomy, of which the last option produces the best long-term results.

Preoperative Preparation

1. Sequential compression stockings and subcutaneous heparin may be used for prophylaxis against deep venous thrombosis. Intravenous antibiotics, usually a first-generation cephalosporin, are administered prophylactically. After induction of general anesthesia, the bladder is emptied with a urinary catheter and the stomach is decompressed with a nasogastric tube.

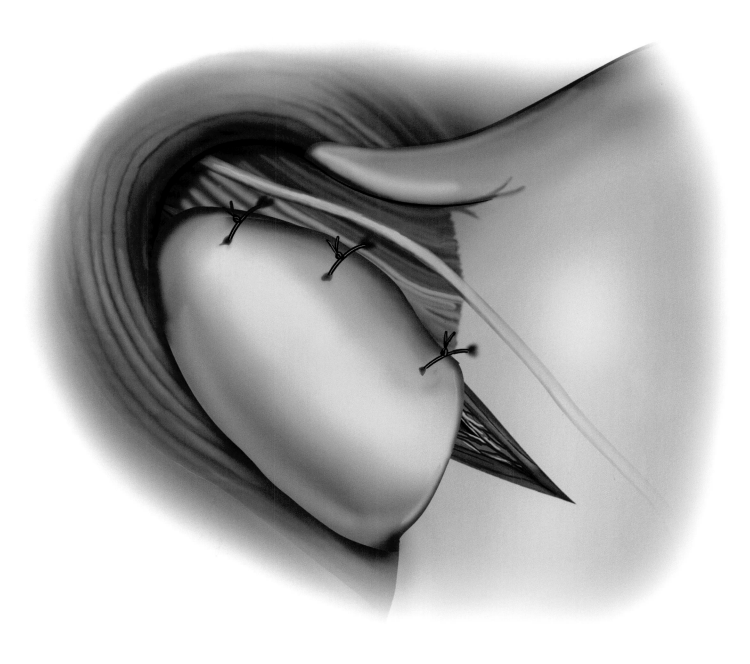

Operating Room Setup

2. The patient is placed on a cushioned bean bag and spreader bars with the surgeon standing between the legs. All pressure points must be adequately padded and the bean-bag device is used to secure the patient's position when rotating the table to facilitate exposure and viewing during the procedure.

3. The assistant is situated to the patient's right, while the camera operator stands on the patient's left side.

4. The video monitors are stationed at both sides of the patient's head to facilitate adequate viewing from either side of the table.

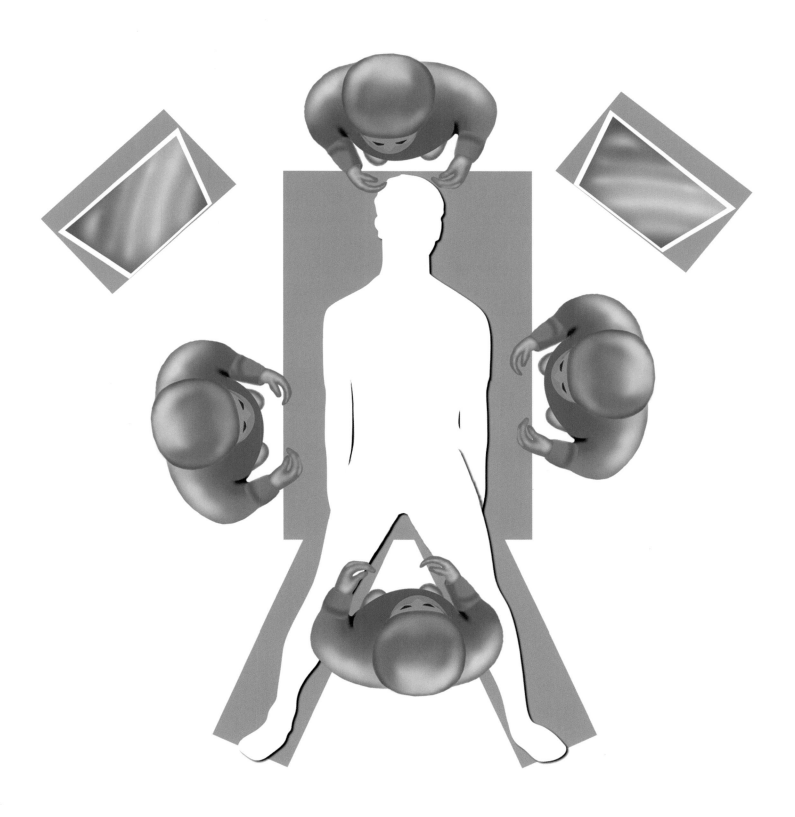

FIGURE B-a,b

Access and Port Placement

5. Pneumoperitoneum is obtained through a left upper subcostal incision with a closed technique using a Veress needle. An optical trocar is used for initial port placement 15 cm beneath the xiphoid process, slightly left of the umbilicus. The 0° scope is switched for a 30° angled laparoscope, and the abdomen is inspected for adhesions or injuries.

6. Next, four radially expanding 11 mm ports are placed under direct vision in the configuration as shown in Figure B-a (alternatively three 5 mm ports and one 11 mm port in the left subcostal area can be used). A slightly altered configuration that can be used as well is depicted in Figure B-b.

7. In general, the most inferior port should be placed no more than 15 cm below the xiphoid process in order to facilitate maximal manipulation and range of motion of the instruments.

FIGURE B-a

FIGURE B-b

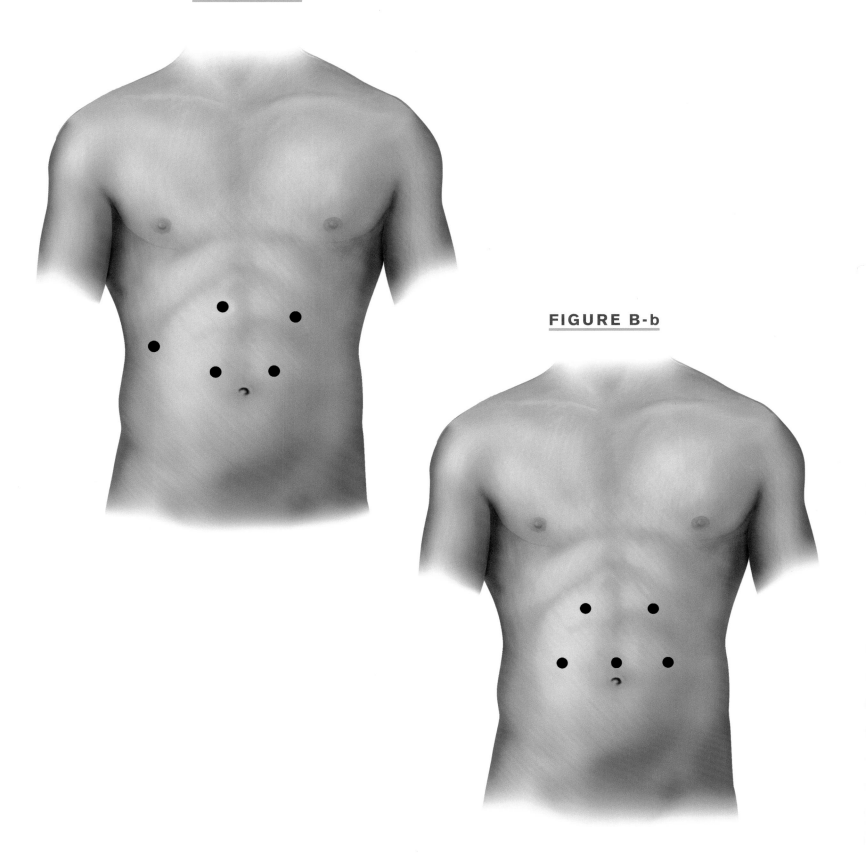

FIGURE C

Exposing the Esophageal Hiatus

8. The patient is placed in the reverse Trendelenburg position to provide gravity retraction. A self-retaining liver retractor is used to displace the left lateral lobe of the liver anterolaterally.

9. The stomach just distal to the gastroesophageal fat pad is grasped with a Babcock grasper and distracted inferiorly to the left while the gastrohepatic and phrenoesophageal ligaments are opened. Both crura of the diaphragm and the anterior vagus nerve are identified after the phrenoesophageal ligament is adequately opened.

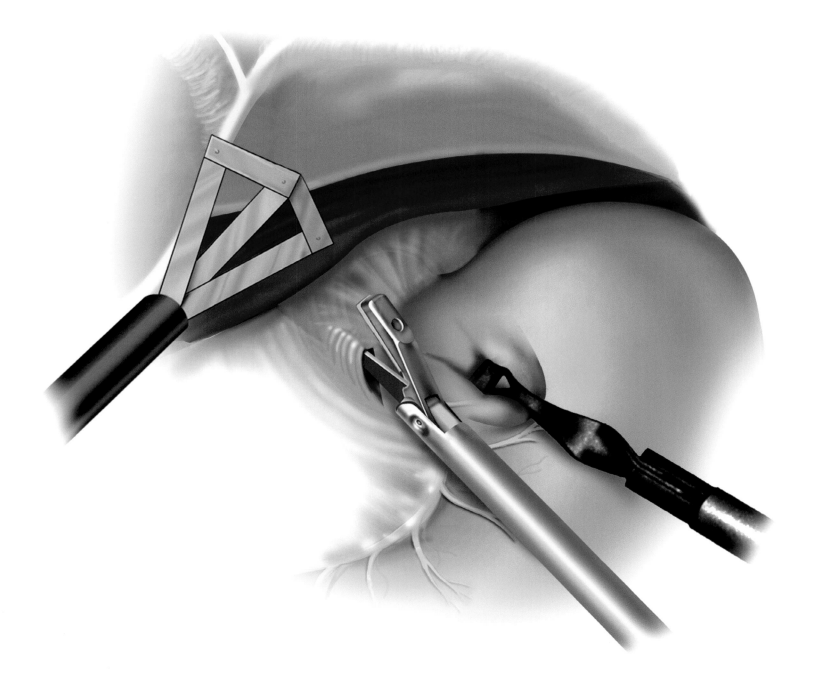

Exposing the Esophageal Hiatus, Part II

10. If a hiatal hernia is present, it is gently reduced into the abdominal cavity by dividing any surrounding adhesions. The right crus is retracted laterally to expose and identify the posterior vagus nerve (Figure D-a). A plane is bluntly developed between the crura and posterior esophageal wall. A Penrose drain is passed through this window and is used to place the esophagus on gentle anterior and caudal traction, facilitating mobilization so that at least 6 cm to 8 cm is below the diaphragmatic hiatus.

11. If partial fundoplication is planned, the gastrosplenic ligament may be divided with an ultrasonic coagulator from a point on the greater curve 8 cm to 10 cm distal to the esophageal junction to the level of the diaphragm (Figure D-b). Yet, many surgeons will not divide the short gastric vessels for partial fundoplication, therefore, eliminating this step.

12. Following dissection, the crura are reapproximated prior to myotomy using the same technique as that described for a laparoscopic Nissen fundoplication.

FIGURE D-a

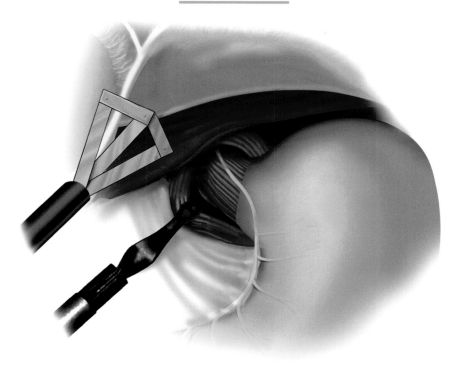

FIGURE D-b

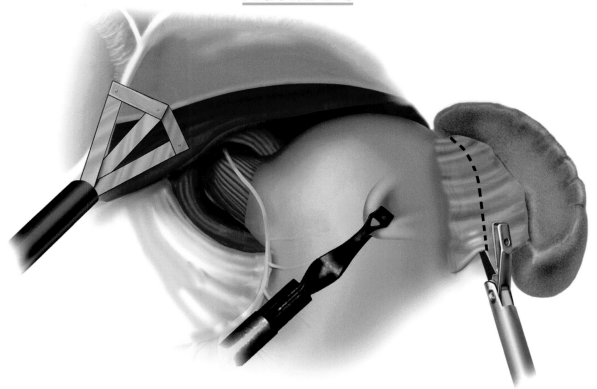

Performing the Myotomy

13. The gastroesophageal junction is identified, thus marking the zone of high pressure. Using either a hook cautery or ultrasonic dissector, the outer esophageal longitudinal muscle over this area is divided for a length of 6 cm to 8 cm along the right anterolateral aspect of the esophagus. Care is taken to avoid the anterior and posterior vagus nerves.

14. Identifying the exact location and extent of the zone of high pressure is facilitated with the use of concurrent upper endoscopy and transillumination. Additionally, endoscopy helps to identify the squamocolumnar junction between the esophagus and stomach. Individual fibers of the circular muscle layer of the LES are then divided with a harmonic scalpel until the submucosal plane is identified and exposed. Once this crucial plane is identified, the circular fibers are divided for the entire length of the myotomy. The myotomy should be extended onto the stomach for approximately 2 cm with meticulous dissection to avoid mucosal perforation. Great care must be taken during the dissection of the muscularis at the level of the gastric fundus, as it is particularly adherent and prone to mucosal injury.

15. The edges of the myotomy should be bluntly separated from each other, thus allowing the mucosa to bulge through the myotomy incision (Figure E-a). Successful division of the entire LES can be confirmed with upper endoscopy (Figure E-b).

16. Once the myotomy is complete, it should be tested with underwater air insufflation to assess for any evidence of inadvertent mucosal perforation. Should a perforation occur, it should be closed primarily with 4-0 absorbable suture using intracorporeal technique. The repair should be buttressed with a partial fundoplication, and an esophagomyotomy can be performed on the contralateral aspect of the esophagus.

FIGURE E-a

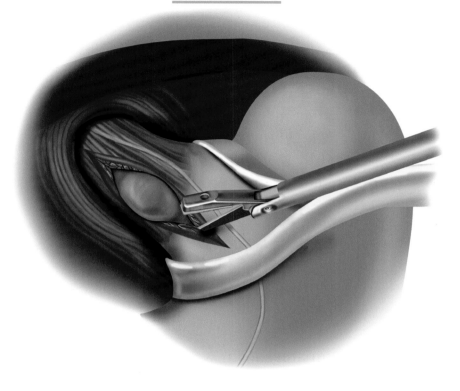

FIGURE E-b

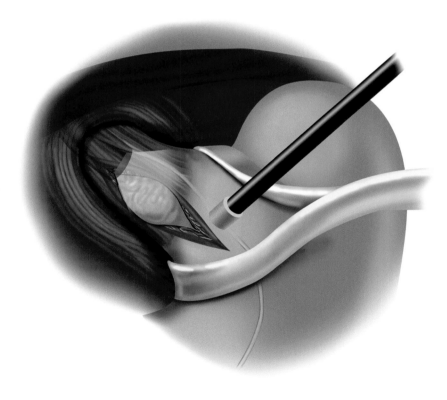

Creating a Partial Fundoplication (Optional)

17. The most common antireflux procedure performed is the Dor fundoplication (Figure F-a,b), which is simply a partial anterior wrap. The anterior portion of the upper stomach is sutured to both cut edges of the myotomy and the right crus, thus bolstering the exposed esophageal mucosa.

18. Toupet fundoplication (Figure G), a partial posterior fundoplication, can also be fashioned to assist with distraction of the two myotomy edges. This reconstruction does not bolster the exposed mucosa.

FIGURE F-a

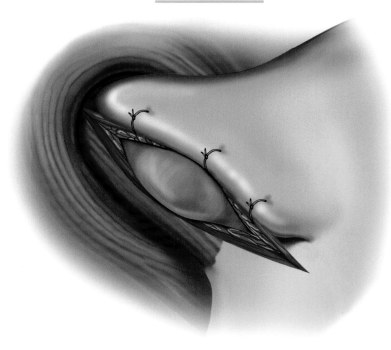

FIGURE F-b

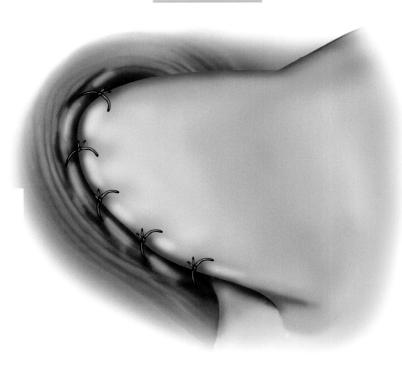

FIGURE G

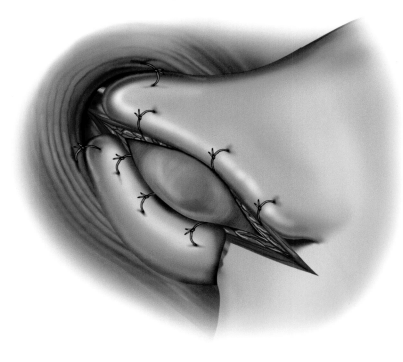

Creating a Partial Fundoplication, Part II (Optional)

19. Alternatively, a Jones-Rege bolstering partial posterior fundoplication, similar to a Toupet fundoplication, can be constructed.

20. The gastric fundus is mobilized and brought posteriorly around the esophagus, similar to that as described for a Nissen fundoplication.

21. The mobilized stomach is sutured (2-0 nonabsorbable) to the crura and to both edges of the myotomy, thus providing protection for the exposed esophageal mucosa (Figure H-a,b). Intracorporeal or extracorporeal knot-tying techniques can be used. This ultimately forms a partial posterior wrap of approximately 270°.

22. A nasogastric tube may be left in place at the discretion of the surgeon. The operative field is inspected for adequate hemostasis and any evidence of leak. The ports are withdrawn under direct vision to ensure hemostasis at each port site. The fascial and skin incisions are closed in the usual manner.

FIGURE H-a

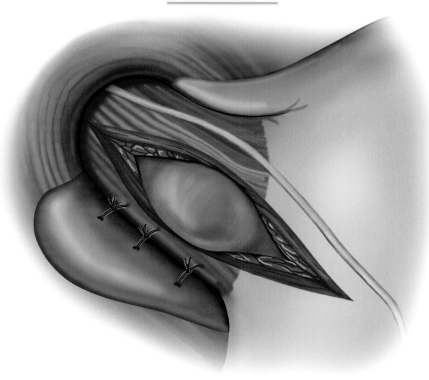

FIGURE H-b

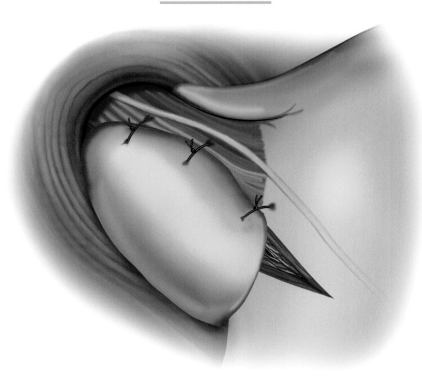

Postoperative Care

Sequential compression devices and/or subcutaneous heparin are continued postoperatively. Postoperative antibiotics may be continued perioperatively at the surgeon's discretion. On the morning of the first postoperative day, the nasogastric tube is removed and oral intake is initiated with clear liquids. A gastrograffin swallow may be performed to rule out leak. The patient is advanced to a full liquid diet and eventually soft mechanical diet as tolerated and maintained for approximately 2 to 4 weeks. Patients are usually discharged from the hospital by postoperative day 2.

Suggested Reading

1. Shiino Y, Filipi C. Awad ZT, et al. Surgery for achalasia. *J Gastrointest Surg*. 1999;3(5):447-455.

2. Urbach DR, Hansen PD, Khajanchee YS, Swanstrom LL. A decision analysis of the optimal initial approach to achalasia: laparoscopic Heller myotomy with partial fundoplication, thoracoscopic Heller myotomy, pneumatic dilatation, or botulinum toxin injection. *J Gastrointest Surg*. 2001;5(2):192-205.

3. Villegas L, Rege RV, Jones DB. Laparoscopic Heller myotomy with bolstering partial posterior fundoplication for achalasia. *J Laparoendosc Adv Surg Tech*. 2003;13(1):1-4.

Commentary

Robert V. Rege, M.D.
University of Texas Southwestern Medical Center

Achalasia, a disease manifest by aperistalsis of the esophageal body, failure of LES relaxation with swallowing, and hypertensive LES, may be treated with drugs, LES botulinim toxin injections, forceful balloon dilatation, or surgical esophageal myotomy. Drugs afford relief in a minority of patients and tachyphylaxis further limits their utility. Botulinim toxin decreases LES pressure about 30%, providing relief in only one-third of patients. Since symptoms return within 6 to 12 months and retreatment is even less effective, it should be reserved for high-risk patients with limited life expectancy. Balloon dilatation relieves symptoms in 80% to 85% of patients. The success and perforation rate increases with balloon size from 30 mm to 40 mm. Although a reasonable alternative to surgical myotomy, the minimally invasive approach afforded by laparoscopic myotomy and excellent outcomes (success rates exceeding 90%) make surgical myotomy quite attractive to patients with achalasia.

Surgical myotomy can be performed using several techniques: transthoracically via thoracotomy or by using video assisted thoracic surgery (VATS), or transabdominally with either an open or laparoscopic technique. Myotomy may be performed alone or combined with an antireflux operation. However, achalasia is a rare disease and it is unlikely that anyone can assemble a large series of patients to determine optimal approaches. Review of the literature and meta-analysis have been helpful and indicate the following:

1. Laparoscopic esophageal myotomy yields the highest success rates.

2. Patients reap the benefits of minimally invasive surgery (less pain, shorter hospital stay, quicker return to full activity, and improved cosmesis).

3. Thoracic approaches produce less symptoms of postoperative acid reflux.

4. Patients with transabdominal approaches appear to benefit from a concomitant antireflux procedure.

5. Disruption of key anatomic relationships during esophageal mobilization may account for reflux after transabdominal surgery. Some surgeons advocate "minimal dissection" myotomy without an antireflux procedure.

6. As illustrated here, partial wraps may be designed to bolster and "protect" the myotomy. A protective wrap is always prudent if perforation is recognized, during myotomy, and repaired.

7. Intraoperative endoscopy improves outcome by ensuring the myotomy is complete. Some surgeons prefer intraoperative manometry. Insufflation of the esophagus at the end of the procedure with the endoscope may reveal unrecognized perforation.

Dr. Jones et al have nicely illustrated the techniques for performance of laparoscopic esophageal myotomy. It should be understood that this procedure requires expert laparoscopic skills. Performance of the myotomy is quite delicate and the consequences of perforation, if not recognized or not repaired adequately when found, are profound. The excellent outcomes with this procedure show that it is a safe and durable operation, and increased numbers of patients with achalasia are choosing surgical therapy since the introduction of the laparoscopic approach.

Jonathan F. Critchlow, M.D., Beth Israel Deaconess Medical Center Harvard Medical School

The advent of laparoscopic and minimally invasive surgery has made the procedure of esophagomyotomy much more popular. It has also greatly increased the number of patients treated surgically, allowing for refinements in technique, which now make it the procedure of choice for both untreated and previously treated achalasia. Treatment with botulinum toxin in fit patients should be discouraged as it merely delays more definitive therapy and may make surgical treatment more difficult.

It now appears that a partial fundoplication does diminish the incidence of postoperative reflux without tremendously affecting the success of relief of dysphagia. The type of fundoplication is left up to the surgeon. An anterior (Dor) has the advantages of being relatively straightforward and also may cover over the esophagus, especially if there are areas that are in question or have been violated. There are at least theoretical considerations of stricture or scar formation to the wrap that could potentially lead to late failure. The Toupet technique requires more fundal mobilization and has the advantage of keeping the myotomy apart. It does not, however, cover the mucosa in situations where one is nervous. It also should be used with caution in patients with an elongated or sigmoid esophagus where the posteriorly placed stomach may over accentuate the anterior angulation of the esophagus, which may lead to kinking and dysphagia. A total fundoplication (Nissen) is contraindicated due to an unacceptably high incidence of postoperative dysphagia.

The myotomy is most easily begun just above the esophagogastric junction as the planes between mucosa and the musculature of the esophagus are more easily identified. The choice of instrument is up to the surgeon. An electric cautery hook may be used but one must be concerned about arcing of electrical current onto the mucosa. The surgeon should also be aware that the Harmonic scalpel blade may stay quite hot for several seconds after use.

The endoscope may be used during the entire procedure to identify position and the adequacy of myotomy. Alternatively, a large bougie may be placed into the esophagus which may stretch some of the fibers around the lower esophageal sphincter. Dissection can be completed to what seems to be the surgeon's satisfaction and then confirmed with the endoscope.

Closure of the hiatus is somewhat debated. As there is some

dissection around the hiatus, it is reasonable to do a posterior closure over a large bougie except in patients with a megaesophagus.

W. Scott Melvin, M.D.
The Ohio State University

Achalasia is an uncommon yet chronic disease. The physician should accurately inform the patient undergoing therapy of the chronicity of their disease. Fortunately, the symptoms of dysphagia attributable to achalasia can be very well controlled using minimally invasive techniques with limited risk of injury and a short recovery period. However, surgical intervention does not cure achalasia; esophageal dismotility remains a problem and it often becomes a lifetime problem. A frank discussion with the patient about the chronicity of their disease prior to surgical intervention will most likely improve patient satisfaction with the operation. Following Heller myotomy, most symptoms are adequately resolved and in many patients symptoms are completely minimized over a long period of time. The relationship between the surgeon and the patient needs to be a long one however, because there still exists a risk of malignant potential and therefore long-term screening is often necessary.

Minimally invasive surgical approaches to achalasia have changed the algorithm for the modern treatment of this disease. Patients with significant dysphagia who after the appropriate work-up are diagnosed with achalasia should be appropriately triaged to surgical intervention as first-line therapy. There exists little role for multiple endoscopic procedures, including injections and dilatations, when the advantages of laparoscopic Heller myotomy have been so well documented.

The use of robotic surgical devices may be applied to laparoscopic surgery and especially to Heller myotomy. Sufficient data exist to demonstrate that the advantages of robotic surgery, such as dissection in an isolated region of the abdomen, three-dimensional imaging, motion scaling, and fine tremor filtration, may improve outcomes in certain surgical procedures.

Achalasia treatment continues to improve based on the technology that has been made available to surgeons and physicians over the last decade. It is important to remember that the application of this technology and a thoughtful treatment process can truly improve patient outcomes, especially for the treatment of achalasia.

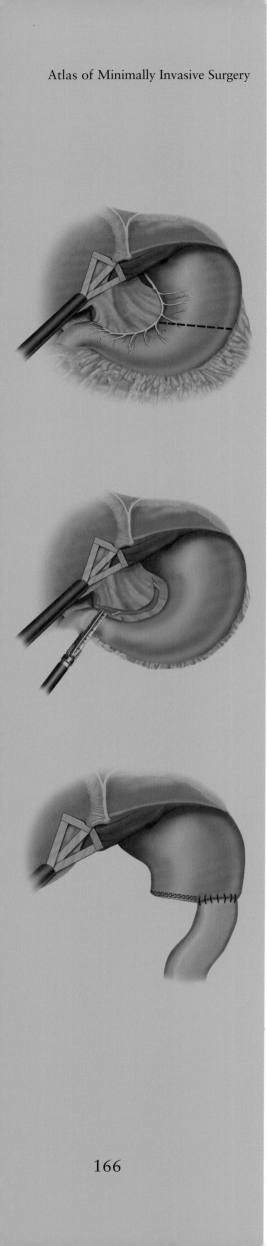

Laparoscopic Partial Gastrectomy

Laparoscopic gastrectomy may be performed for gastrointestinal stromal tumors (GIST), complications of peptic ulcer disease (obstruction, bleeding, intractable pain), lymphoma, and adenocarcinoma. It is imperative to adhere to oncologic priniciples when performing minimally invasive resections for malignant disease, such as including the omentum in the specimen.

Billroth I Gastrectomy

Preoperative Preparation

1. Sequential compression stockings and subcutaneous heparin are used for prophylaxis against deep venous thrombosis. Intravenous antibiotics are administered prophylactically. After induction of general anesthesia, the bladder is emptied with a urinary catheter and the stomach is decompressed with a nasogastric tube. Intraoperative endoscopy may be performed to confirm anatomic relationships.

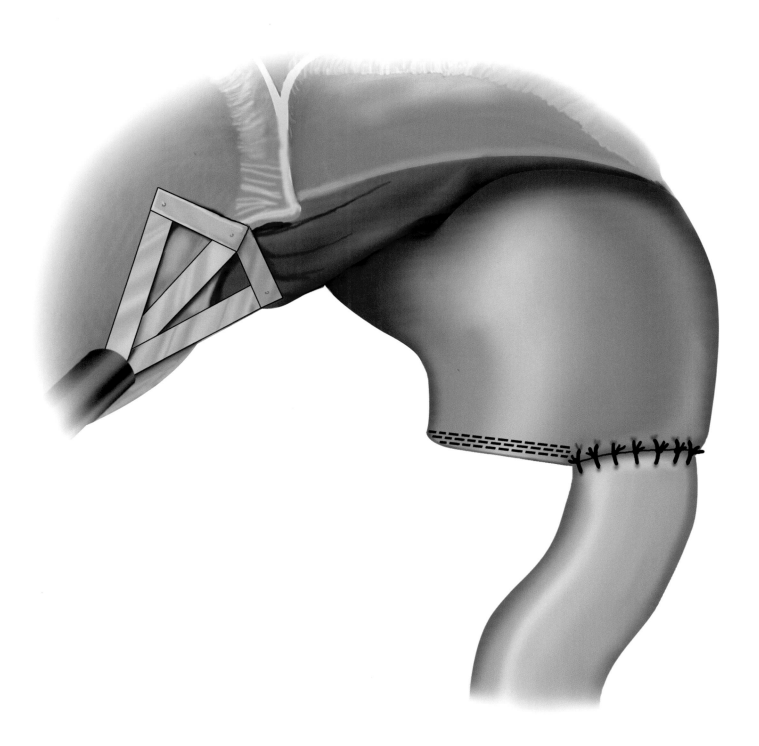

Operating Room Layout

2. The patient is placed in a modified lithotomy position with the legs in stirrups, being careful to appropriately pad all prominences as to avoid pressure injuries. The abdomen is prepared and draped in a sterile fashion. We prefer the surgeon to stand between the patient's legs, while the camera operator is situated to the patient's left and the assistant surgeon on the right. Monitors are positioned at the head of the table as shown.

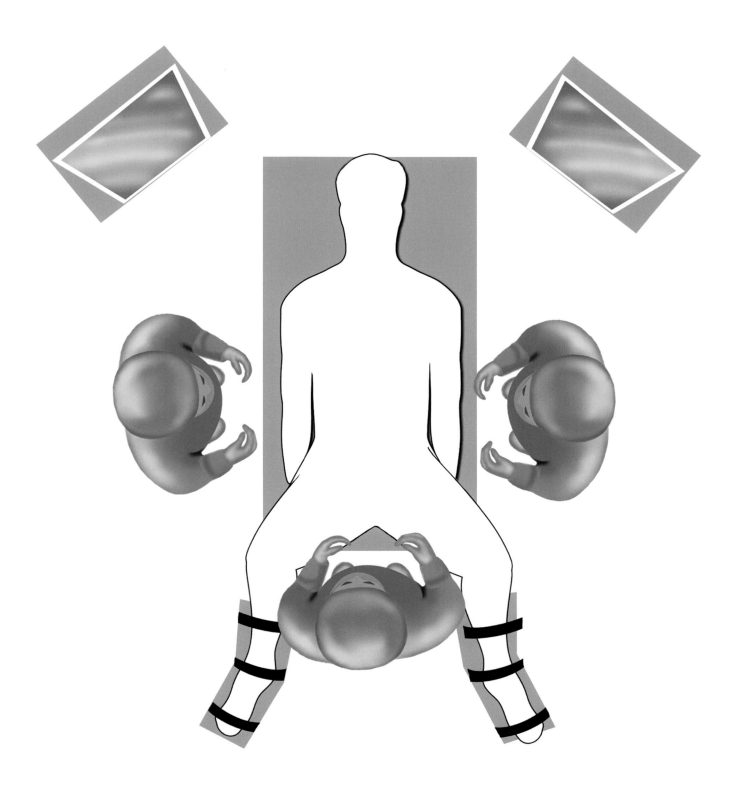

Access and Port Placement

3. An infraumbilical incision is used to establish pneumoperitoneum, setting a maximum pressure limit of 15 mm Hg. This is established either with an open or closed technique. A 10/11 mm port is placed here and a 30° angled laparoscope is inserted. A careful exploration is performed to ensure that no injury occurred during port insertion and that no other abnormalities are present. Five additional ports (four 10 mm and a 12 or 18 mm) are inserted under direct vision.

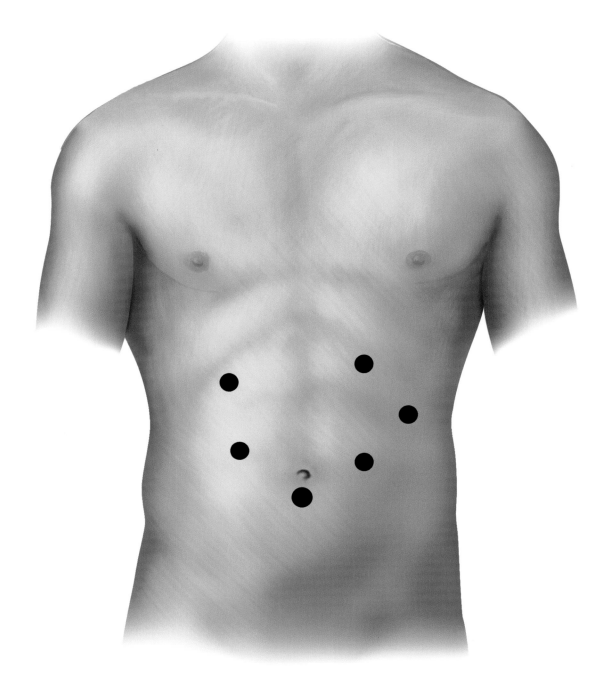

FIGURE C

Determining the Proximal Resection Margin

4. The liver edge is retracted superiorly and laterally to provide adequate exposure of the lesser curve.

5. The anterior surface of the stomach is inspected and the area of the crow's foot is identified at the incisura of the lesser curve. The confluence of the right and left gastroepiploic arteries is also identified along the greater curve, and the stomach's serosa is scored using cautery along a line that connects this area with the incisura of the lesser curve.

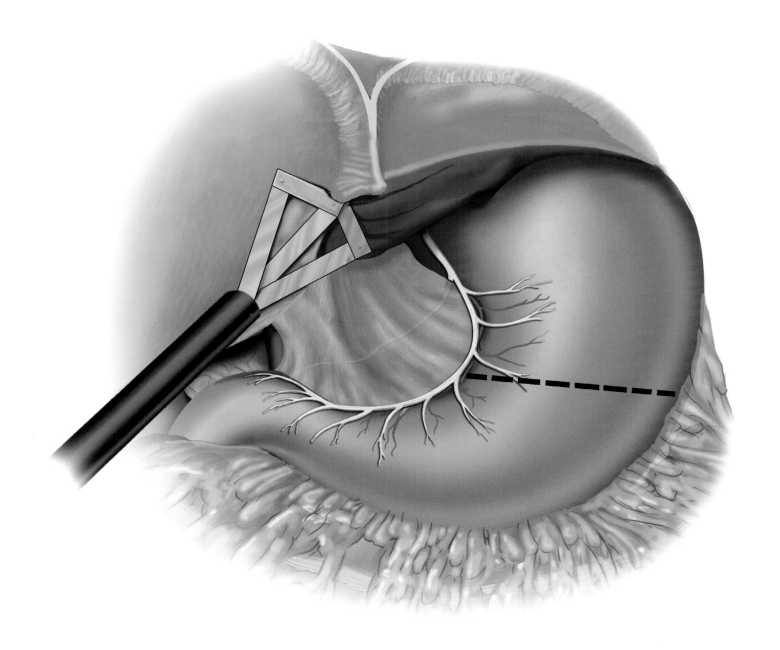

Devascularizing the Stomach

6. The portion of the stomach that is intended for resection is devascularized by dividing the left gastric artery. Typically, this is performed either with sutures or surgical clips.

7. Next, branches of the right gastric and right gastroepiploic arteries and veins are also ligated using sutures, surgical clips, or a harmonic scalpel.

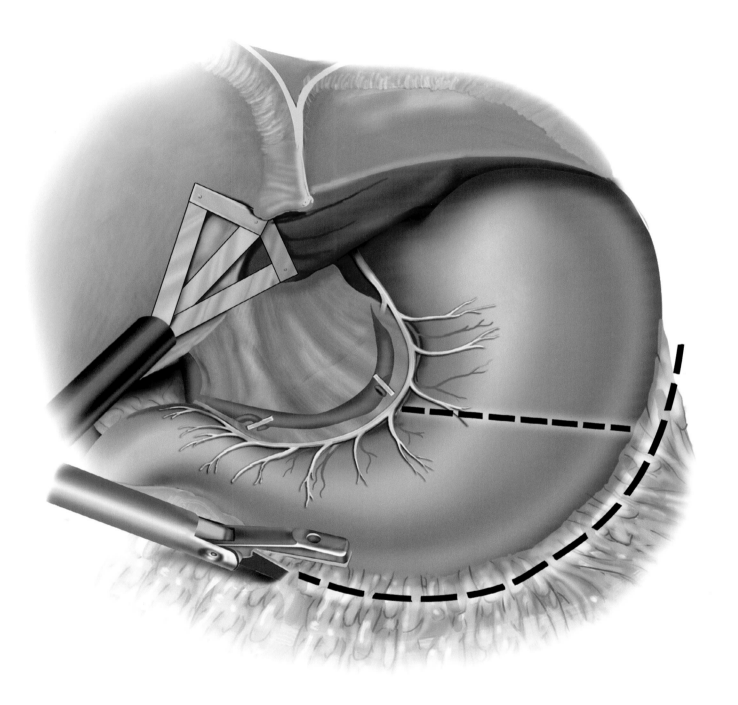

FIGURE E

Kocherizing the Duodenum

8. Using a combination of cautery and blunt dissection, a generous Kocher maneuver is performed that will allow creation of a tension-free gastroduodenostomy.

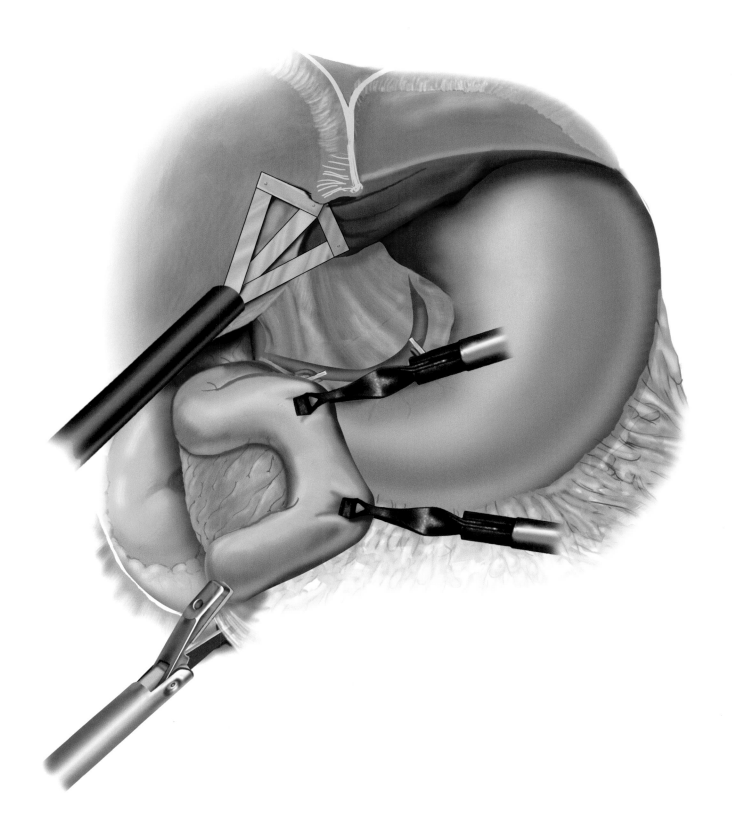

Dividing the Duodenum

9. The duodenum is transected approximately 1 cm distal to the pylorus using an endoscopic linear stapling device (3.5 mm staples). The distal end is controlled with atraumatic graspers and mobilized to ensure a tension-free anastomosis. The Kocher maneuver may need to be extended.

FIGURE F-a

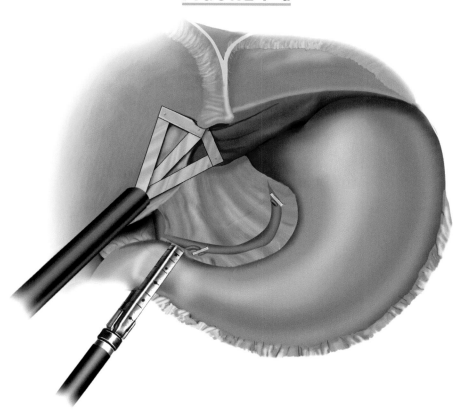

FIGURE F-b

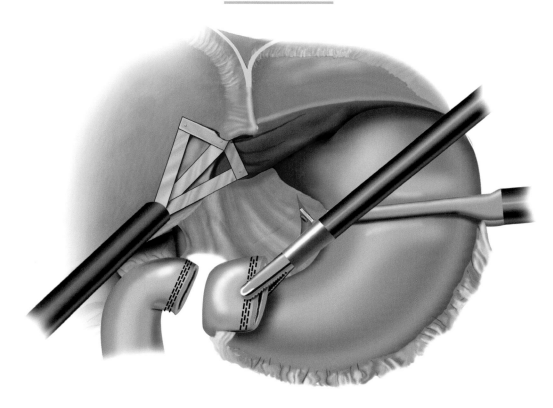

Dividing the Stomach

10. Division of the stomach begins at the lesser curve using repeated applications of a 60 mm Endo-GIA (3.5-4.8 mm staples). The stapler can be left engaged after the final firing to act as a retractor. The stomach is flipped cephalad and a gastrotomy is created along the posterior aspect, being careful to match the size of the duodenal stump.

11. Alternatively, after separating the greater omentum from the stomach, the duodenum can be stapled and then the lesser curve approached. With more mobilization of the stomach, the left gastric vessel can then be divided using a linear stapler.

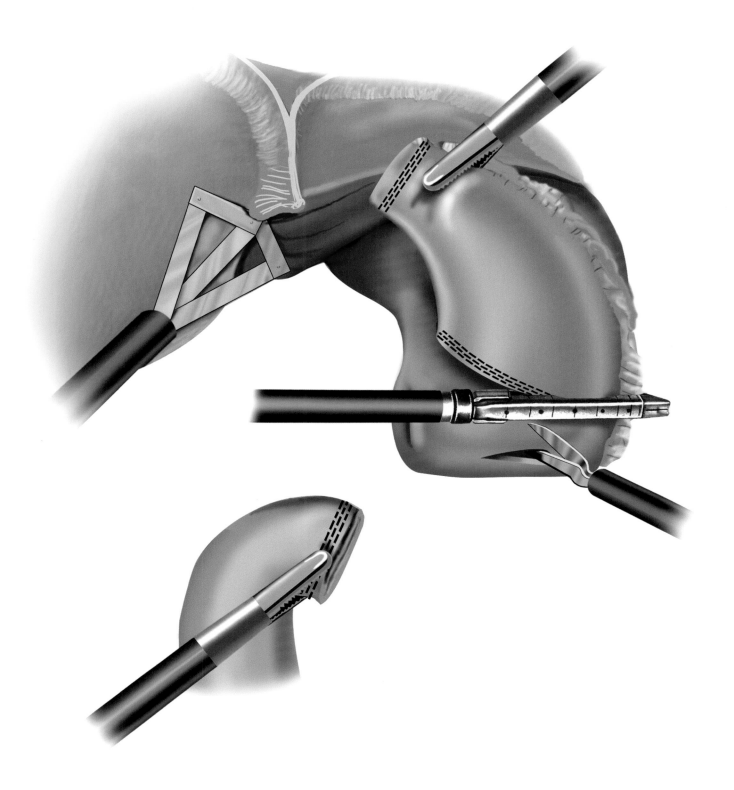

FIGURE H, I-a,b

Creating the Gastroduodenostomy

12. A hand-sewn, single-layer anastomosis is fashioned between the stomach and duodenum. Stay sutures are placed at each corner (Figure H).

13. The posterior suture line is completed with interrupted full-thickness stitches, with the knots placed intraluminally. Next, the stay sutures are tied down and the anterior suture line is completed using a similar technique. Additional Lembert stitches may be applied to any sites of concern.

14. Alternatively, the stomach can be completely transected and a portion of the gastric staple line can be excised to create the gastroduodenostomy in a similar fashion as described above (Figure I-a,b).

15. Consider adding truncal vagotomy as part of the procedure of distal gastrectomy.

FIGURE H

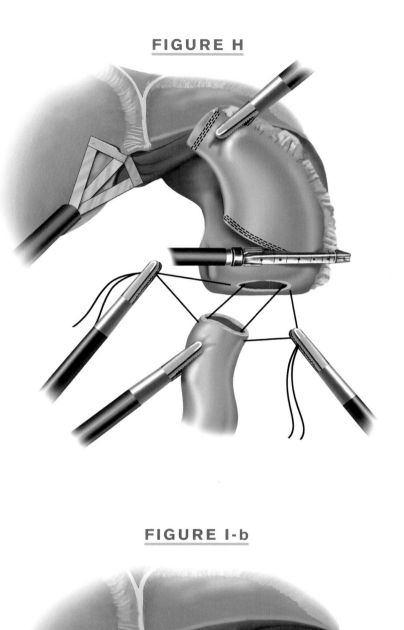

FIGURE I-a

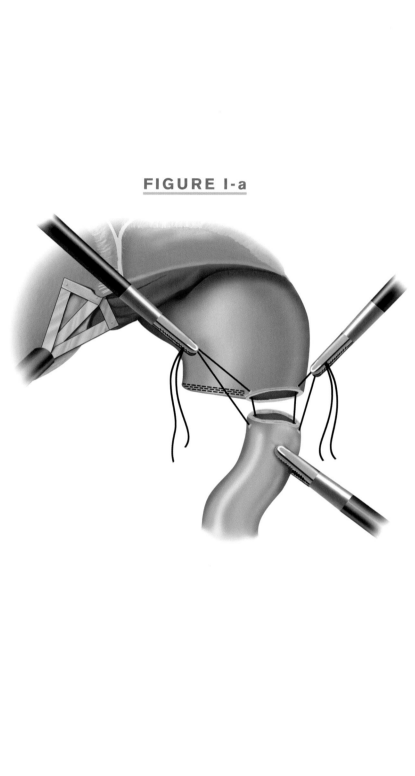

FIGURE I-b

Removing the Specimen

16. The specimen is placed in an entrapment sac (Figure J) and is removed through one of the port sites, which usually needs to be enlarged to retrieve the specimen (Figure K).

17. The abdomen is inspected, irrigated, and aspirated dry. A closed suction drain may be left exiting the abdomen via one of the port sites. The fascia and skin are closed in the standard fashion.

FIGURE J

FIGURE K

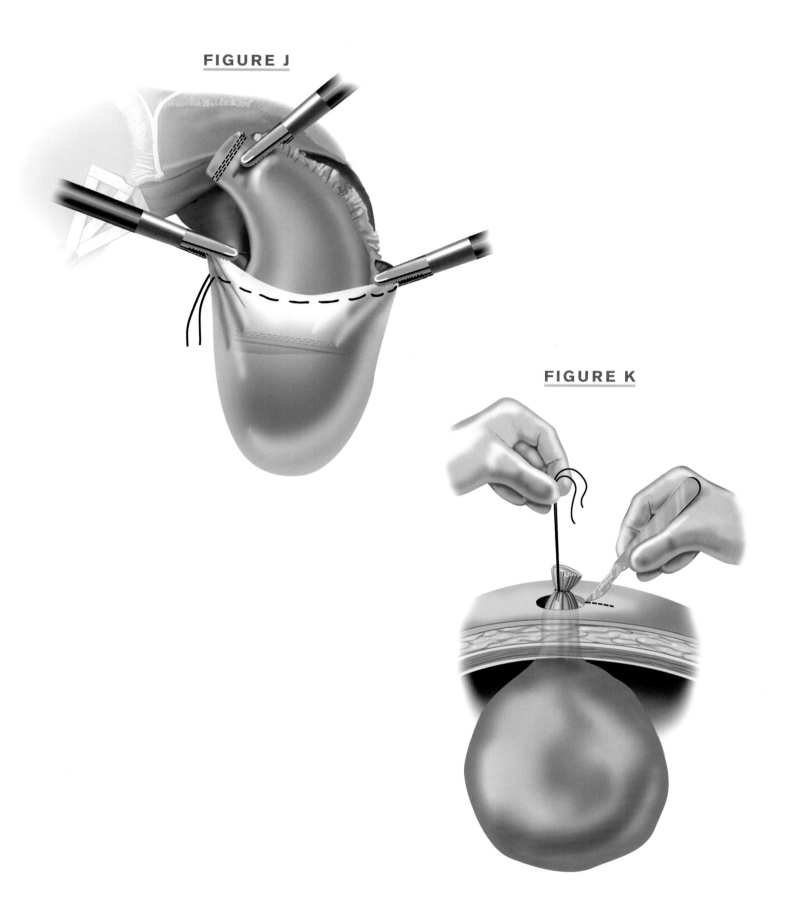

Billroth II Gastrectomy

The preoperative preparation, operating room setup, dissection, specimen removal, and closure are identical to a Billroth I procedure. The difference lies in the reconstruction. Furthermore, the duodenal stump staple line may be reinforced with 3-0 silk Lembert stitches.

FIGURE L

Creating the Gastrojejunostomy

1. The stomach is divided as described for the Billroth I procedure. Again, the stapler can be left engaged after the last firing to facilitate retraction.

2. A loop of jejunum approximately 20 cm to 30 cm distal to the ligament of Treitz is brought up via either an ante- or retrocolic approach to approximate the posterior aspect of the gastric remnant.

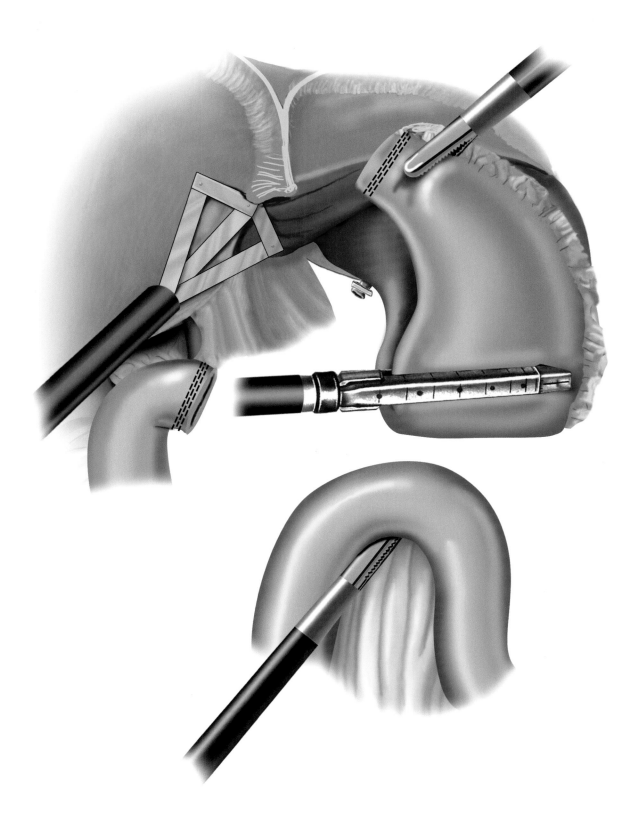

Creating the Gastrojejunostomy, Part II

3. A gastrotomy is made in the posterior aspect of the gastric remnant, approximately 1 cm to 2 cm proximal to the staple line. Similarly, an enterotomy is made along the antimesenteric edge of the jejunum. A 60 mm stapled anastomosis is fashioned in the usual manner (Figure M-a).

4. The enterotomies are closed with a second firing of the stapler to complete the anastomosis (Figure M-b). Lembert stitches are used to reinforce as needed. Alternatively, a hand-sewn anastomosis can be fashioned in a similar manner as described for a Billroth I procedure.

FIGURE M-a

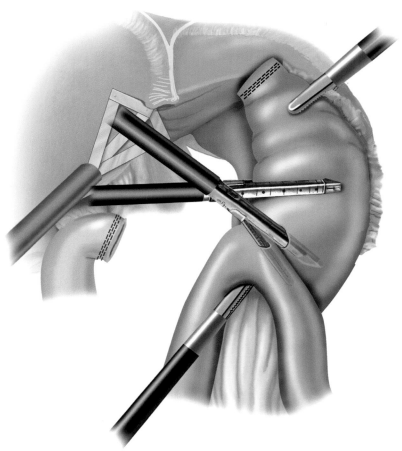

FIGURE M-b

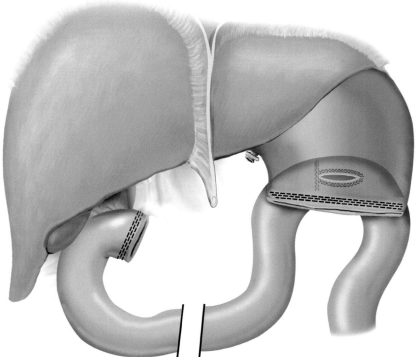

Gastric Wedge Resection

The setup is similar to that as described for a Billroth I procedure, except that only three trocars are generally required. The lesions can be localized with endoscopic tattoo.

Excising the Lesion

1. If the lesion can be grasped, it is elevated from the gastric wall and multiple firings of a retriculating endoscopic GIA (4.5-4.8 mm staples) are used to resect the specimen. Occasionally, seromuscular stay sutures need to be placed proximal and distal to the lesion to facilitate elevating it, and a GIA stapler is fired below the lesion (Figure N). If the lesion cannot be localized easily, an endoscope can be inserted using CO_2 gas insufflation to transilluminate the exact location of the lesion.

2. For lesions lying near the greater curvature of the stomach, the omentum is detached and the lesion can be excised with sequential full-thickness firings of a reticulating linear stapler (4.5–4.8 mm staples, Figure O).

3. Care must be taken when resecting lesions near the pylorus or cardia, as a wedge resection in these locations may cause excessive narrowing of the lumen. An endoscope may be placed through the pylorus for resection of a lesion near the pylorus so that the patency of the pylorus is protected. If patency is not ensured, a formal gastric resection may be the better surgical option.

FIGURE N

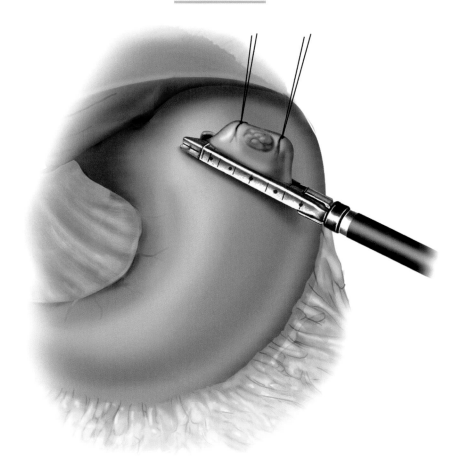

FIGURE O

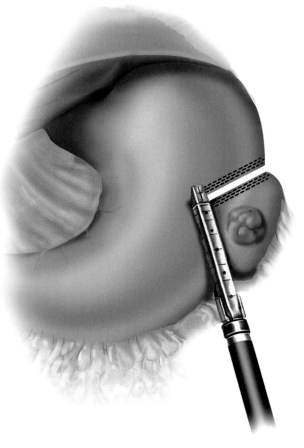

Postoperative Care

Sequential compression devices and subcutaneous heparin are continued postoperatively. The duration of antibiotics is at the discretion of the surgeon, however, 24 hours will usually suffice. A nasogastric tube is left in place until return of bowel function, at which time it is removed and oral intake is slowly advanced as tolerated. Routine upper GI contrast studies are not necessary unless there is clinical concern for an anastomotic leak.

Suggested Reading

1. Reyes CD, Weber KJ, Gagner M, Divino CM. Laparoscopic vs open gastrectomy. A retrospective review. *Surg Endosc.* 2001;15:928-931.

2. Shimizu S, Noshiro H, Nagai E, et al. Laparoscopic wedge resection of gastric submucosal tumors. *Dig Surg.* 2002;19:169-173.

3. Wilkiemeyer MB, Bieligk SC, Asnfaq R, Jones DB, et al. Laparoscopy alone is superior to peritoneal cytology in staging of gastric and esophageal carcinoma. *Surg Endosc.* 2004;18(5):852-857.

Commentary

W. Scott Melvin, M.D.
The Ohio State University

Almost all gastric surgery can be accomplished using a variety of minimally invasive surgical techniques. The development of multiple linear stapling devices and energy devices for hemostasis have allowed a wide variety of resections to be performed along with complex reconstructive procedures. While the incidence of operations for complications of peptic ulcer disease has decreased over time, the significance of this disease process in a variety of patients remains important. Pyloric stenosis and nonhealing gastric ulcers remain the primary indication for gastric resection in patients with peptic ulcer disease. Truncal vagotomy should be added to a distal gastrectomy in many patients because of this complication. Truncal vagotomy can easily be accomplished by exposing the vagus nerve at the level of the crura with minimal dissection. Laparoscopic techniques work quite nicely to provide this exposure with minimal retraction of the rib cage and decreased incidence of pulmonary complications. The addition of vagotomy for patients undergoing partial gastrectomy for other reasons remains controversial. It may not be necessary in a wide variety of patients but many authors continue to suggest prophylactic vagotomy at the time of gastrectomy and reconstruction be considered because the increased incidence of marginal ulcerations. A highly selective vagotomy can be accomplished laparoscopically, although this operation is rarely indicated.

A variety of reconstructive techniques can be accomplished using minimally invasive techniques. Billroth I or Billroth II reconstructions are useful as outlined in this chapter. Alternatively, a Roux-en-Y reconstruction can be created using many of the techniques similar to bariatric surgery. Gastrojejunostomy can be created using a circular endoluminal stapling device, linear stapling devices, or laparoscopic suturing. Using similar techniques, gastrojejunostomy without resection should be considered as palliative treatment for patients with obstructing lesions, and should be considered as first-line therapy, rather than open laparotomy.

As minimally invasive approaches have been adapted to more complex procedures, potential advantages for minimally invasive approaches to malignant diseases have been identified. Now with adequate experience and appropriate techniques, curative operations can be accomplished for gastric adenocarcinoma. En bloc resection of the omentum and lymph-node–baring tissue around the stomach should be accomplished adhering to strict oncological principles. Containment of the specimen in an impermeable membrane prior to tissue extraction is important. Reconstruction can be performed in a variety of different techniques as outlined. The fear of malignant disease should not preclude the laparoscopic approach. Even in patients with malignancy, decreased morbidity is seen with minimally invasive techniques for gastric resection.

Namir Katkhouda, M.D.
University of Southern California

Laparoscopic gastrectomy can be finished as a B1 or B2 gastrojejunostomy as described in this chapter. My preference goes to a B2, as there is likely less scarring than in the duodenal area, especially if the procedure is performed for duodenal ulcers

One trick is to stay away from the gastroepiploic arcade and open quickly the gastrosplenic ligament with the ultrasonic shears. Also, the retroduodenal dissection requires special attention. I advise to place a right-angled dissector in the subxyphoid trocar and place the stapler from above. It is much easier than from below.

Once the duodenum is closed, the staple line is inspected and if there is an issue, it should be reinforced with intracorporeal suturing.

The B2 reconstruction following resection will expose the patient to the risk of bile reflux and severe gastritis. The best way to remedy this would be to connect a Roux-en-Y to the gastric stump. This can be done stapled or hand sewn.

Finally, if a large specimen is to be removed, one can use a hand-assisted technique. An incision the length of the glove size is made in the right upper quadrant of the abdomen for the nondominant hand. A lap disk or other device is placed to keep the pneumoperitoneum. This will allow for a faster operation and the specimen can be exteriorized and the anastomosis performed quickly and safely outside the abdomen. The specimen is then transected outside. The wound has to be protected to avoid any infection.

Laparoscopic Management Of Peptic Ulcer Disease

Operative management of ulcer disease is directed at reducing acid secretion and is primarily reserved for patients refractory to medical therapy or for treating complications such as bleeding and perforation. The decision of whether or not to simultaneously perform an acid-reducing procedure at the time of operative treatment of bleeding and/or perforation is dependent on each individual patient's clinical state and presentation.

Gastric ulcers must be biopsied to assess for the presence of malignancy.

Parietal cell acid production is stimulated by three different mechanisms that include vagus nerve input, gastrin (secreted by the antrum) stimulation, and histamine-2 receptor activation. Operative procedures are directed primarily at the first two pathways, specifically performing some level of vagotomy and/or antrectomy, respectively. Truncal vagotomy has a lower rate of recurrence compared to a highly selective vagotomy, although it requires a drainage procedure and is associated with greater morbidity, including dumping syndrome and diarrhea. Highly selective, or parietal cell, vagotomy, on the other hand, may cause ischemic necrosis of the lesser curvature. Thus, some advocate performing a combined procedure that consists of a posterior truncal vagotomy and an anterior highly selective vagotomy, which is described in detail here.

Preoperative Preparation

1. Sequential compression stockings and subcutaneous heparin may be used for prophylaxis against deep venous thrombosis. Intravenous antibiotics, usually a first-generation cephalosporin, are administered prophylactically. After induction of general anesthesia, the bladder is emptied with a urinary catheter and the stomach is decompressed with a nasogastric tube.

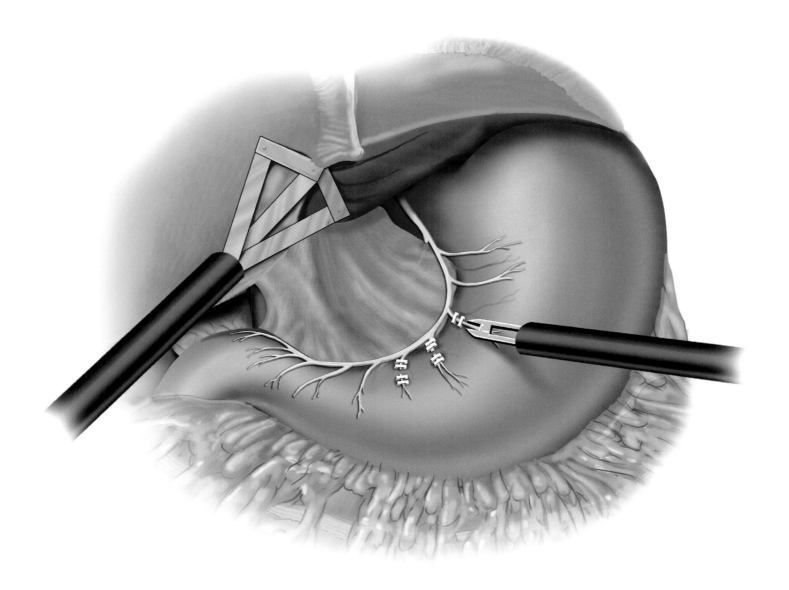

Operating Room Setup

2. The patient is placed in a modified lithotomy position. All pressure points must be adequately padded and a bean-bag device is used to secure the patient's position when rotating the table to facilitate exposure and viewing during the procedure.

3. The surgeon stands between the patient's legs, the assistant is situated to the patient's right, and the camera operator stands on the patient's left side. Alternatively, the patient can be placed supine with the surgeon standing to the patient's right.

4. The video monitors are stationed at both sides of the patient's head to facilitate adequate viewing from either side of the table.

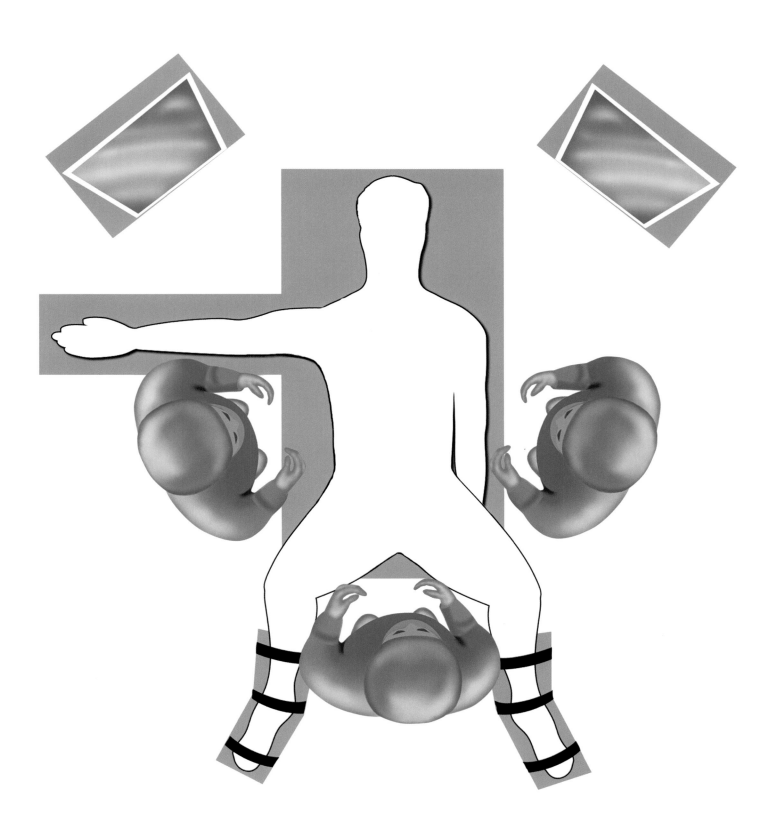

Access and Port Placement

5. Pneumoperitoneum is obtained through a supraumbilical incision with either an open or closed technique (Veress needle). Using a 30° angled laparoscope, the abdomen is inspected for adhesions or injuries.

6. Four additional trocars are inserted under direct vision in the configuration depicted. The periumbilical trocar should be a 10/12 mm port, while the other three can be 5 mm in size and enlarged if necessary.

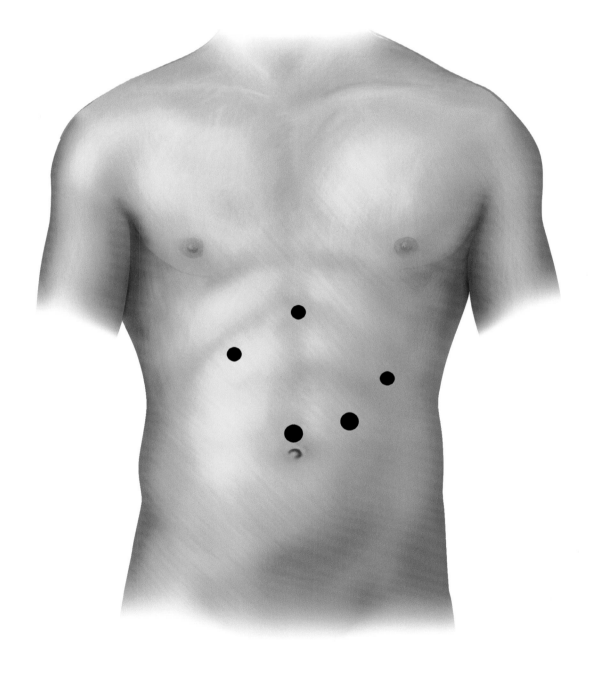

FIGURE C

Exposing the Esophageal Hiatus

7. The patient is placed in the reverse Trendelenburg position to provide gravity retraction. A self-retaining liver retractor is placed through the subxiphoid port to displace the left lateral lobe of the liver anterolaterally.

8. The stomach is grasped with a Babcock grasper and retracted inferiorly while the lesser sac is entered through the gastrohepatic ligament or pars flaccida. Both crura of the diaphragm and the anterior vagus nerve are identified after the phrenoesophageal ligament is adequately opened. The right crus is retracted laterally to expose and identify the posterior vagus nerve. Prior to performing any vagotomy, both anterior and posterior trunks, their hepatic and celiac branches, respectively, and both nerves of Latarjet should be clearly identified.

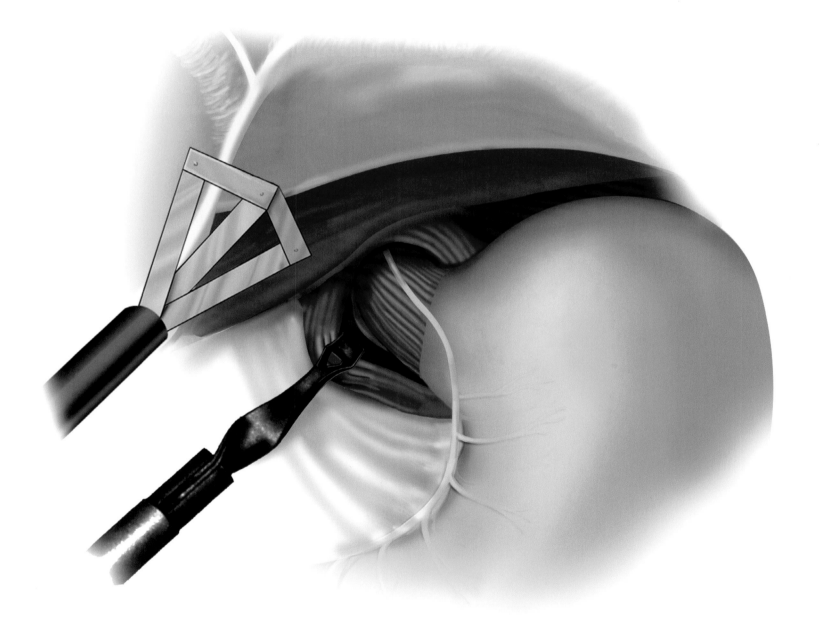

Posterior Truncal Vagotomy

FIGURE D

Performing a Posterior Truncal Vagotomy

9. The posterior vagal trunk is bluntly mobilized away from the esophagus. A short segment measuring approximately 1 cm is resected between surgical clips and is sent to pathology for frozen section confirmation of neural tissue.

10. An anterior truncal vagotomy may also be performed using this same technique, but this will necessitate performance of a drainage procedure such as a pyloroplasty.

11. Alternatively, a posterior highly selective vagotomy may also be performed using a similar technique as that subsequently described for an anterior highly selective vagotomy. All proximal branches to the right of the esophagus and posterior branches to the stomach must be divided, being careful to preserve innervation to the pylorus, thus avoiding a drainage procedure.

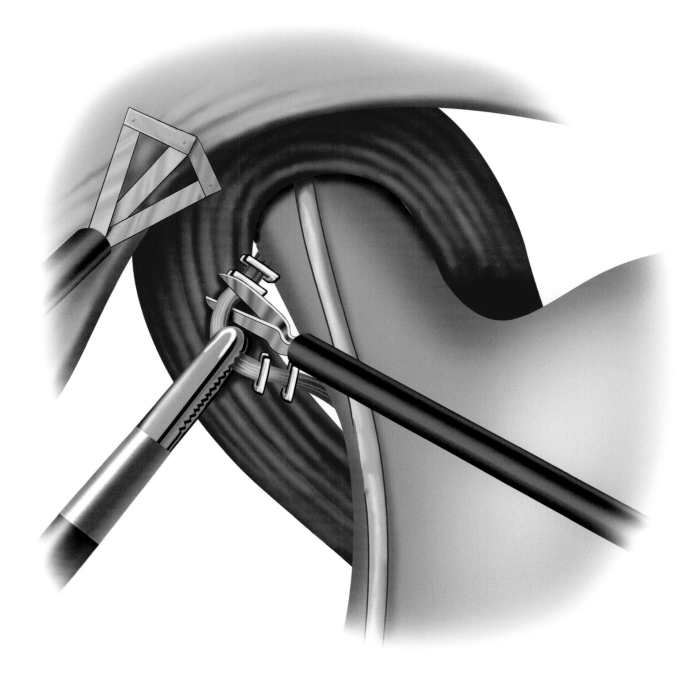

Options of Anterior Highly Selective Vagotomy Performed in Conjunction With a Posterior Truncal Vagotomy

Anterior Highly Selective (Parietal Cell) Vagotomy

12. The previously identified anterior (left) vagal trunk is bluntly dissected free from the esophageal wall. The proximal branches of the anterior vagal trunk are identified, which usually requires mobilization of the abdominal esophagus.

13. All branches to the left of the esophagus should be divided between surgical clips, including the criminal nerve of Grassi. The hepatic branch of the anterior vagal trunk is spared from division.

14. Distal dissection begins approximately 5 cm to 7 cm proximal to the pylorus. This ensures preservation of the "crow's foot" branches of the nerve of Latarjet, thus maintaining innervation to the pylorus and avoiding the need for a drainage procedure. The gastric branches are sequentially divided between clips to the level of the gastroesophageal junction. Prior to initiating nerve division, the proximal and distal margins may be marked with a loosely tied suture in order to preserve orientation should any bleeding occur that inhibits adequate visibility of each nerve branch.

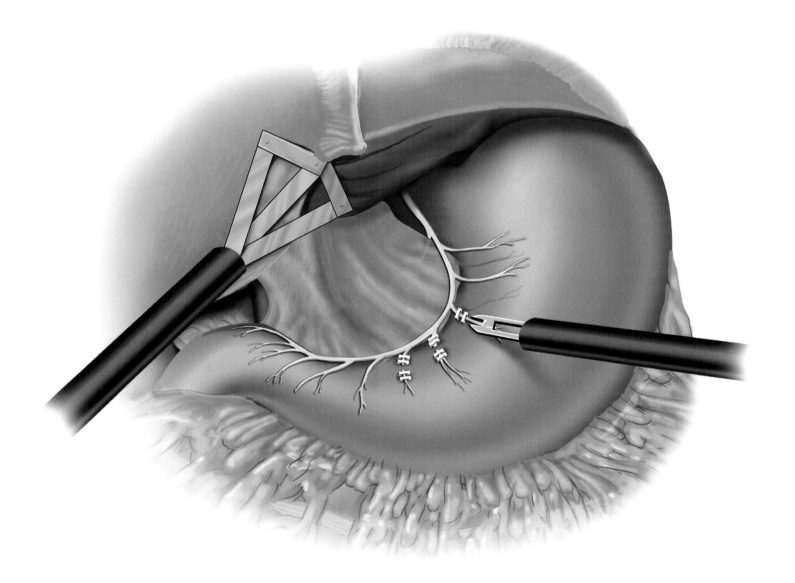

Anterior Gastric Seromyotomy (Taylor Procedure)

15. A seromyotomy is performed using either hook electrocautery or an ultrasonic coagulator to dissect along the anterior gastric wall parallel, and 1.5 cm inferior, to the lesser curvature. The myotomy is extended from the posterior aspect of the angle of His down to the first branch of the crow's foot (5-7 cm proximal to the pylorus), thus once again preserving innervation to the pylorus and avoiding a drainage procedure (Figure F-a). Using a similar technique as that described for performing a Heller myotomy, the muscular layers are sequentially divided until the bluish-hued gastric mucosa is noted to bulge through the wound. Careful and controlled dissection will usually prevent inadvertent gastric perforation. A suspected perforation can be detected by injecting air and/or methylene blue through the nasogastric tube.

16. Once the seromyotomy is complete, having divided the anterior gastric vagal branches, the edges are reapproximated using a running suture in such a manner as to prevent vagal reinnervation (Figure F-b).

FIGURE F-a

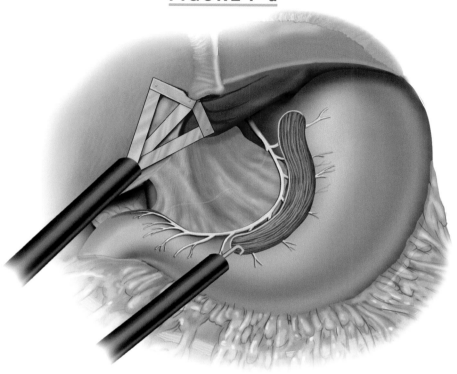

FIGURE F-b

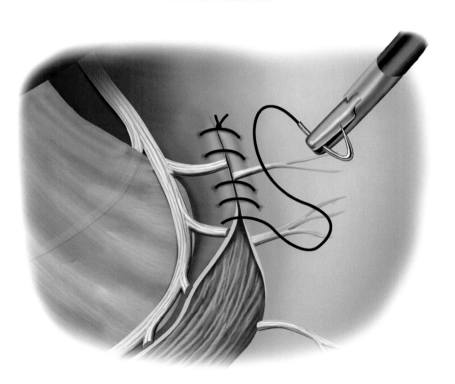

Anterior Stapled Linear Gastrectomy

17. Alternatively, a stapled technique may be used instead of a seromyotomy. Using atraumatic graspers, an anterior fold of gastric tissue is elevated approximately 1 cm and an endoscopic linear stapler (4.5-4.8 mm staples) is fired across its base, thus excising a full thickness segment of gastric tissue and dividing the anterior gastric vagal branches (Figure G-a). The staple line is extended along the same line as that described for performing a seromyotomy, being careful to preserve pyloric innervation (Figure G-b).

18. The operative field is irrigated and inspected for adequate hemostasis. The ports are withdrawn under direct vision to ensure hemostasis at each port site. The fascial and skin incisions are closed in the usual manner.

Postoperative Care

Sequential compression devices and/or subcutaneous heparin are continued postoperatively. Postoperative antibiotics are usually not necessary, but may be continued for 24 hours at the surgeon's discretion. The nasogastric tube can usually be removed within 24 hours. Oral intake is initiated with clear liquids and is advanced as tolerated.

FIGURE G-a

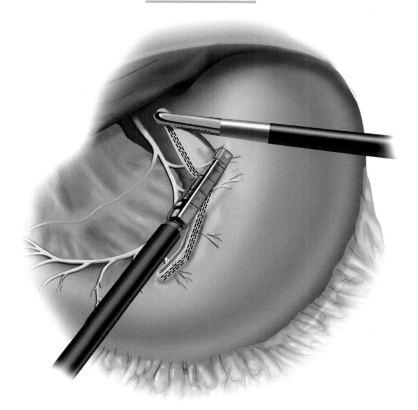

FIGURE G-b

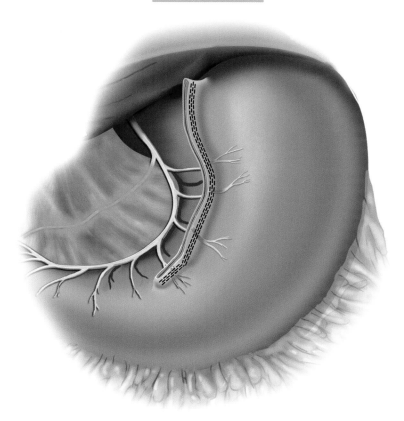

Laparoscopic Repair of a Perforated Duodenal Ulcer

Peptic perforation usually involves the duodenum or pylorus and, less commonly, the stomach. Treatment usually involves a combination of primary closure of the defect, an omental patch to buttress the repair, pharmacologic acid-suppression therapy, and antibiotics to address the peritonitis and probable *Helicobacter pylori* infection.

FIGURE H

Identifying a Perforated Duodenal Ulcer

1. The abdomen is carefully inspected and any abscess or soilage is irrigated and suctioned. A sample of the fluid should be sent for Gram's stain and culture.

2. The left lobe of the liver is elevated and retracted anterolaterally with either a Nathanson retractor or paddle device to adequately expose the perforation site.

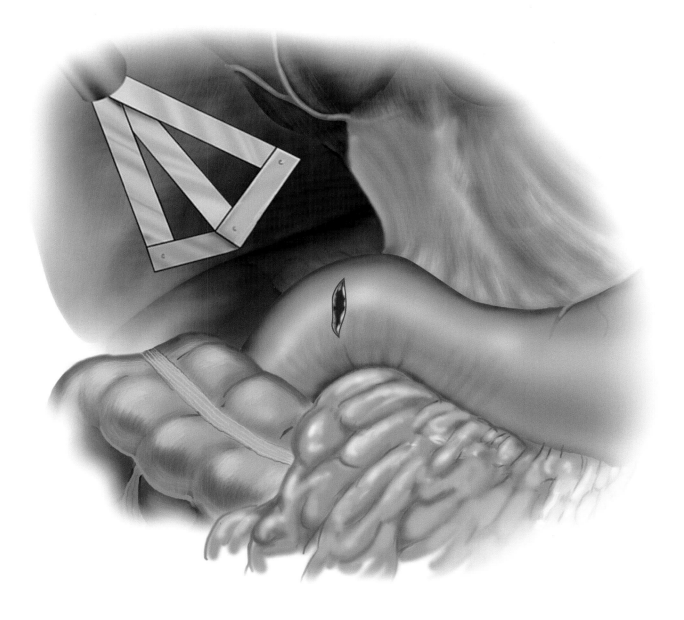

FIGURE I-a,b

Primary Closure of a Duodenal Perforation

3. The identified perforation is closed with full-thickness interrupted 3-0 silk sutures. The closure should be performed in a transverse fashion so as not to narrow the duodenal lumen (Figure I-a).

4. The tails of the sutures are left long such that a tongue of omentum may be secured over the repaired site (Figure I-b).

FIGURE I-a

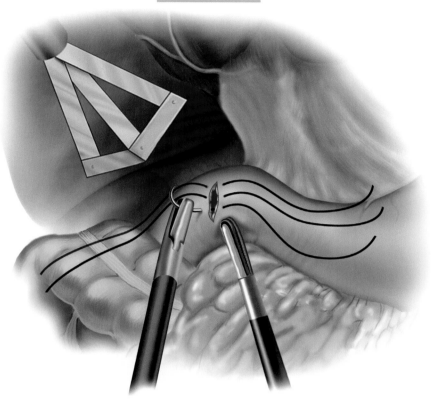

FIGURE I-b

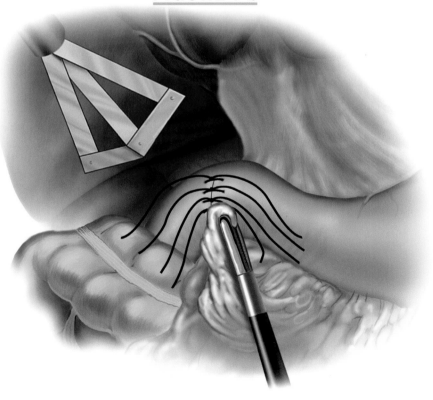

Securing an Omental Patch

5. A piece of omentum is placed over the repair site and is secured in position by tying the ends of the sutures over the omental patch. Intraoperative endoscopic evaluation may be used to confirm the absence of leak at the repair site.

6. A closed suction drain should be left in the right upper quadrant.

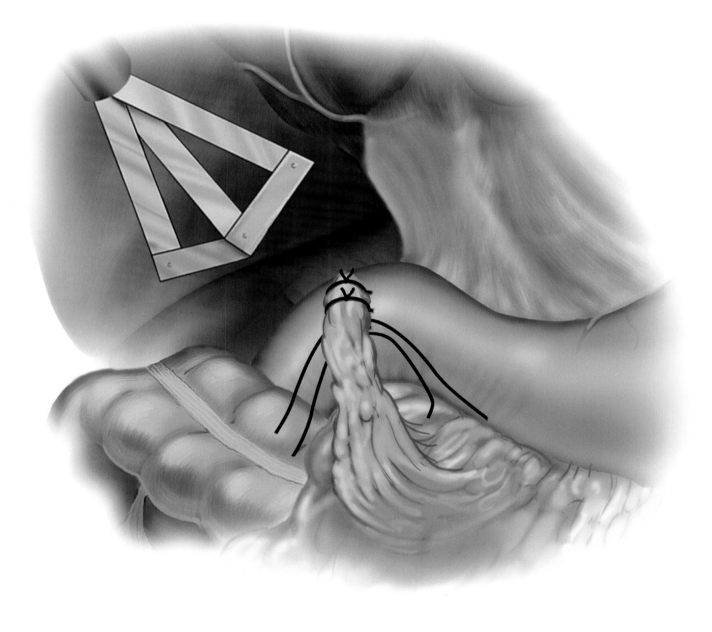

Postoperative Care

Sequential compression devices and/or subcutaneous heparin are continued postoperatively. Broad spectrum antibiotics are continued for 5 to 14 days, depending on the amount of soilage and the patient's clinical status. Gastric decompression with a nasogastric tube is usually maintained for approximately 5 days, after which an upper GI contrast study is obtained to assess for any residual leak. If no leak is present, the nasogastric tube can be removed and oral intake is initiated with clear liquids.

Suggested Reading

1. Katkhouda N, Mouiel J. Laparoscopic treatment of peptic ulcer disease. In: Hunter JG, Sackier J, eds. *Minimally Invasive Surgery*, New York: McGraw-Hill. 1993;123-130.

2. Casas AT, Gadacz TR. Laparoscopic management of peptic ulcer disease. *Surg Clin North Am*. 1996;76:515-522.

3. Jones DB, Rege RV. Operations for peptic ulcer and their complications. In: Feldman M, Friedman LS, Sleisenger MH, eds. *Sleisenger and Fordtan's Gastrointestinal and Liver Disease*. 7th ed. New York: WB Saunders. 2002;797-809.

4. Taylor TV, Lythgo JP, McFarland JB, et al. Anterior lesser curve seromyotomy and posterior truncal vagotomy versus truncal vagotomy and pyloroplasty in the treatment of chronic duodenal ulcer. *Br J Surg*. 1990;77:1007-1009.

Commentary

Steven Schwaitzberg, M.D., Cambridge Hospital
Harvard Medical School

The discovery that many patients with duodenal ulcer were actually suffering from *Helicobacter* infection has greatly reduced the need for surgery for peptic ulcer disease. That said, there are acid-hypersecreting patients who are not infected creating a need for minimally invasive approaches to this disease.

House officers of a bygone era could recite litany and verse when it came to the complications of, and recurrence rates for, the various surgical approaches to duodenal ulcer disease. I look back with great fondness discussing the vagaries of the truncal vagotomy with "B1" versus "B2" reconstructions or engaging in debates of the merits of these resective procedures as opposed to highly selective vagotomy or vagotomy and pyloroplasty. As the laparoscopic era has blossomed, old dogma has fallen in many arenas. Surgical pioneers attempting minimally invasive approaches to ulcer disease of the mid-1990's did not have the extensive experience with laparoscopic gastrojejunostomy that we do today. Thus posterior truncal vagotomy coupled with methods of transecting the branches of the anterior nerve of Latarjet emerged, avoiding the need to get involved with anastomoses or resections. The authors have nicely illustrated three methods for accomplishing this. Five-year data are emerging, validating the soundness of these approaches. Do we even need to remember the "criminal" nerve of Grassi, which we once thought was so important to avoid failed vagotomy?

For patients with a very long torso, choosing a preinsufflation length 13 cm caudad to the xiphoid will avoid the camera from being too low or too flat to the horizon to visualize the esophageal hiatus and posterior vagus nerve well. In order to well visualize the nerves of Latarjet, avoid disturbing the area along the lesser curve of the stomach as the nerves become somewhat obscured with extensive manipulation in that area.

As dogmas fall, one wonders about the need for drainage procedures. Would a pyloromyotomy do just as well? Endoscopic balloon dilatation of the pylorus has been reported in association with truncal vagotomy to avoid the need for formal drainage procedures.

Treatment of acute perforation by omental patch rather than by gastric resection/vagotomy has become more popular in this era of *Helicobacter* infection and ubiquitous nonsteroidal anti-inflammatory drugs. Often it is not practical to actually suture the perforation closed since the edges tend to be friable. (In fact, some surgeons are taught not to close the hole since doing so may lead to stenosis). Fortunately, a well-secured omental patch over the hole as illustrated combined with nasogastric decompression will allow for adequate healing of the perforation. In more seriously ill patients, cultures ascertaining the presence of *Candida* contamination should be considered. In addition, a laparoscopic feeding jejunostomy can be performed at the time of omental patch creation if needed.

The modern foregut surgeon should definitely have these techniques available to him/her for the surgical treatment of peptic diseases. Complex cases of esophageal reflux and peptic ulcer disease can be treated by combined procedures aimed at treating both problems.

Robert V. Rege, M.D.
University of Texas Southwestern Medical Center

The instrumentation and techniques available today allow the surgeon to accomplish laparoscopically any of the operations for peptic ulcer disease formerly performed by open techniques—from simple closure of perforations to gastric resection. However, the need for elective operative treatment of peptic ulcer disease has become vanishing small. The introduction of effective medications to control acid secretion, first H2-receptor antagonist and later proton pump inhibitors, and the recognition of *H pylori* as a contributing factor in ulcer disease, has lead to effective nonoperative therapy in the large majority of patients. Today, surgical therapy is largely limited to treatment of the complications of ulcers, such as perforation, hemorrhage, or obstruction. Patients often present with a complication as their first sign of ulcer disease. Patients are more likely to be older and to have ulcers related to nonsteroidal anti-inflammatory drug usage. Since control of gastrointestinal bleeding with the laparoscope is difficult, laparoscopic management of peptic ulcer disease is largely delegated to treatment of perforation or obstruction.

The techniques presented here, therefore, must be largely taken in the context of an emergency situation. A laparoscopic approach to perforated duodenal ulcer is technically possible; experienced laparoscopic surgeons today certainly have the knowledge and skills to expose, suture, and reinforce a perforated duodenal ulcer. Likewise, performance of a pyloroplasty and vagotomy or highly selective vagotomy can easily be accomplished. Dr. Jones et al illustrate techniques for the performance of vagotomy suturing or patching of perforated ulcers.

The key to outcome then is not the technique, but rather judgment about when a minimally invasive approach should and should not be undertaken. The principles are similar to those used during open operations for perforation. Closure of early perforations (within 6-12 hours) and vagotomy can easily be accomplished, but late perforations with marked inflammation and friability of tissues are best dealt with expeditiously by Graham patching of the ulcer. In fact, there is a growing consensus that vagotomy is rarely, if ever, needed, since medical control of acid secretion and ulcers associated with *H pylori* is so effective.

The small number of patients requiring operative therapy for peptic ulcer disease make it unlikely that series of patients will ever be assembled to determine the efficacy of laparoscopic versus open approaches to peptic ulcer disease. However, experience to date indicates that laparoscopic surgery for peptic ulcer disease can be performed effectively and safely, and patients usually benefit from the minimally invasive approach.

Robert Bailey, M.D., Miami Laparoscopic Center
University of Miami

The authors and editors are to be commended for an excellent presentation of a very complex and, unfortunately, less commonly encountered surgical disease. Although the decline in the incidence of peptic ulcer disease appears to have begun prior to the introduction of H2-blockers and proton pump inhibitors, the subsequent recognition of the role of *H pylori* in peptic ulcer disease has dramatically reduced the prevalence of this disease. Nonetheless, the practicing general and laparoscopic surgeon should be familiar with the current surgical options for the management of peptic ulcer disease and its complications.

The artwork provided in this chapter is exquisite and provides an intricate and easily comprehended anatomic description of the pertinent surgical maneuvers. The organization and presentation of the topic is simple, straightforward and very educational. As is true with most surgical conditions, there may be different conceptual approaches and procedural variations that are adopted by different surgeons. Some of these differences are explained below.

The preoperative evaluation should include, of course, a recent endoscopic evaluation of the upper GI tract. Gastric analysis, once an important diagnostic tool, is now mostly of historical importance only. The availability and clinical indication for this test has declined in proportion with the overall incidence of peptic ulcer disease. It should also be mentioned that the preoperative evaluation will vary greatly depending on whether the presentation is that of chronic peptic ulcer disease or as an acute emergency, such as with a perforated or bleeding ulcer. The choice of operation, especially for acute perforation or bleeding, should be determined according to well-established criteria that include consideration of the duration of illness (acute versus chronic peptic ulcer disease), the stability of the patient, his or her age, and the duration and severity of perforation and its associated contamination. Additional perioperative measures should also include the routine use of proton pump inhibitors during the surgical procedure and for up to 1 week afterwards.

Similar to the authors, we prefer a modified lithotomy position but we have increasingly utilized a supine approach. As with gastric bypass procedures, access to the stomach can be easily accomplished without the trouble of placing the patient in a lithotomy position. The surgeon may utilize this approach according to patient habitus and personal preference. Variations in trocar location are readily accommodated according to surgeon preference and experience. Intraoperatively, once the stomach is decompressed, we typically remove the nasogastric tube as it tends to hinder and limit retraction of the stomach during the operative procedure.

The authors provide a very thorough description of the surgical options to achieve an acid-reducing outcome. Although we initially subscribed to one or more of these so-called "combined anterior/posterior" procedures, our current procedure of choice is a standard highly selective vagotomy. We cannot overemphasize the degree of diligence and perseverance that is required when performing this operation. Surgeons who have pre-existing experience with an open approach are quite familiar with the meticulous dissection and patience that is required to complete an effective acid-reducing operation. We would humbly suggest that some of the initial laparoscopic variations/modifications to a standard highly selective vagotomy were adopted due to a lack of adequate instrumentation and laparoscopic experience with the technique. These concerns, combined with the relatively rare presentation of patients with peptic ulcer disease, lead surgeons to consider alternatives that might shorten the operative time by minimizing operative dissection. As the instruments have improved and as our laparoscopic experience has grown, we have abandoned these alternative approaches in favor of a more traditional approach.

If the surgeon does decide to perform a more traditional highly selective vagotomy, he or she may consider an alternative starting point to the operative dissection. Instead of exposing the esophageal hiatus as the first step, the surgeon may commence the dissection just above the crow's foot. This location, as mentioned in the text, is typically 5 cm to 7 cm proximal to the pylorus. Identification of this area may be assisted by identifying the first one or two vascular pedicles going to the antrum. Dissection may be safely begun at or just above the second major pedicle. In addition, anatomic inspection of the contour of the stomach should aid the surgeon in this process. It is also recommended to actually measure the distance from the pylorus using the open end of a grasper as a "measuring tape." All laparoscopic graspers open to an exact width that can be measured extracorporeally and then used to estimate distance intracorporeally.

During the operative dissection, the surgeon should be aware of certain "dissection" pitfalls. First, the presence of wandering branches of the vagus nerve, such as the criminal nerve of Grassi, should be appreciated and actively sought for during the operative dissection. Such branches may arise from the main vagal trunks at locations somewhat remote (2-3 cm) from the actual area of dissection. The surgeon should also be aware that the branches arising from the main vagal trunks along the lesser curvature do so at varying levels in an "anterior-posterior" direction. That is to say, there is not a single anterior or posterior leaflet that contains all of the small vagal branches. Rather, there are multiple branches that enter the lesser curvature across the entire anterior-to-posterior aspect of the lesser curvature. Therefore, it is important that the entire anterior-to-posterior aspect of the lesser curvature be cleared of all neurovascular branches during the operative dissection. This typically requires sequential rotation and mobilization of the medial aspect of the stomach wall during the operative dissection. Atraumatic Babcock forceps are best suited to provide the necessary retraction during this portion of the procedure.

Although the surgeon should be aware of the various "combined" procedures available, these options are not being utilized or reported in the literature with substantial frequency. Options such as anterior seromyotomy (stapled or otherwise), by definition, are associated with the additional risks of gastric leakage, staple-line dehiscence, vagal trunk injury, and incomplete vagotomy. As mentioned, we now advocate a traditional highly selective vagotomy as the procedure of choice.

Postoperatively, the patients typically recover quite rapidly and are usually discharged home within 24 hours. As such, we now routinely remove the nasogastric tube intraoperatively, unless there is evidence of persistent gastric distension or other concerns over gastric viability as a result of the operative procedure. Postoperative gastric distension has not been an issue in our patients.

In summary, even though peptic ulcer disease has begun a less commonly encountered surgical disease, a minimally invasive approach remains a viable and highly recommended approach to this condition. A general familiarity with the surgical options and techniques is recommended.

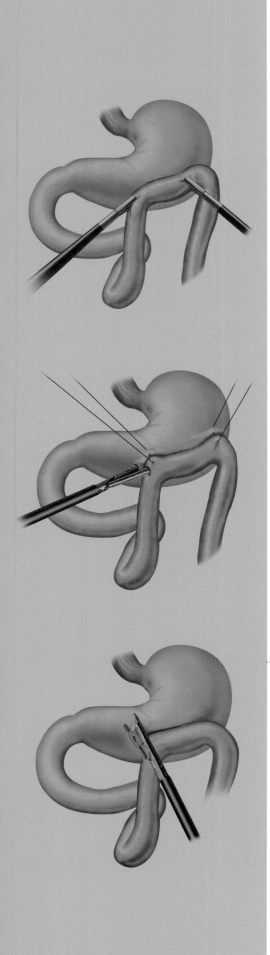

Laparoscopic Gastrojejunostomy

Periampullary tumors are often unresectable at the time of diagnosis due to local invasion and/or metastatic spread. An enteric bypass procedure with a gastrojejunostomy may be required to relieve duodenal obstruction. If a concurrent biliary bypass procedure is being performed, a 40 cm Roux limb fashioned distal to the loop gastrojejunostomy should be utilized for the biliary bypass. Each procedure can be performed with either a Roux-en-Y jejunal limb or a jejunal loop reconstruction.

Preoperative Preparation

1. Sequential compression stockings and subcutaneous heparin may be used for prophylaxis against deep venous thrombosis. Intravenous antibiotics, usually a first-generation cephalosporin, are administered prophylactically. After induction of general anesthesia, the bladder is emptied with a urinary catheter and the stomach is decompressed with a nasogastric tube.

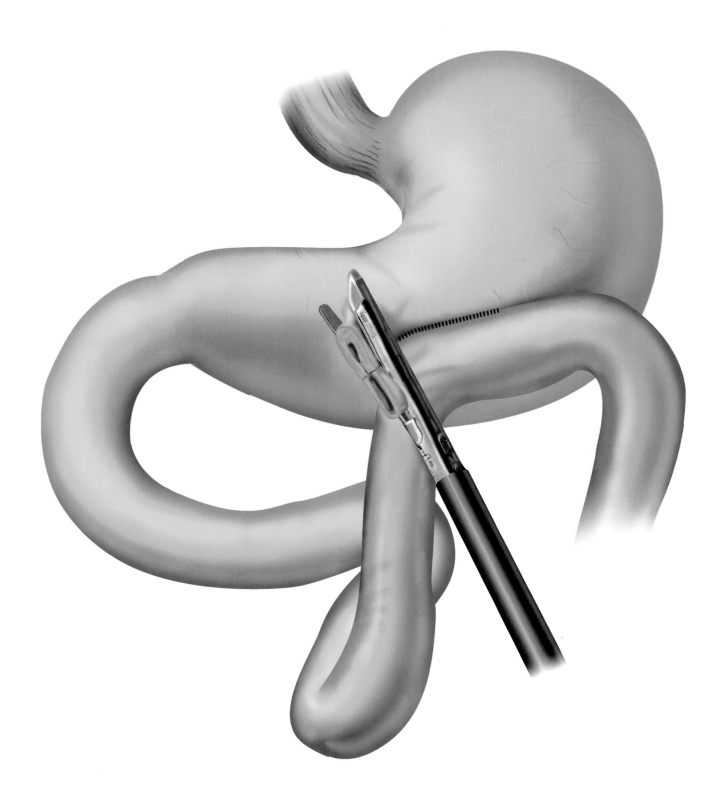

Operating Room Setup

2. The patient is placed in the supine position. All pressure points must be adequately padded.

3. The surgeon stands to the patient's right, while the assistant stands to the left.

4. A video monitor is stationed at each side of the patient's head to provide adequate viewing from both sides of the table.

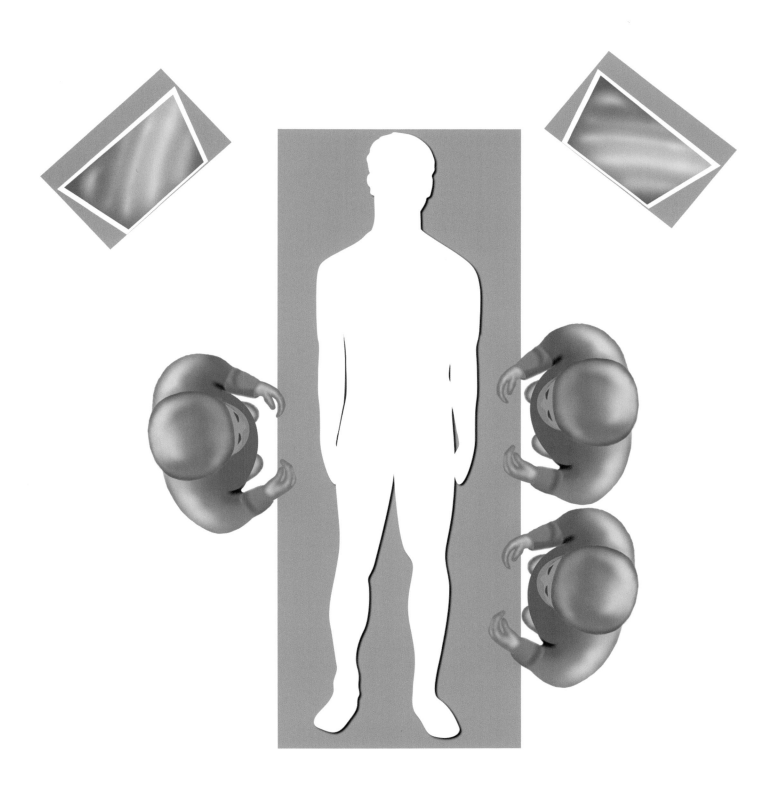

Access and Port Placement

5. The same port placement utilized for performing a cholecystojejunostomy biliary bypass can be used to perform a gastrojejunostomy as well.

6. An infraumbilical incision is used to establish pneumoperitoneum, setting a pressure limit of 15 mm Hg. This is established either with an open or closed technique. A 10/11 mm port is placed here and the laparoscope is inserted. A 30° angled scope facilitates visualization during the operation. A careful exploration is performed to ensure that no injury occurred during port insertion and that no other abnormalities are present.

7. A 5 mm trocar is placed under direct vision below the right costal margin in the anterior axillary line. A second 5 mm port is placed in the left midclavicular line below the costal margin. Finally, a 12 mm port is placed above the right iliac crest.

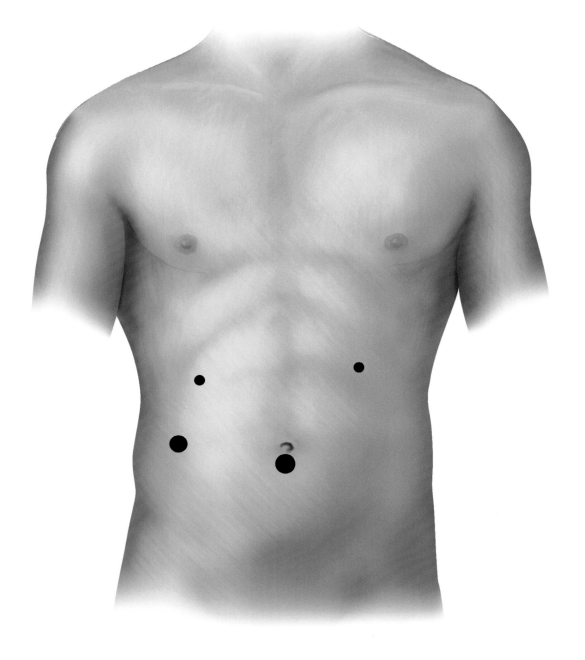

FIGURE C

Approximating the Stomach and Jejunum

8. Atraumatic graspers are used to approximate a loop of jejunum located 40 cm distal to the ligament of Treitz to the anterior (shown) or posterior aspect of the stomach in either an ante- or retrocolic fashion.

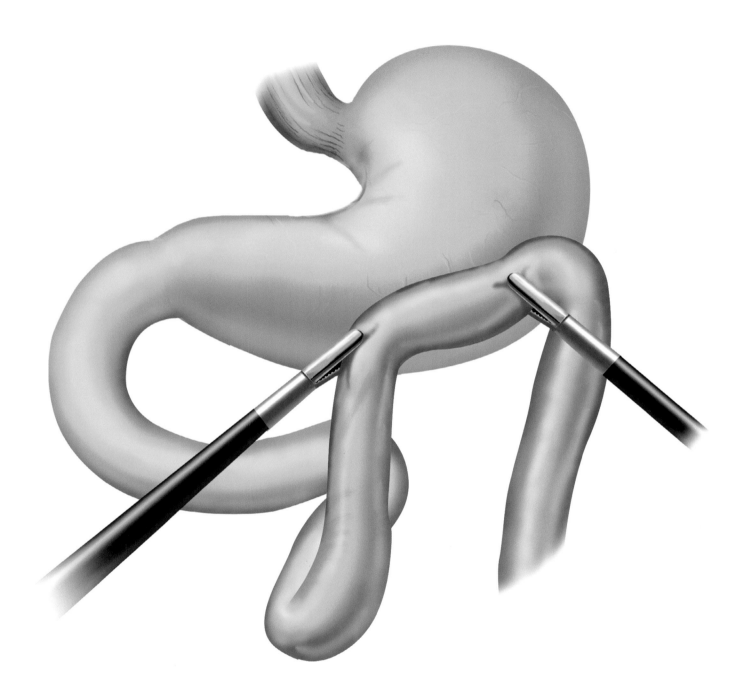

Approximating the Stomach and Jejunum, Part II

9. The loop of jejunum and stomach are anchored together using a
    3-0 silk suture and an extracorporeal technique. The suture is
    placed on slight traction, thus promoting apposition of the
    jejunum to the gastric wall. Alternatively, two stay sutures can be
    placed at either end of the intended anastomotic site.

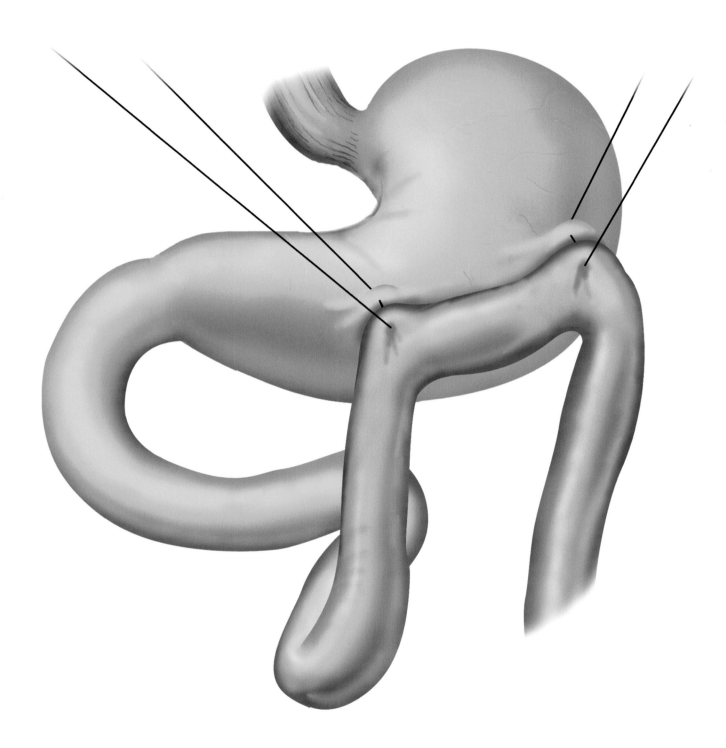

Creating a Stapled Gastrojejunostomy

10. A 1 cm long gastrotomy and enterotomy are created using electrocautery scissors. The enterotomy is created on the antimesenteric side of the jejunum. Hemostasis is obtained with electrocautery.

11. An endoscopic linear stapler (3.5 mm staples) is introduced in line with the long axis of the stomach and loop of jejunum. One jaw of the device is inserted into each of the openings. The stapling device is closed and fired to form the anterior and posterior walls of the stapled anastomosis.

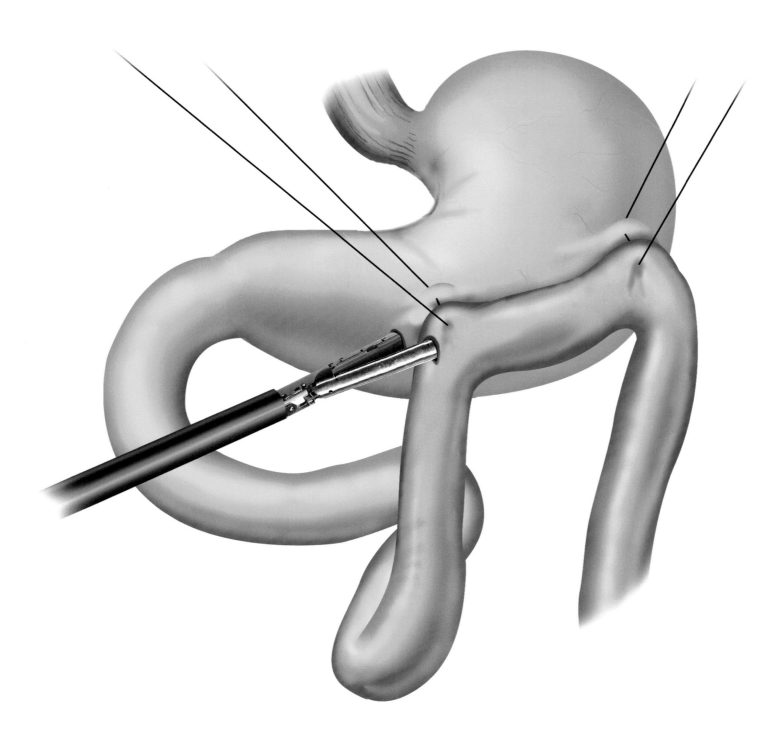

Closing the Enterotomy and Completing the Anastomosis

12. The remaining enterotomy is closed with a second firing of the stapler in a transverse orientation, so as not to narrow the anastomosis.

13. Alternatively, the entire anastomosis can be constructed using a hand-sewn technique as previously described.

14. The operative field is again inspected for hemostasis and the ports are removed under laparoscopic visualization to ensure hemostasis at each of the port sites as well. Each incision is infiltrated with a solution of 0.5% bupivacaine and irrigated with saline solution. The fascia of each incision greater than 10 mm is closed with an absorbable suture. The skin incision at each port site is closed with a subcuticular absorbable suture.

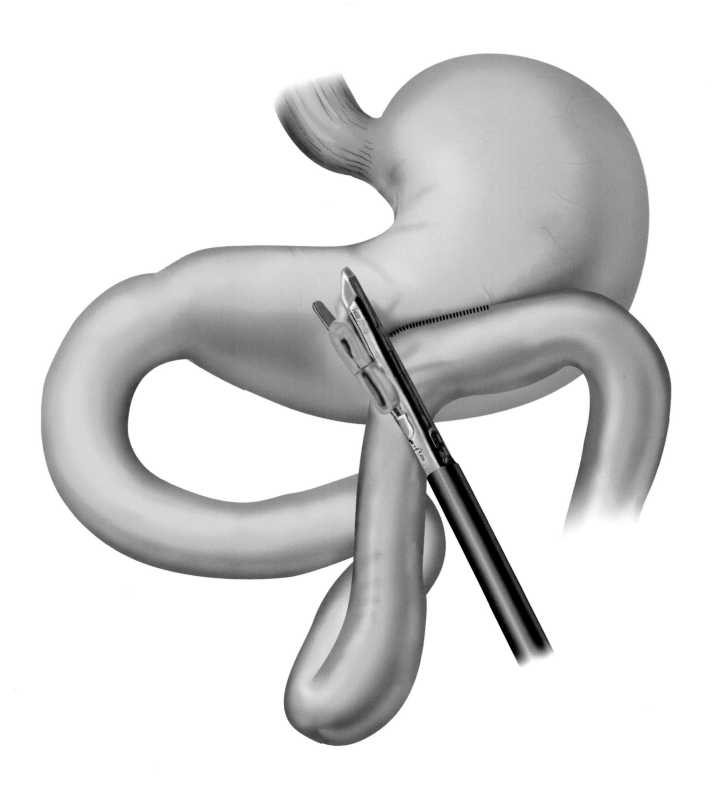

Postoperative Care

Pneumatic compression devices and/or subcutaneous heparin are continued postoperatively. Antibiotics are usually continued for 24 hours after the operation at the discretion of the surgeon. The nasogastric tube is removed after return of bowel function. Oral intake is initiated with clear liquids and advanced as tolerated. Patients are usually discharged within 3 to 4 days after the operation.

Suggested Readings

1. Chekan EG, Clark L, Wu J, Pappas TN, Eubanks S. Laparoscopic biliary and enteric bypass. *Semin Surg Oncol.* 1999;16:313-320.

2. Mittal A, Windsor J, Woodfield J, Casey P, Lane M. Matched study of three methods for palliation of malignant pyloroduodenal obstruction. *Br J Surg.* 2004;91:2005-2009.

3. O'Rourke N, Nathanson L. Laparoscopic biliary-enteric bypass. In: Paterson-Brown S, Garden J, eds. *Principles and Practice of Surgical Laparoscopy.* London: WB Saunders. 1994:179-189.

Commentary

Michael A. Edwards, M.D., Beth Israel Deaconess Medical Center
Harvard Medical School

Advanced gastric, duodenal, periampullary and pancreatic cancers are not uncommon causes of gastric outlet obstruction (GOO). GOO occurs in 15% to 20% and 10% to 20% of patients with unresectable pancreatic and periampullary cancers, respectively. The goal of management is the early reintroduction of enteral feeding and early hospital discharge. GOO is still managed most effectively by palliative surgical gastrojejunostomy (GJ), traditionally performed via an open technique. Open gastrojejunostomy carries a low perioperative mortality, but a significant risk of morbidity. Postoperative complications occur in 25% to 37% of patients. Common complications include wound infection (10%) and delayed gastric emptying (8-30%). Hospital length of stay (LOS) is often prolonged (10-15 days).

The risks inherent in operating on these patients, who are by definition in a poor state of health with expected poor long-term survival, have encouraged much interest in minimal access surgery. Alternatives to open palliative GJ include endoscopic/fluoroscopic endoluminal self-expanding metallic stents and laparoscopic gastrojejunostomy.

Palliative endoscopic treatment of malignant gastric outlet obstruction with endoluminal self-expanding metallic stents is a well-established procedure. It is successful in over 95% of patients and relieves symptoms in greater than 90% of cases. Minor complications occur in 11% of patients, compared to up to 37% in open gastrojejunostomy. Hospital LOS and return to oral intake is reported to be 3 days and 2 days, respectively. Delayed gastric emptying (DGE) occurs in 11%. Compared to surgical GJ, endoscopic stenting is cheaper and more effective with respect to operative time, restoration of oral intake and median hospitalization. Complications of endoluminal stents remain a significant drawback. These include bleeding and perforation (1.2%), stent migration (5%), and obstruction due to tumor infiltration (18%).

Laparoscopic palliative gastrojejunostomy (LGJ) is a feasible, safe, and effective technique for GOO, with associated low mortality, and morbidity and greater long-term patency. The antecolic, isoperistaltic technique is most commonly performed and is described in this atlas. There is no significant difference in mortality compared to other techniques. DGE occurs in 6% of patients. Compared to open GJ, LGJ is associated with a lower morbidity (DGE, wound infections), shorter hospital LOS, earlier return to diet and earlier return to daily activitiees. There is no significant difference in mortality and morbidity between LGJ and endoluminal stents (ES). ES is associated with earlier return to diet and shorter LOS. ES is associated with a significantly higher recurrence of GOO due to stent obstruction by infiltrated tumor.

Palliative gastrojejunostomy remains the standard of care for malignant gastric outlet obstruction. The laparoscopic approach can achieve excellent results. The advantages of LGJ include lower morbidity, earlier recovery, return to diet and hospital discharge, with improvement in quality of life. Endoscopically placed metal stents offer an effective alternative to surgical palliation in patients with unresectable malignant strictures, and laparoscopic gastrojejunostomy is contraindicated.

Michael D. Holzman, M.D., M.P.H.
Vanderbilt University Hospital

For patients with a functional gastrointestinal tract, enteral feedings provide the most effective and safest method for nutritional support. If a patient is unable to eat due to illness, placement of enteral access may be necessary. In considering placement of feeding tubes, one needs to consider the condition for which enteral access is necessary and options which might be available. For many patients, endoscopic placement can provide a safe and effective access to the gastrointestinal tract. However, there are situations (patients who have had gastric resections or restrictive procedures) in which endoscopic access is not amenable.

The steps provided in this section on minimally invasive surgery for the placement of gastrostomy (temporary and permanent) and jejunostomy feeding tubes provides a simple and succinct overview of the procedure.

These procedures are particularly useful as an adjunct to other minimally invasive surgical procedures (esophagectomy, gastrectomy, or staging laparoscopy).

Though technically easily, the minor details of these procedures, as outlined in this atlas, are important for their success. For both the gastrostomy and jejunostomy tubes, the bowel needs to be secured to the abdominal wall in order to minimize potential for leaks. However, pulling the organs to the abdominal wall with too much tension can lead to ischemic ulcerations and erosions. I have elected to place the nylon suture from the T-fasteners through the skin disk and tie them together. This eliminates having extra suturing for the skin disk as well and the sometimes bulky cotton pledgets and crimps. With the jejunostomy tube, I attempt to have a short submucosal tract when placing the initial 18-gauge needle. This will provide more of a Witzel-type procedure.

When added to other laparoscopic procedures, minimally invasive gastrostomy and jejunostomy tubes can be performed quickly and safely and provide an excellent route for enteral nutrition.

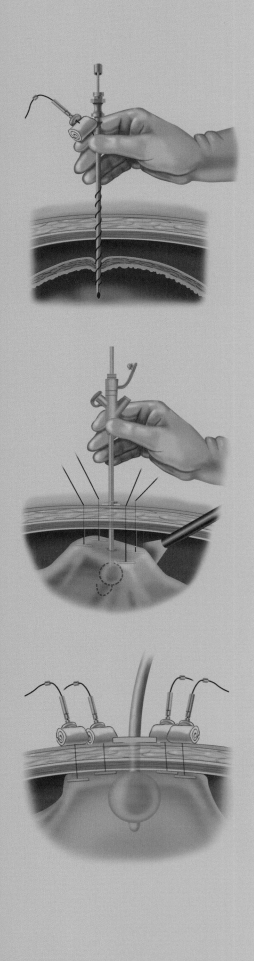

Laparoscopic Gastrostomy (T-Fasteners Technique)

Enteral feeding is the preferred method of delivering nutrition to patients. For those patients unable to feed themselves, gastrostomy and jejunostomy tubes provide an alternate route. When possible, a gastrostomy, rather than a jejunostomy, tube is the preferred route for providing long-term enteral nutrition. Gastrostomy allows for bolus tube feeding and may be associated with fewer complications than jejunostomy.

Preoperative Preparation

1. Sequential compression stockings and subcutaneous heparin may be used for prophylaxis against deep venous thrombosis. Intravenous antibiotics are administered prophylactically. After induction of general anesthesia, the bladder is emptied with a urinary catheter and the stomach is decompressed with a nasogastric tube.

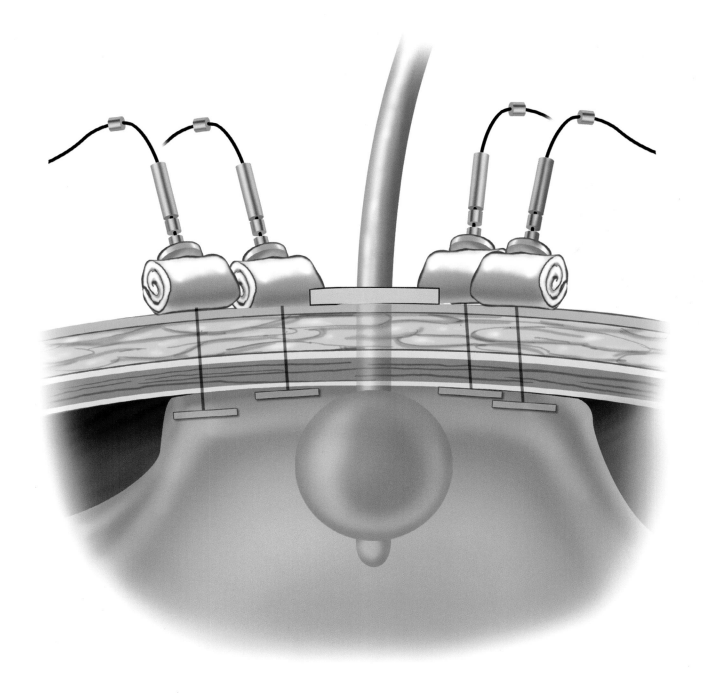

Operating Room Setup

2. The patient is placed in the supine position.

3. The surgeon stands to the patient's left, while the assistant stands to the right.

4. A video monitor is stationed at both sides of the table.

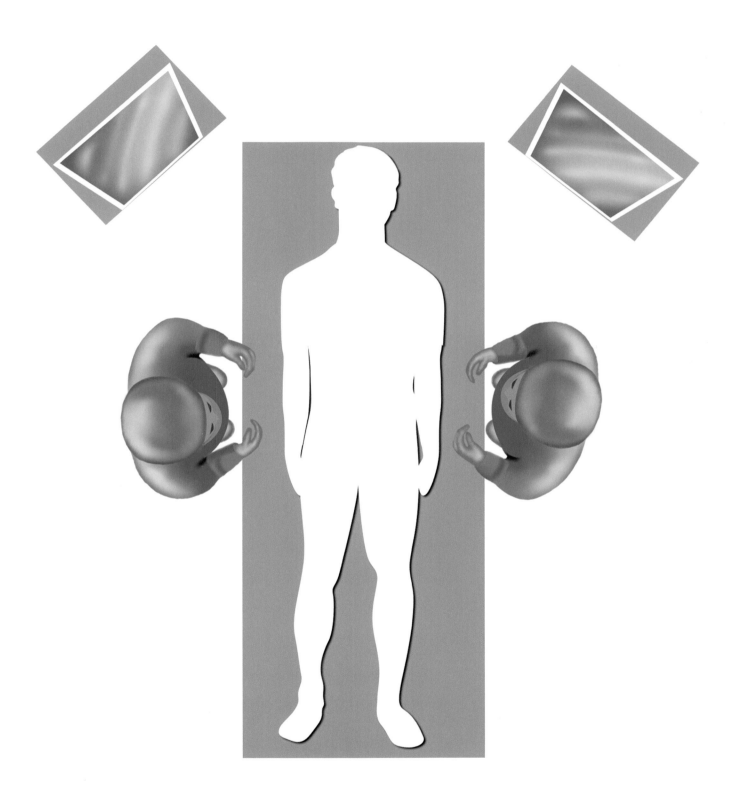

Access and Port Placement

5. A supraumbilical or infraumbilical incision can be used to establish pneumoperitoneum with either an open or closed technique. A 10/11 mm port is placed and a 30° angled laparoscope is inserted. A careful exploration is performed to ensure that no injury occurred during port insertion and that no other abnormalities are present.

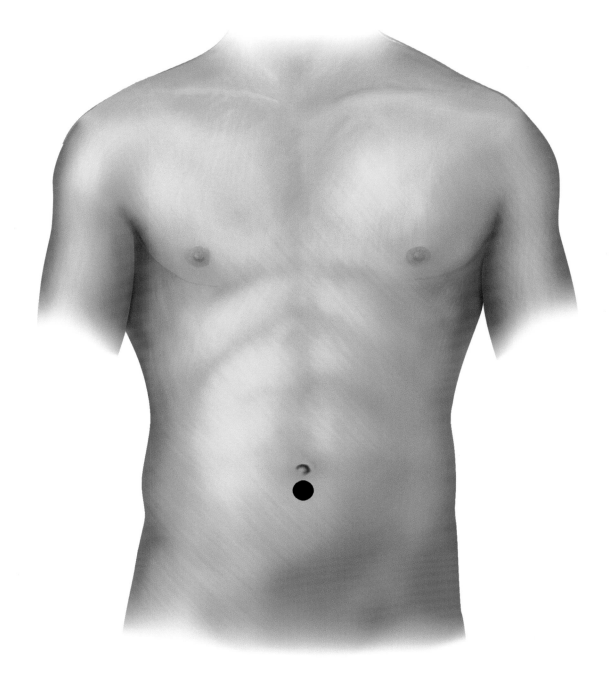

FIGURE C

The T-Fastener Apparatus

6. The Flexiflo Lap G Kit (Ross Product Division, Abbott Laboratories, Columbus, Ohio), which includes a Brown/Mueller T-Fastener Set, is utilized for this technique. As depicted in Figure C, the T-fastener consists of a one centimeter stainless steel T-shaped piece attached to a nylon suture. The mechanism by which to secure the T-fastener to the skin consists of a cotton pledget, nylon washer, two aluminum crimps, a 4 Fr sleeve, followed by a final aluminum crimp. The T-piece is loaded inside an 18 gauge needle, through which it will be inserted into the peritoneal cavity and gastric lumen.

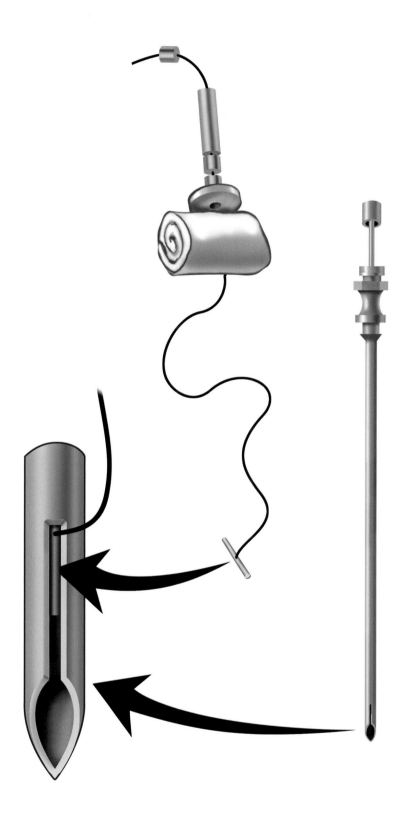

Preparing for T-Fastener Insertion

7. The stomach is insufflated through the nasogastric tube. Using digital palpation and laparoscopic viewing, the site for gastrostomy tube placement is selected. The tract should ideally traverse the rectus muscle and should be at least a few centimeters caudal to the costal margin. The site for gastrostomy tube placement in the stomach should be along the greater curvature.

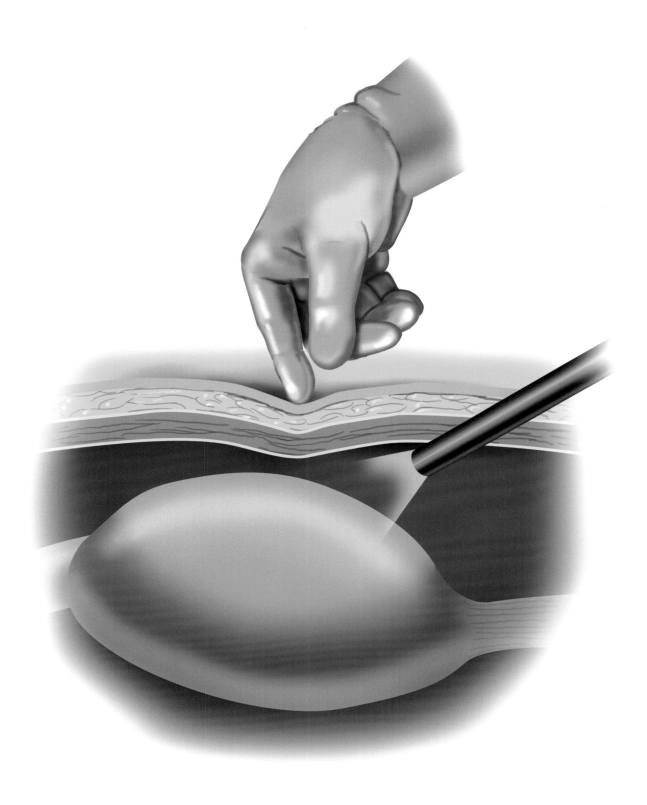

Inserting the T-Fasteners

8. After pneumoperitoneal pressure is decreased from 15mm Hg to 7 mm Hg, the T-fastener, loaded on the 18 gauge needle, is inserted into the peritoneal cavity and gastric lumen under laparoscopic guidance at the previously selected site (Figure E-a). An atraumatic grasper placed through a 5 mm port in the right upper quadrant or left lower quadrant can facilitate puncture of the anterior gastric wall.

9. Once the T-piece is inside the gastric lumen, it is dislodged from the needle using a stylet (Figure E-b). Gentle upward traction is applied on the T-fastener to mobilize the anterior gastric wall to the abominal wall (Figure E-c).

10. Three more T-fasteners should be similarly inserted approximately 2 cm away from each other, forming a diamond or square pattern. To facilitate viewing, the first T-fastener should be inserted furthest from the laparoscope, with each subsequent insertion moving closer to the camera. Once all four T-fasteners are in place, they are placed on anterior traction to hold the gastric wall close to the abdominal wall.

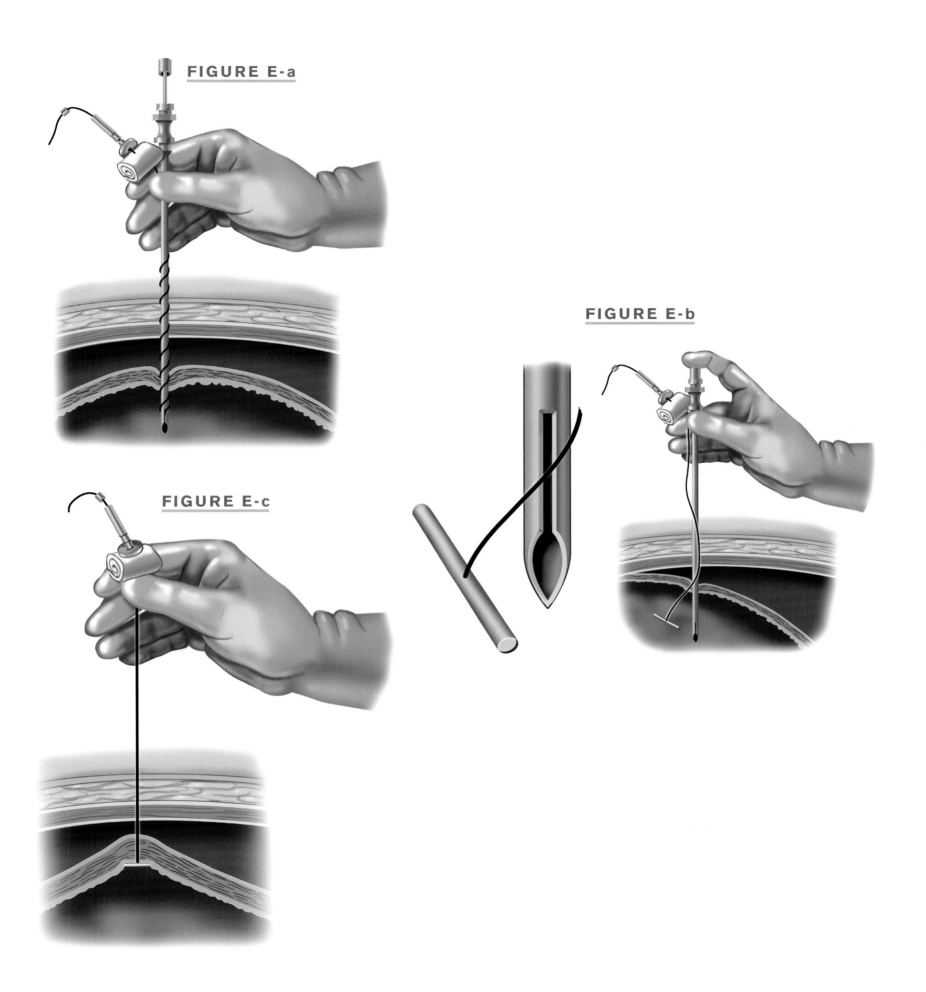

FIGURE E-a

FIGURE E-b

FIGURE E-c

Placing the Gastrostomy Tube

11. An 18 gauge needle is percutaneously inserted into the gastric lumen through the middle of the square created by the four T-fasteners. A J guide wire is threaded through the needle and the needle is withdrawn (Figure F). Proper placement of the needle and guide wire is confirmed with direct laparoscopic visualization.

12. A 5 mm skin incision is made at the guide wire insertion site and is extended down to the level of the fascia. This tract is serially dilated with lubricated dilators over the guide wire ranging from 12 Fr to 20 Fr. An 18 Fr balloon-tipped gastrostomy tube is placed over a stylet and inserted into the gastric lumen over the J guide wire. The balloon is inflated with sterile water (Figure G). Placement is confirmed with direct laparoscopic visualization by loosening traction on the T-fasteners and allowing the stomach to slightly fall away from the abdominal wall. Alternatively, contrast injected through the gastrostomy tube under fluoroscopy will also help to confirm proper placement.

FIGURE F

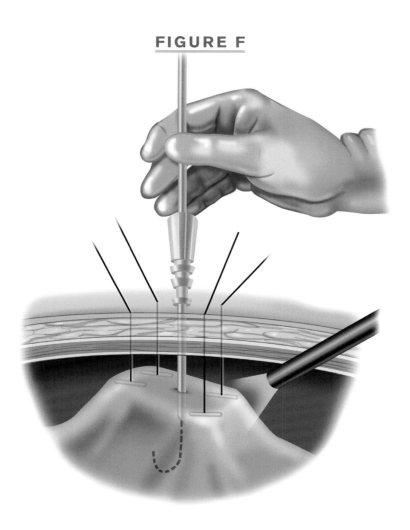

FIGURE G

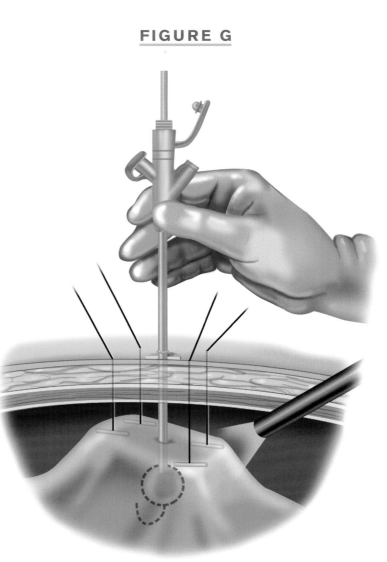

Securing the Gastrostomy Tube

13. The stylet and J guide wire are removed. All four T-fasteners are retightened by sliding the aluminum crimps and nylon washer down on the cotton pledget (Figure H-a). This maneuver secures the anterior surface of the stomach to the abdominal wall, thus creating a water-tight seal. The gastrostomy tube is further secured by suturing an external skin disk to the skin (Figure H-b).

14. The peritoneal cavity is examined for hemostasis and any evidence for leakage around the gastrostomy insertion site. After the laparoscope is removed, the umbilical fascia and skin incisions are closed in the usual manner. The T-fastener sutures may be cut after 2 weeks, allowing the T-pieces to pass in the stool.

FIGURE H-a

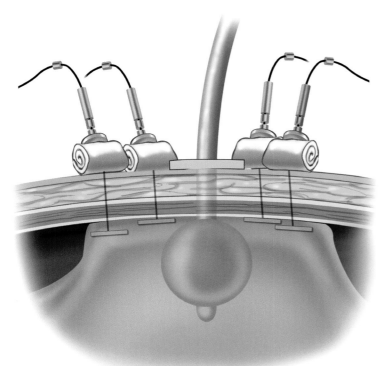

FIGURE H-b

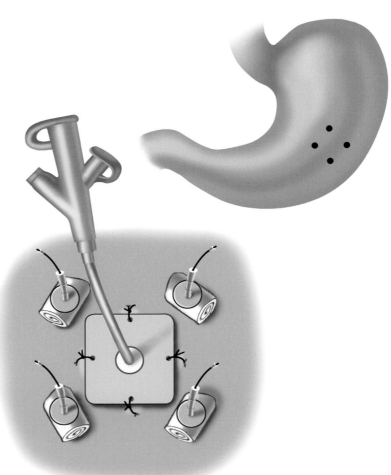

Postoperative Care

Pneumatic compression devices and/or subcutaneous heparin are continued postoperatively. Antibiotics are usually continued for 24 hours after the operation at the discretion of the surgeon. Tube feeds are usually started the morning after surgery, although the catheter can be used immediately for feeding. The feeding tube should be regularly irrigated with 30 mL to 50 mL of saline to maintain its patency.

Suggested Readings

1. Brown AS, Mueller PR, Ferruci JT Jr. Controlled percutaneous gastrostomy: nylon T-fastener for fixation of the anterior gastric wall. *Radiology*. 1986;158:543-545.

2. Duh QY, Senokozlieff AL, Choe YS, Siperstein AE, Rowland K, Way LW. Laparoscopic gastrostomy and jejunostomy. *Arch Surg*. 1999;134:151-156.

3. Wu J, Soper NJ, Gastrostomy and jejunostomy. In: Jones DB, Wu J, Soper NJ, eds. *Laparoscopic Surgery: Principles and Practice*. New York: Marcel Dekker. 2004;219-241.

Commentary

Steven Schwaitzberg, M.D., Cambridge Hospital
Harvard Medical School

Laparoscopic gastrostomy is a valuable method of creating enteral access, particularly when conventional percutaneous techniques are not feasible such as in near obstructing esophageal malignancy. The lack of a substantial incision needed to access the abdomen is a potential advantage of this technique that avoids potential wound-healing problems (especially dehiscence) in a generally debilitated population. The T-fastener technique is simple, quick, and requires minimal instrumentation. In carefully selected patients, we have performed this technique in the intensive care unit.

Reducing the pneumoperitoneum is a subtle but important trick that the authors have pointed out that facilitates apposition of the stomach to the abdominal wall. Insufflation of the stomach with air (not oxygen) via the nasogastric tube can facilitate T-fastener placement by creating a lumen. If the esophagus is obstructed preventing nasogastric tube placement, a long needle may be placed through the abdominal wall and into the stomach and then connected to the insufflator tubing. This will gently inflate the stomach and allow for safe placement of T-fasteners.

When securing the gastrostomy to the abdominal wall, it is important to avoid excessive traction on the balloon, which could potentially cause gastric necrosis and subsequent leakage. Surgeons who routinely provide enteral access should have this technique in their armamentarium.

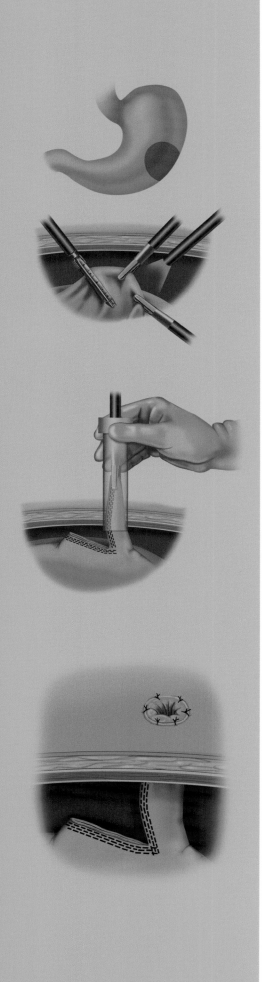

Laparoscopic Janeway Permanent Gastrostomy

A permanent gastrostomy can also be constructed for those patients with no prospect of being able to feed themselves.

Preoperative Preparation

1. Sequential compression stockings and subcutaneous heparin may be used for prophylaxis against deep venous thrombosis. Intravenous antibiotics are administered prophylactically. After induction of general anesthesia, the bladder is emptied with a urinary catheter and the stomach is decompressed with a nasogastric tube.

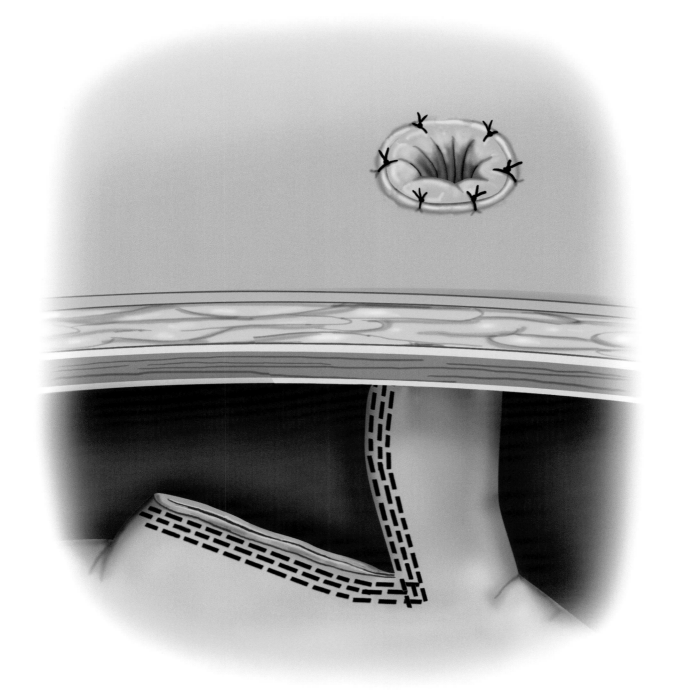

FIGURE A

Operating Room Setup

2. The patient is placed in the supine position.

3. The surgeon stands to the patient's left, while the assistant stands to the right.

4. A video monitor is stationed at both sides of the table.

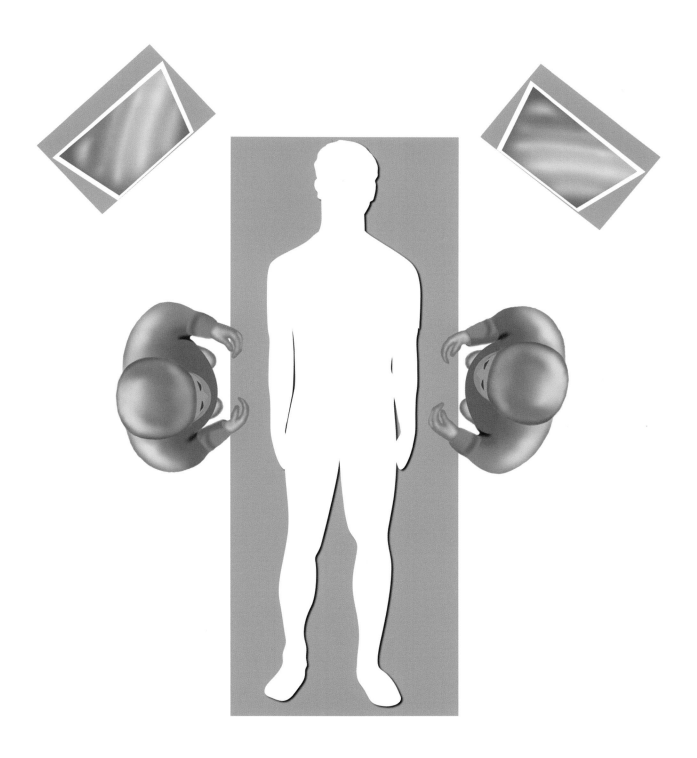

Access and Port Placement

5. An infraumbilical incision is used to establish pneumoperitoneum with either an open or closed technique. A 10/11 mm port is placed and a 30° angled laparoscope is inserted. A careful exploration is performed to ensure that no injury occurred during port insertion and that no other abnormalities are present.

6. Two 5 mm ports are placed under direct vision in the right and left midclavicular lines above the level of the umbilicus.

7. Atraumatic graspers are used to identify a section of stomach along the greater curvature that can be mobilized to the abdominal wall without any tension. A corresponding area on the skin is marked for gastrostomy insertion site. A 12 mm port is inserted under direct visualization at this site.

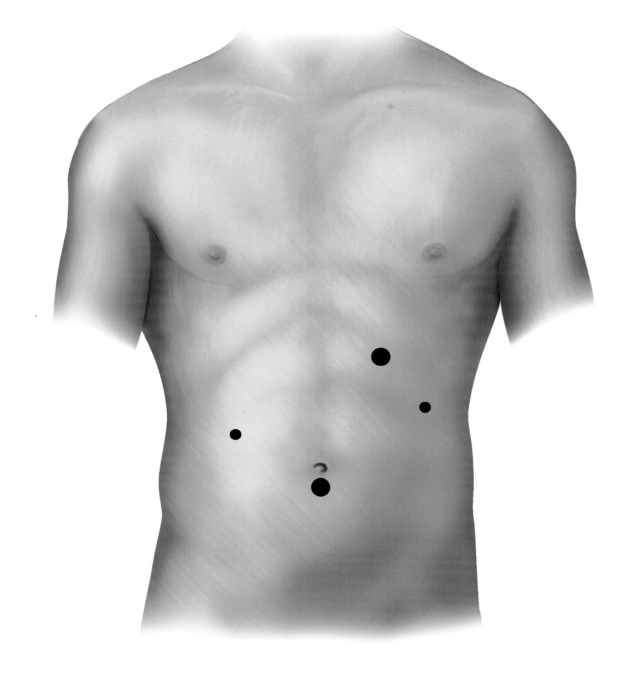

FIGURE C-a,b

Creating a Gastric Diverticulum

8. Using two graspers to lift and expose a section of stomach, an endoscopic linear stapler (loaded with 4.5 mm-4.8 mm staples) is inserted through the 12 mm port and is fired to create a 3 cm wide gastric diverticulum (Figure C-a).

9. The length of the diverticulum is adjusted to facilitate a tension-free gastrostomy (Figure C-b).

FIGURE C-a

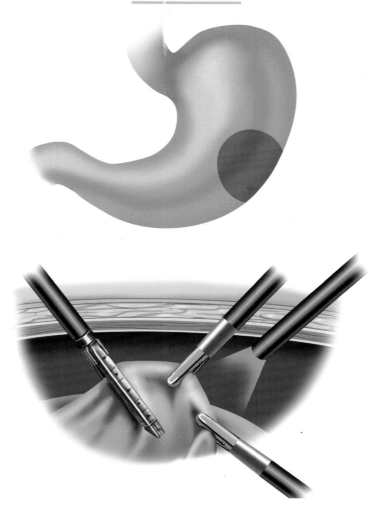

FIGURE C-b

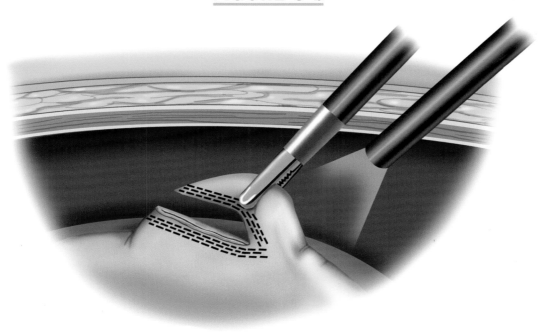

Delivering the Gastric Diverticulum

10. A grasper is inserted through the 12 mm port and the diverticulum is retrieved into the port. The grasper, port, and diverticulum are extracted as one unit, thus delivering the gastric diverticulum to the level of the skin.

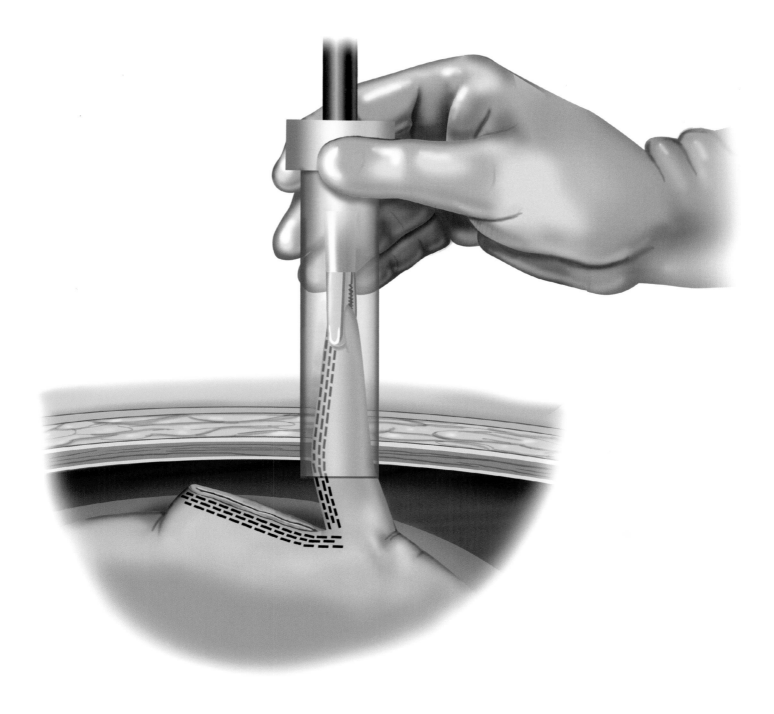

FIGURE E

Maturing the Gastrostomy

11. The gastric diverticulum is opened using electrocautery and is circumferentially sutured to the skin using 3-0 absorbable sutures.

12. A 24 Fr gastrostomy tube is inserted through the diverticulum into the gastric lumen and the bulb is inflated. The gastrostomy tube is pulled up until the bulb is snug against the abdominal wall. Proper placement is confirmed by laparoscopic visualization or with a fluoroscopic contrast injection study.

13. The peritoneal cavity is examined for hemostasis and any evidence for leakage around the gastrostomy insertion site. After the laparoscope is removed, the umbilical fascia and skin incisions are closed in the usual manner.

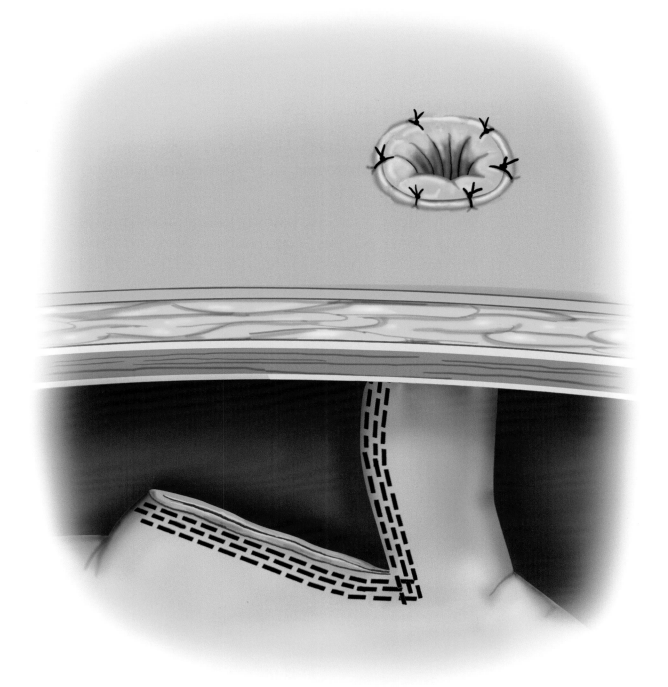

Postoperative Care

Pneumatic compression devices and/or subcutaneous heparin are continued postoperatively. Antibiotics are usually continued for 24 hours after the operation at the discretion of the surgeon. Tube feeds are usually started the morning after surgery, although the catheter can be used immediately for feeding. The feeding tube should be regularly irrigated with 30 mL to 50 mL of saline to maintain its patency.

Suggested Readings

1. Duh QY, Senokozlieff AL, Choe YS, Siperstein AE, Rowland K, Way LW. Laparoscopic gastrostomy and jejunostomy. *Arch Surg.* 1999;134:151-156.

2. Wu J, Soper NJ, Gastrostomy and jejunostomy. In: Jones DB, Wu J, Soper NJ, eds. *Laparoscpoic Surgery: Principles and Practice.* New York: Marcel Dekker;2004:219-241.

Commentary

Steven Schwaitzberg, M.D., Cambridge Hospital
Harvard Medical School

The creation of a permanent gastrostomy for chronically ill or institutionalized patients has many advantages. The mucosa-lined stoma will not close when the tube is removed. For patients who have a tendency to remove feeding tubes, this feature can avoid a return to the emergency room or clinic for tube replacement.

When creating the gastric diverticulum, pay close attention to creating a base at the junction with the stomach wide enough to allow for an adequate blood supply to the entire structure. If the patient has a particularly thick abdominal wall, the diverticulum can be lengthened with a second firing of the linear stapler although there is a practical limit to how well the blood supply can be maintained to reach the stoma. If there is any question concerning arterial blood supply at the stoma, a Doppler probe can be placed directly on the mucosa to confirm the presence of a biphasic signal.

If there is any tendency for the stomach to pull away from the abdominal wall causing traction on the stoma, laparoscopic sutures should be placed securing the gastric body to the abdominal wall. Alternatively, T-fasteners could be used as well to accomplish this.

An element of continence can be added to the stoma by placing the 12 mm port at a gentle angle from the perpendicular with the skin. In some cases, a simple dressing is all that is needed in between feedings. The stoma is intubated as needed, eliminating the problems and discomfort associated with securing the feeding tube.

The diverticulum will be healed in about 2 weeks. At that time, the initial feeding tube can be replaced. Low-profile feeding appliances can be used if the abdominal wall is not too thick.

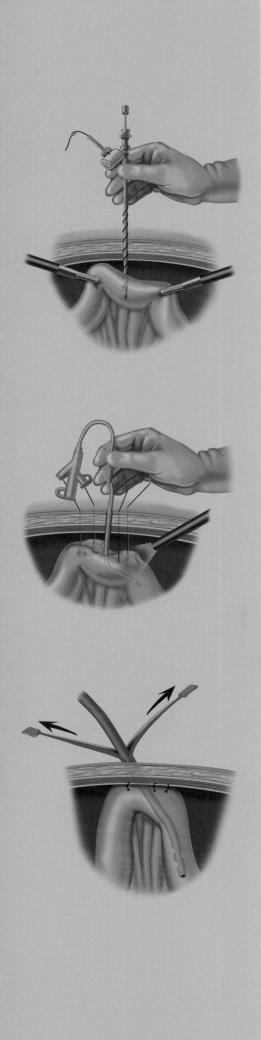

Laparoscopic Jejunostomy

T-Fasteners Technique

A jejunostomy tube can be placed laparoscopically by using the Flexiflo Lap J Kit (Ross Product Division, Abbott Laboratories, Columbus, Ohio), which is similar to the kit previously described in detail for inserting a gastrostomy tube.

Preoperative Preparation

1. Sequential compression stockings and subcutaneous heparin may be used for prophylaxis against deep venous thrombosis. Intravenous antibiotics are administered prophylactically. After induction of general anesthesia, the bladder is emptied with a urinary catheter and the stomach is decompressed with a nasogastric tube.

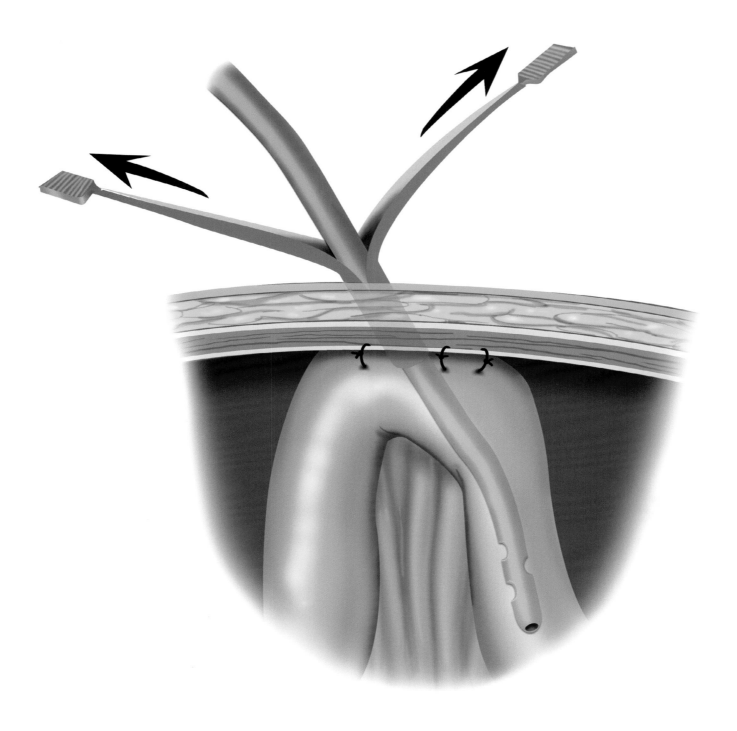

Operating Room Setup

2. The patient is placed in the supine position.

3. The surgeon stands to the patient's left, while the assistant stands to the right.

4. A video monitor is stationed at both sides of the table.

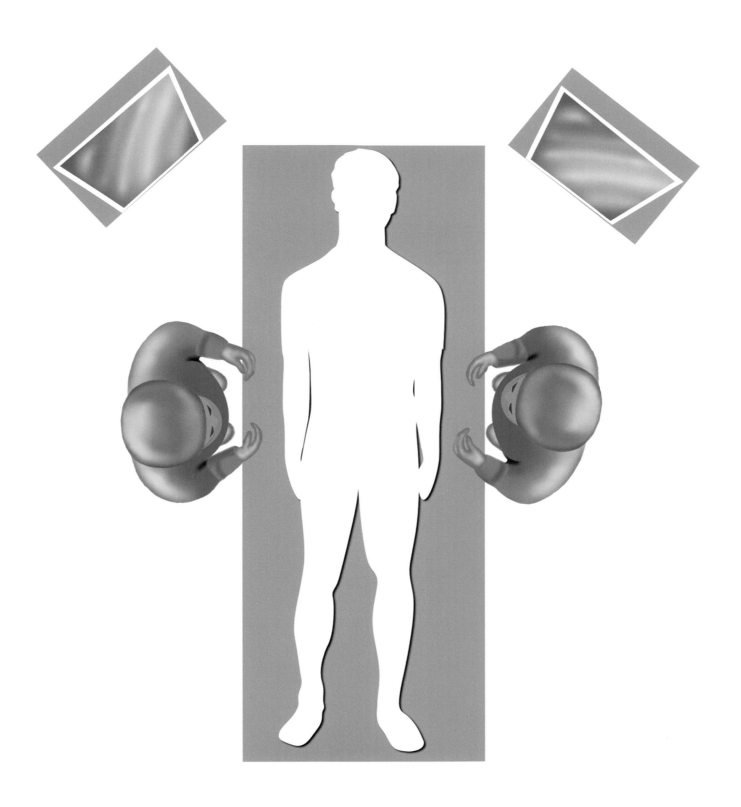

FIGURE B

Access and Port Placement

5. An infraumbilical incision is used to establish pneumoperitoneum with either an open or closed technique. A 10/11 mm port is placed and a 30° angled laparoscope is inserted. A careful exploration is performed to ensure that no injury occurred during port insertion and that no other abnormalities are present.

6. Two 5 mm trocars are placed under direct vision in the right upper and lower quadrants in the midclavicular line.

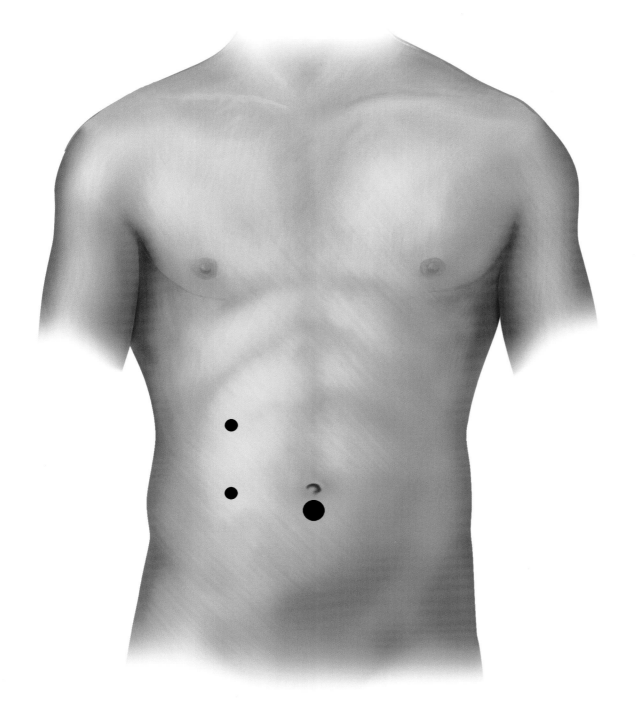

FIGURE C-a,b

Inserting the T-Fasteners

7. Atraumatic graspers are used to identify the ligament of Treitz and a section of jejunum approximately 30 cm distally is selected for jejunostomy tube placement. The proximal jejunum is insufflated with air through the nasogastric tube.

8. Graspers are used to position the segment of bowel close to the abdominal wall, and a T-fastener is inserted into the antimesenteric border of the jejunum, using a similar technique to that as described for gastrostomy tube placement (Figure C-a).

9. Three additional T-fasteners are inserted in a diamond pattern, and the jejunum is held close to the abdominal wall by placing traction on the T-fasteners (Figure C-b).

FIGURE C-a

FIGURE C-b

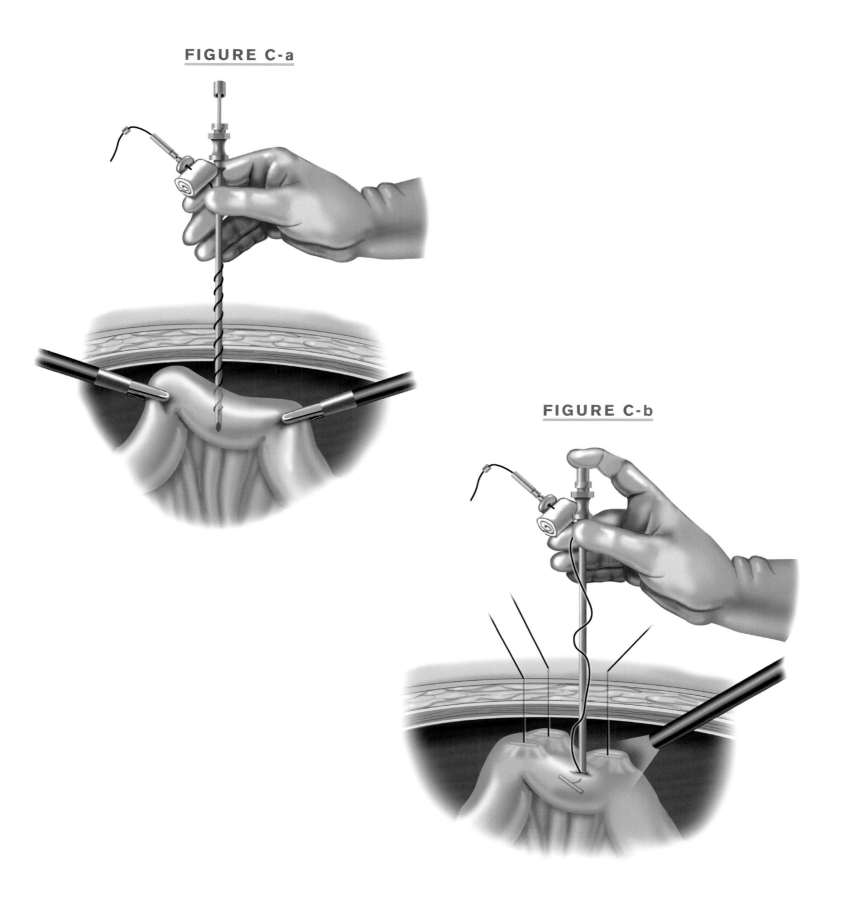

Inserting the Jejunostomy Tube

10. A J guide wire is inserted into the jejunal lumen through an 18 gauge needle inserted in the middle of the diamond pattern created by the four T-fasteners. The distal bowel is angled away from the abdominal wall during needle placement to prevent posterior wall penetration (Figure D-a).

11. After a 5 mm skin incision is made at the guide wire insertion site down to the level of the fascia, the tract is dilated with an 11 Fr peel-away sheath/dilator. The dilator and guide wire are removed.

12. A 10 Fr jejunostomy tube is inserted into the jejunal lumen through the introducer sheath. The tip of the jejunostomy tube is inserted approximately 10 cm to 15 cm distal to the bowel insertion site (Figure D-b). The sheath is peeled away and removed. Proper placement is confirmed with laparoscopic visualization and/or a fluoroscopic contrast injection study.

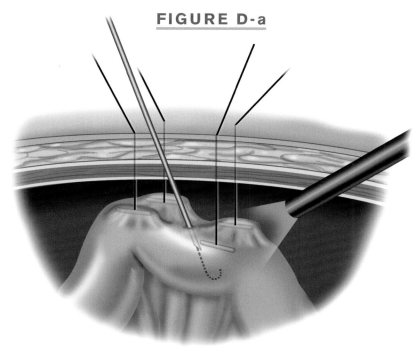

FIGURE D-a

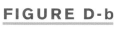

FIGURE D-b

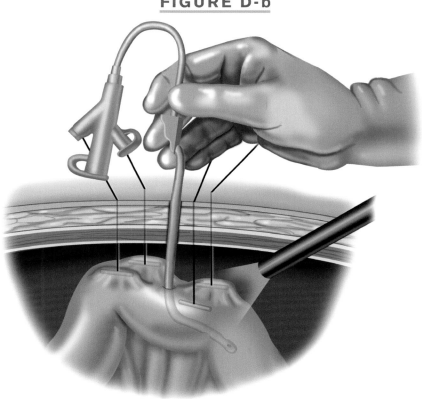

Securing the Jejunostomy Tube

13. All four T-fasteners are retightened by sliding the aluminum crimps and nylon washer down on the cotton pledget. This maneuver secures the segment of jejunum to the abdominal wall, thus creating a water-tight seal. The jejunostomy tube is further secured by suturing an external skin disk to the skin.

14. The peritoneal cavity is examined for hemostasis and any evidence for leakage around the jejunostomy insertion site. After the laparoscope is removed, the umbilical fascia and skin incisions are closed in the usual manner. The T-fastener sutures may be cut after 2 weeks, allowing the T-pieces to pass in the stool.

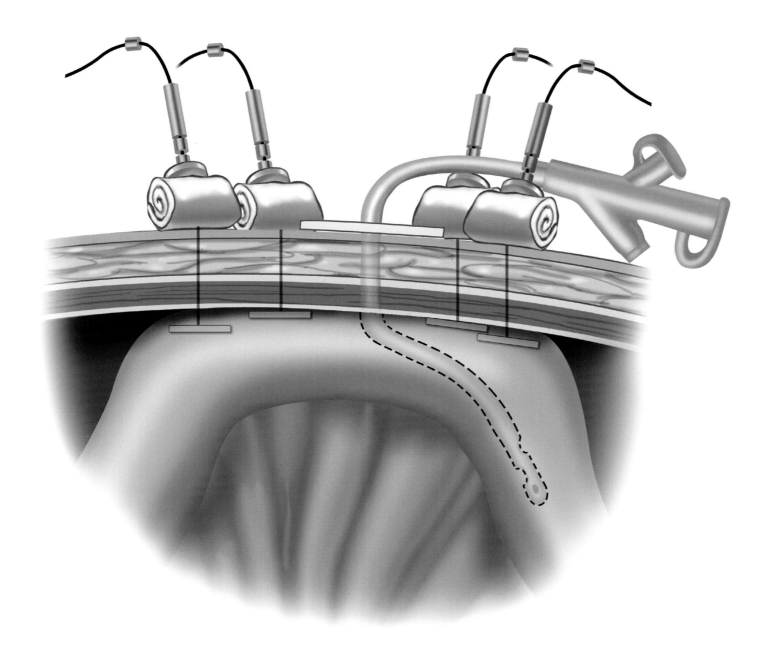

Suturing Technique

The patient's positioning and operating room setup are similar to that as described for the T-fasteners technique, except that the surgeon usually stands to the patient's right and the assistant to the left.

FIGURE F

Access and Port Placement

1. Pneumoperitoneum is obtained via a periumbilical incision. A 5 mm trocar is placed in the midepigastrium and a 10 mm trocar is placed in the right lower quadrant. The camera is then transferred to the right lower-quadrant port.

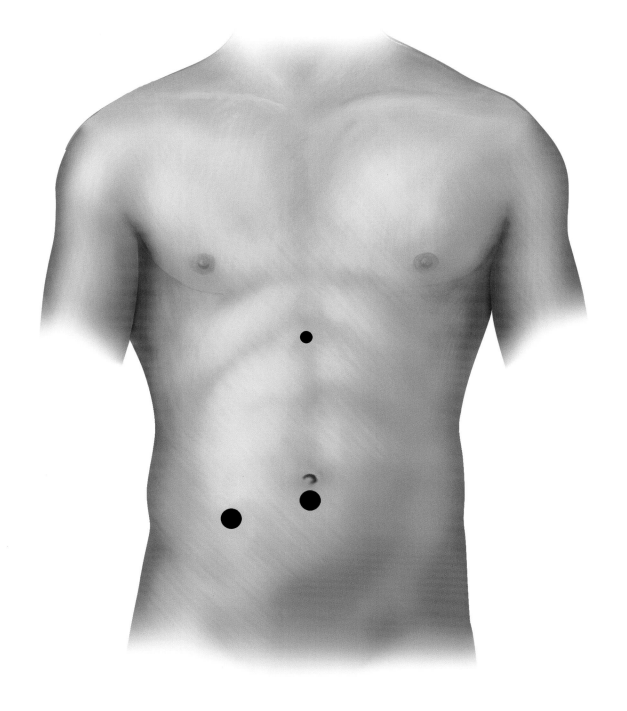

Suturing the Jejunum to the Abdominal Wall

2. A point 30 cm distal to the ligament of Treitz is selected as the jejunostomy tube insertion site.

3. Three 3-0 nonabsorbable seromuscular sutures placed in a triangular pattern are used to anchor the antimesenteric side of the jejunum to the abdominal wall. Either intracorporeal or extracorporeal knot tying techniques can be used. Alternatively a trocar closure device may be used to retrieve the ends of the suture in a transabdominal fashion.

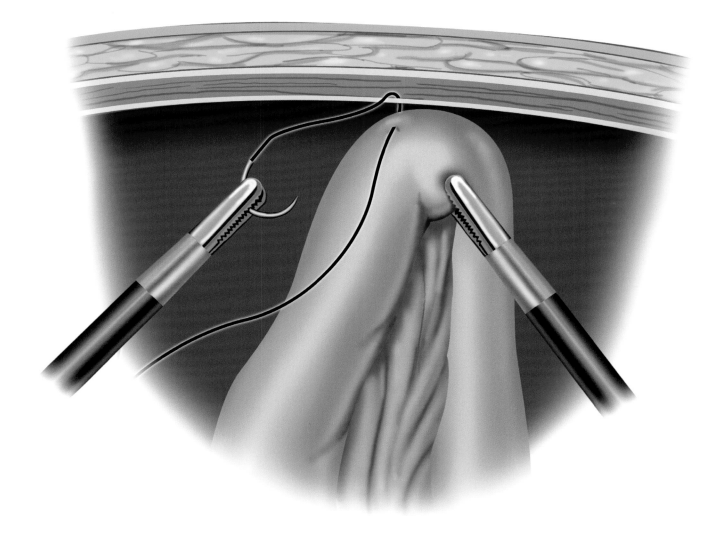

Placing the Jejunostomy Tube

4. Using laparoscopic visualization, the jejunal lumen is accessed using a standard 12 Fr venous introducer kit. A J guide wire is introduced into the lumen via an 18 gauge needle (Figure H-a).

5. The needle is removed and a dilator is inserted over the guide wire and through a peel-away sheath to dilate the tract (Figure H-b). The dilator and guide wire are then removed.

6. Finally, a 10 Fr jejunostomy tube (red rubber catheter) is passed through the introducer sheath 10 cm distal to the jejunal insertion site. The edges of the introducer are peeled apart and removed (Figure H-c).

7. Proper tube placement is confirmed with laparoscopic visualization and/or a fluoroscopic contrast injection study. The jejunostomy tube's position is secured by suturing it to the skin, being careful to not obstruct the lumen with an excessively tight knot.

8. The peritoneal cavity is examined for hemostasis and any evidence for leakage around the jejunostomy insertion site. After the laparoscope is removed, the fascial and skin incisions are closed in the usual manner.

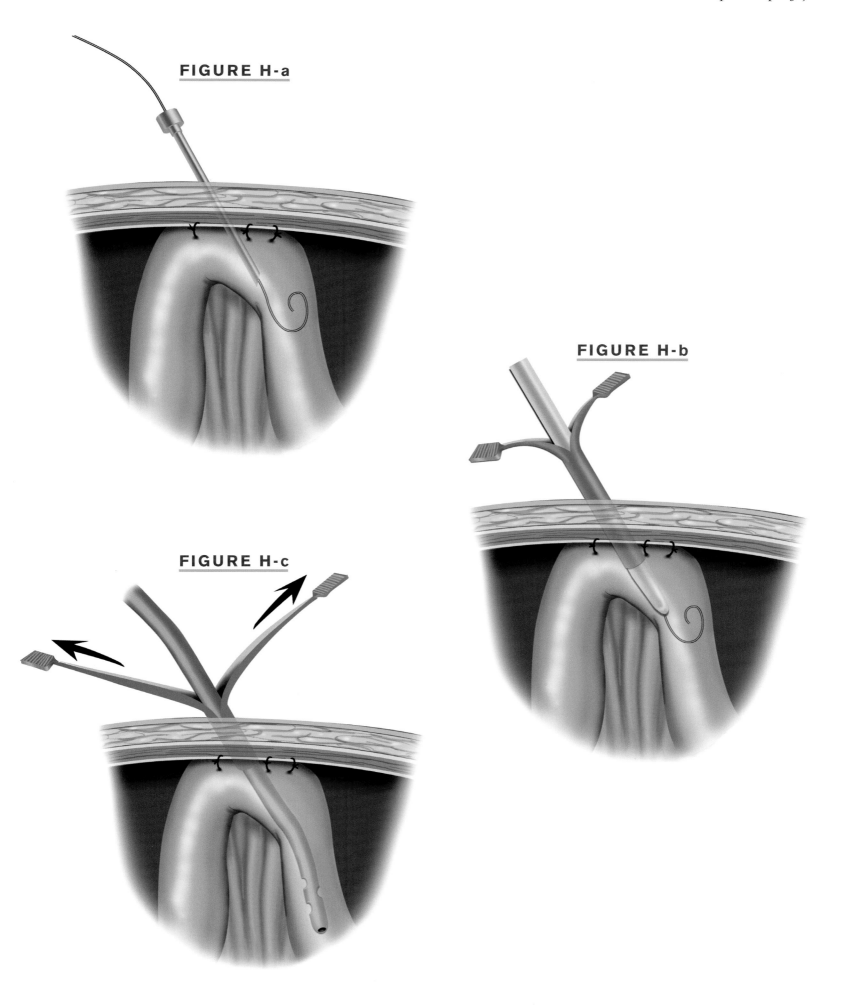

FIGURE H-a

FIGURE H-b

FIGURE H-c

Postoperative Care

Pneumatic compression devices and/or subcutaneous heparin are continued postoperatively. Antibiotics are usually continued for 24 hours after the operation at the discretion of the surgeon. Tube feeds are usually started the morning after surgery, although either catheter can be used immediately for feeding. The feeding tube should be regularly irrigated with 30 mL to 50 mL of saline to maintain its patency.

Suggested Readings

1. Duh QY, Senokozlieff AL, Choe YS, Siperstein AE, Rowland K, Way LW. Laparoscopic gastrostomy and jejunostomy. *Arch Surg.* 1999;134:151-156.

2. Wu J, Soper NJ, Gastrostomy and jejunostomy. In: Jones DB, Wu J, Soper NJ, eds. *Laparoscpoic Surgery: Principles and Practice.* New York: Marcel Dekker; 2004:219-241.

Commentary

Steven Schwaitzberg, M.D., Cambridge Hospital
Harvard Medical School

Feeding via jejunostomy clearly has specific advantages over enteral access through the stomach and is the procedure of choice in selected circumstances. The authors illustrate two different methods for performing this procedure totally laparoscopically. The real beauty of the laparoscopic approach to jejunostomy is the ease by which the proximal jejunum is definitively located. Those who perform open feeding jejunostomy through small upper midline or left transverse incisions can attest to the challenge of clearly identifying the ligament of Treitz, especially in heavier patients. Laparoscopically, this process is fairly straightforward. By lifting the transverse colon anteriorly and cephalad with an atraumatic grasper, the proximal jejunum is readily identified. (For those who prefer a classical Witzel approach to tube placement within the jejunum, consider laparoscopy and jejunal mobilization/identification prior to skin incision.)

When performing laparoscopic jejunostomy secured with intra-abdominal sutures, it can be difficult to place the guide wire in the center of the three sutures. Some surgeons prefer to place the guide wire after the first suture is placed so that precise triangulation is achieved by placing the next two sutures under direct visualization with relation to the guide wire. This is less of a problem when using the T-fasteners since they can be kept loose until the wire and feeding tube are placed. As with laparoscopic approaches to gastrostomy, the authors' approach to feeding jejunostomy minimizes the length of abdominal wall incision in a population potentially vulnerable to wound infection and dehiscence, making it a valuable tool in the surgeon's armamentarium.

Michael A. Edwards, M.D., Beth Israel Deaconess Medical Center
Harvard Medical School

Enteral feeding is the preferred choice of nutritional support for patients with a functioning gastrointestinal tract but for whom oral intake is not possible. Percutaneous endoscopic gastrostomy (PEG) was introduced in 1980 by Gauderer and Ponsky, and has been established over the last 2 decades as the standard of care for long-term enteral nutritional access because it is less invasive, less expensive and, can be performed without general anesthesia in a minor procedure room. The procedure is not without limitations, including : 1) risk for aspiration, which occurs in up to 30% of patients, and 2) contraindication in patients with gastric outlet obstruction, gastroparesis, or gastric resection. As a result, new endoscopic techniques for long-term feeding access in the jejunum evolved, including percutaneous endoscopic gastrojejunostomy (PEG/J) and direct percutaneous endoscopic jejunostomy (DPEJ) tube placements. The success and complications with PEG/J and DPEJ have been variable. Reported successful placement for DPEJ and PEG/J are 86% to 92% and 88% to 100%, respectively. DPEJ has a reported 3% to 11% risk of aspiration.

Any barrier to endoscopy should be considered a contraindication to a PEG. These barriers include obstructing tumors or strictures of the head and neck, esophagus, stomach, or duodenum. Barriers to transillumination, such as colon or liver overlying the stomach, obesity, and adhesions, can increase complication rates with PEG, and should be a relative contraindication. When an endoscopic means of obtaining long-term enteral access is contraindicated or problematic, a minimally invasive approach is desirable. In 1991, Edelman et al published the first method of laparoscopic gastrostomy tube placement using the Russell percutaneous technique. This technique has since been applied to jejunal feeding access. With experience and developing technology, there has been further advancement in laparoscopic techniques. The different techniques include laparoscopic assisted, laparoscopic needle catheter, transabdominal suturing techniques, and use of Brown/Mueller T-fasteners. In this atlas, the authors describe the commonly used T-fasteners and transabdominal suturing techniques and acknowledge that there are other evolving techniques.

Similar to open and endoscopic techniques, laparoscopic gastrostomy is preferred to laparoscopic jejunostomy. Gastrostomy tubes are larger bore, easier to care for, and patients are able to better tolerate bolus feeds, which are more physiological and cost effective. Laparoscopic gastrostomy is indicated for patients who are candidates for long-term gastric feeding or decompression. A laparoscopic jejunostomy is indicated in patients with long-term feeding access requirements and, in whom a laparoscopic gastrostomy is contraindicated (e.g., outlet obstruction, gastroparesis).

Laparoscopic gastrostomy and jejunostomy are preferred over open techniques in patients requiring a surgical feeding access. The advantages of the minimally invasive approach include less pain, post-operative ileus, earlier recovery, better cosmesis and lower incidence of wound infection.

**Justin Wu, M.D., Kaiser Permanente Medical Center
University of California, San Diego**

Enteral feeding has clearly been demonstrated to be the preferred choice of nutritional supplementation for patients with a functioning gastrointestinal tract. This can best be provided through a gastric or jejunal tube, which has traditionally been surgically placed via a laparotomy. Since its introduction in 1980 by Gauderer and Ponsky, percutaneous endoscopic gastrotomy has replaced Stamm gastrostomy in most patients because it is less invasive and less expensive. The endoscopic-assisted technique, however, has not been as successful for jejunostomy, so most have been performed via a laparotomy. In 1984, Russell et al described a new endoscopically assisted insertion of a percutaneous tube gastrostomy adapting the Seldinger's vascular technique. The authors emphasized only a single passage of the endoscope to observe intraluminally the insertion of a needle, guide wire, dilator, sheath, and gastrostomy (Foley) tube. In 1991, the laparoscopic method of gastrostomy tube insertion, using the Russell percutaneous technique, was first published by Edelman et al. Subsequently, the use of Brown/Mueller T-fasteners to anchor the stomach or jejunum to the abdominal wall during laparoscopic gastrostomy or jejunostomy has been a further advancement of the technique.

The authors of this chapter have clearly and succinctly demonstrated the techniques of laparoscopic gastrostomy and jejunostomy using T-fasteners, suturing technique for the latter, and the laparoscopic stapling for the Janeway gastrostomy. The illustrations are clear, vivid, and easy to follow.

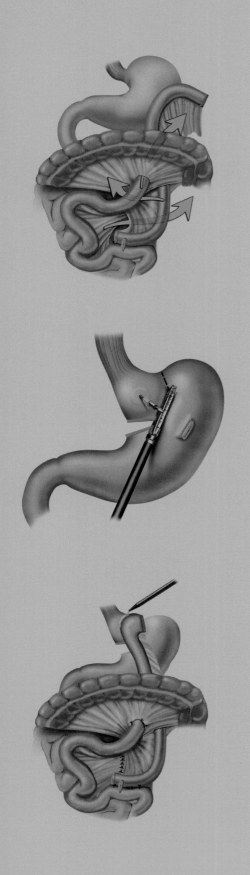

Laparoscopic Roux-en-Y Gastric Bypass

In the United States, one third of Americans are overweight and one fifth are obese. According to the National Institutes of Health Consensus Development Panel, candidates for Roux-en-Y gastric bypass should have a body mass index (BMI) greater than 40 kg/m², or a BMI > 35 kg/m² with associated comorbidity. Furthermore, an experienced surgeon should perform procedures in a setting capable of preoperative assessment, management, and long-term follow-up.

Preoperative Preparation

1. Sequential compression stockings and subcutaneous heparin are used for prophylaxis against deep venous thrombosis. A first-generation cephalosporin is administered prophylactically. After induction of general anesthesia, the bladder is emptied with a urinary catheter and the stomach is decompressed with a nasogastric tube.

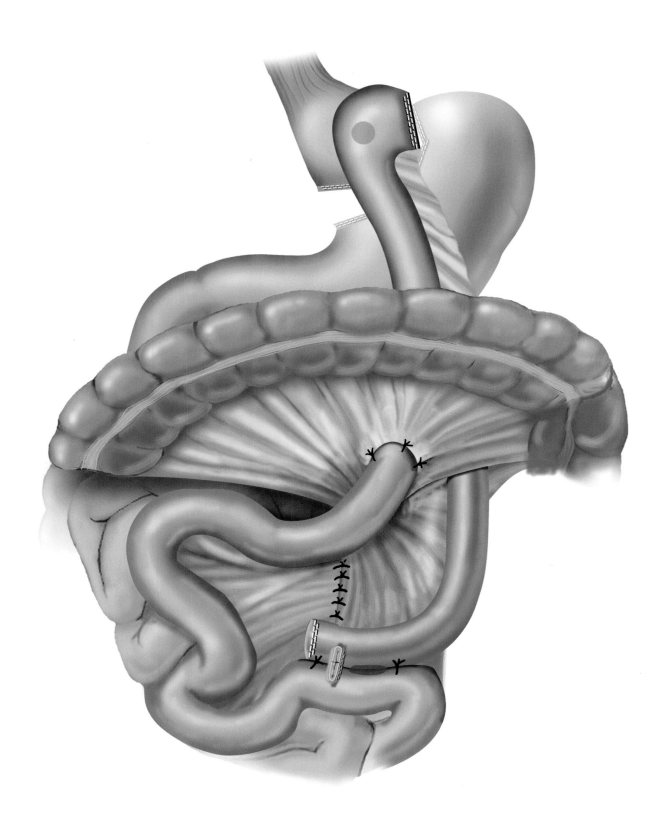

Operating Room Layout

2. The patient is positioned supine on a beanbag cushion. A footboard is placed on the table and the patient is appropriately padded and secured with a safety strap. Arms are abducted and secured on padded arm boards.

3. We prefer the surgeon and camera operator to be situated on the patient's right with the assistant surgeon on the left. Monitors are positioned at the head of the table as shown. Standing stools may be more comfortable and reduce wrist strain.

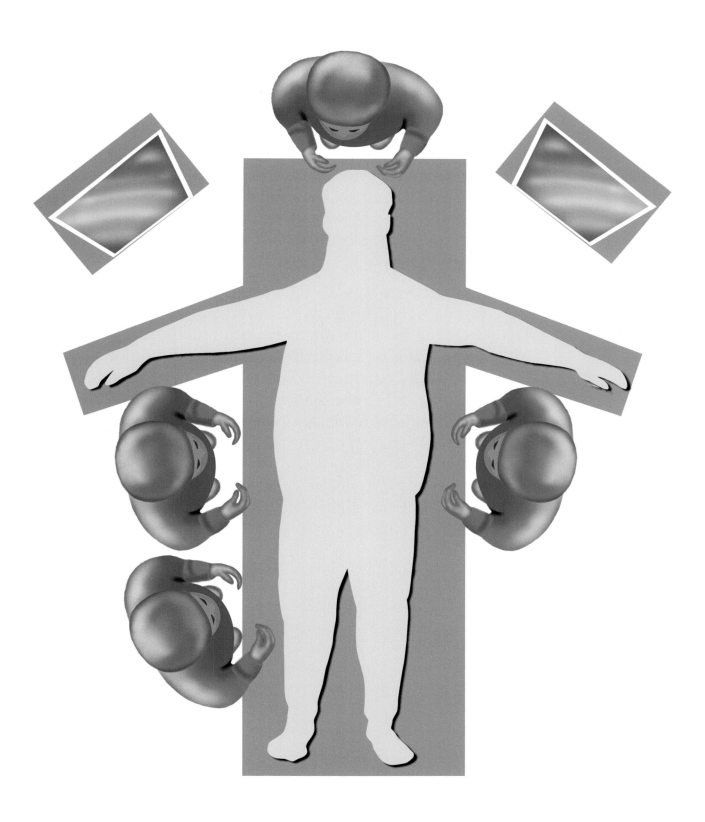

Access and Port Placement

4. A total of five to six ports are placed, including three 5 mm and three 12 mm ports. Pneumoperitoneum of 15 mm Hg is established via a Veress needle through a small nick in the left upper quadrant after a drop test is performed with saline. An optical trocar may be used for intitial access from a left paramedian 12 mm skin incision. After initial access, the abdomen is explored for adhesions before remaining ports are placed under direct visualization. Radially expanding extra-long ports minimize port slippage. A second insufflator may be used to ensure that adequate pneumoperitoneum is maintained in the event of port site leaks.

5. To improve access to the upper abdomen, the patient is placed in a reverse Trendelenburg position, and the falciform ligament may be detached from the anterior abdominal wall using an ultrasonic shears. If a retrocolic Roux limb configuration is planned, the gastrocolic omentum is divided and an opening in the mesocolon is made lateral to the ligament of Treitz, creating a passage between the upper and lower abdomen.

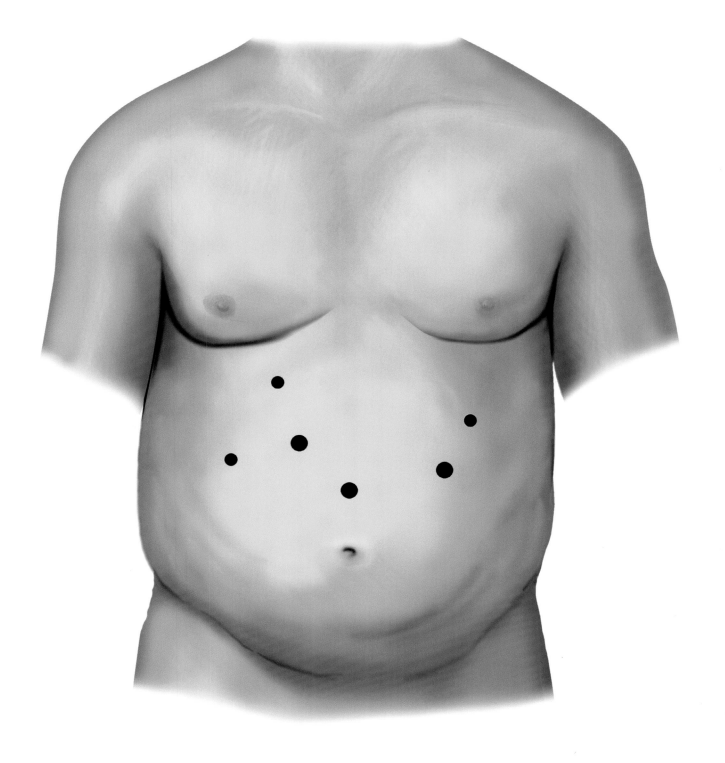

FIGURE C-a,b,c,d

Creating the Jejunojejunostomy

6. A 30 cm to 50 cm length of jejunum is measured from the ligament of Treitz and marked proximally with a suture to maintain orientation. The jejunum is divided with a 60 mm endoscopic GIA stapler (3.5 mm staples); its mesentery is divided twice with a 45 mm endoscopic GIA stapler (2.5 mm staples).

7. The distal jejunum is measured for a distance of 75 cm to 100 cm for use as the Roux limb. The Roux and biliopancreatic limbs are then sutured together with a long traction suture, and a side-to-side jejunojejunostomy is created using a 60 mm endoscopic GIA stapler (3.5 mm staples). Hemostasis is confirmed.

8. We prefer to close the enterotomy using three interrupted stay sutures to approximate the wound edges, after which an endoscopic GIA is applied transversely. Alternatively, a running suture can be performed.

9. An "anti-obstruction stitch" approximates the divided end of the proximal jejunum to the Roux limb.

FIGURE C-a

FIGURE C-b

FIGURE C-c

FIGURE C-d

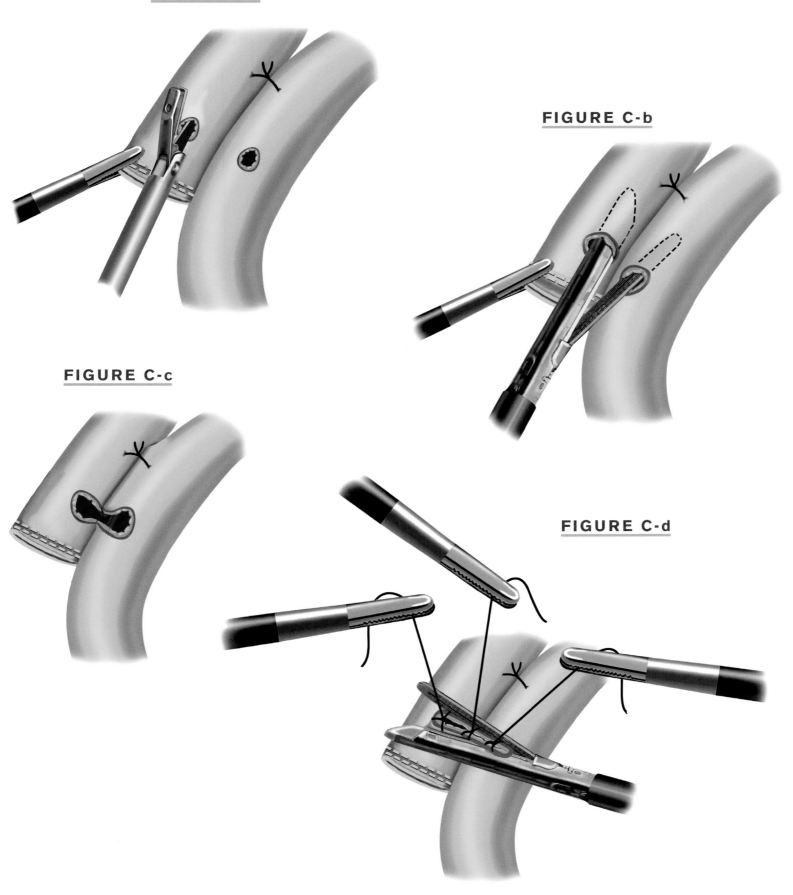

Mobilizing the Roux Limb to the Stomach

10. Next, the Roux limb is carried through the transverse colon's mesenteric defect in a retrocolic antegastric fashion with care taken to avoid twisting of the Roux limb. The three mesenteric defects created with this maneuver, which are illustrated with arrows, will be closed with silk suture at the end of the procedure.

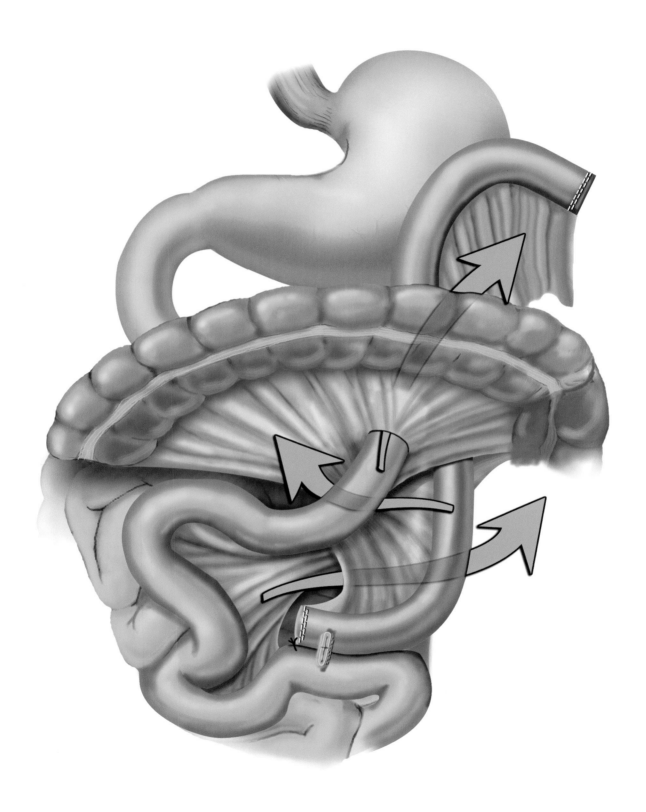

Sizing the Gastric Pouch

11. The left lateral lobe of the liver is elevated using a liver retractor paddle or Nathanson retractor to expose the hiatus. The epigastric fat pad and angle of His are mobilized using ultrasonic shears.

12. The gastric pouch is sized by inflating an orally inserted gastric balloon with 20 mL of saline. The balloon is then brought back to the gastroesophageal (GE) junction. Alternatively, many surgeons use a bougie or approximate the pouch division site using the second gastric vessel on the lesser curvature as a landmark.

13. The harmonic shears are used to create a retrogastric window, which is completed bluntly along the lesser curvature. We preserve the vagus nerve and left gastric artery (optional).

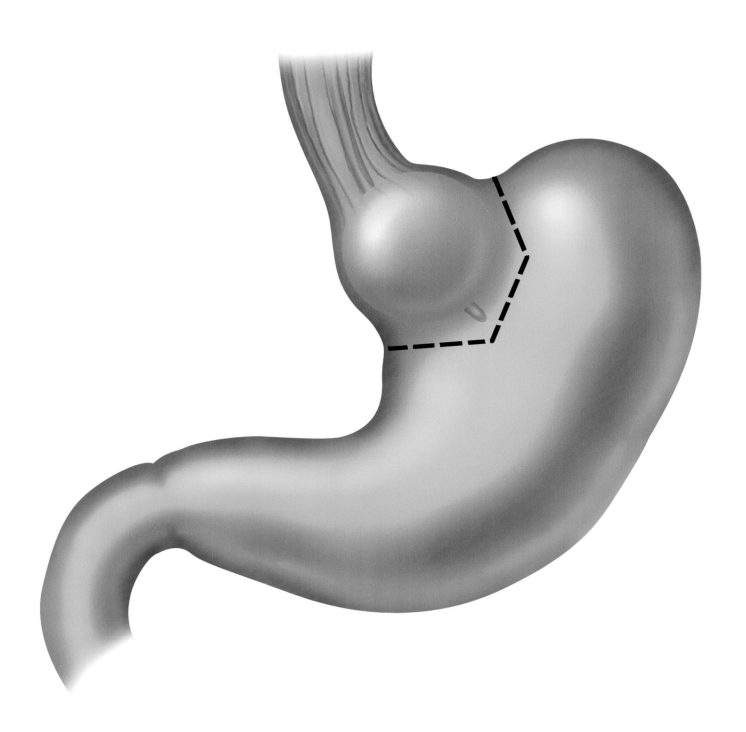

Transgastric Anvil Approach

14. Through the nasogastric tube (NGT), the stomach is again aspirated and all tubes (NGT, gastric balloon, temperature probe) are removed by the anesthesiologist. A 1 cm gastrotomy is performed on the anterior wall of the stomach 5 cm distal to the intended site of gastric division.

15. A looped 10 cm–long suture is tied to the anvil of a 21 mm circular stapler. The operating table is returned to the neutral position and the working port is digitally dilated allowing passage of the EEA anvil into the abdomen.

16. Using our transgastric approach, a pointed Provost-Jones Perforator grasper (Access Surgical) is used to advance the suture through the gastrotomy and to penetrate the anterior gastric wall at the site of the intended gastrojejunostomy (Figure F).

17. Alternatively, the anvil may be passed via a standard NGT using transesophageal technique (Figure G).

FIGURE F

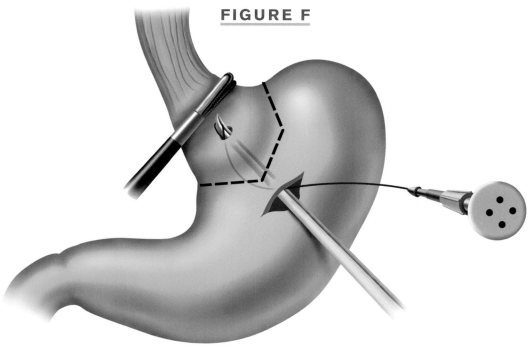

FIGURE G

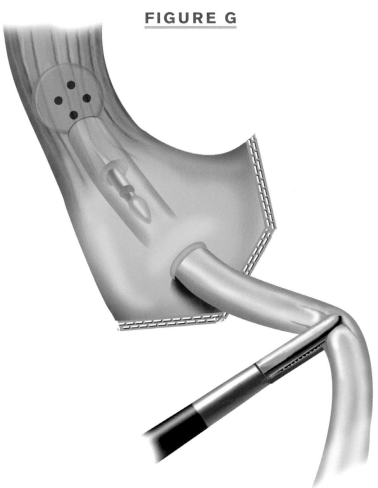

Creation of the Gastric Pouch

18. Three applications of a 60 mm endoscopic GIA (3.5-4.8 mm staples) are used to create the gastric pouch. The gastrotomy used for introduction of the anvil is also closed with an endoscopic GIA (3.5-4.8 mm staples). Surgeons may elect to use staple line buttress materials (optional).

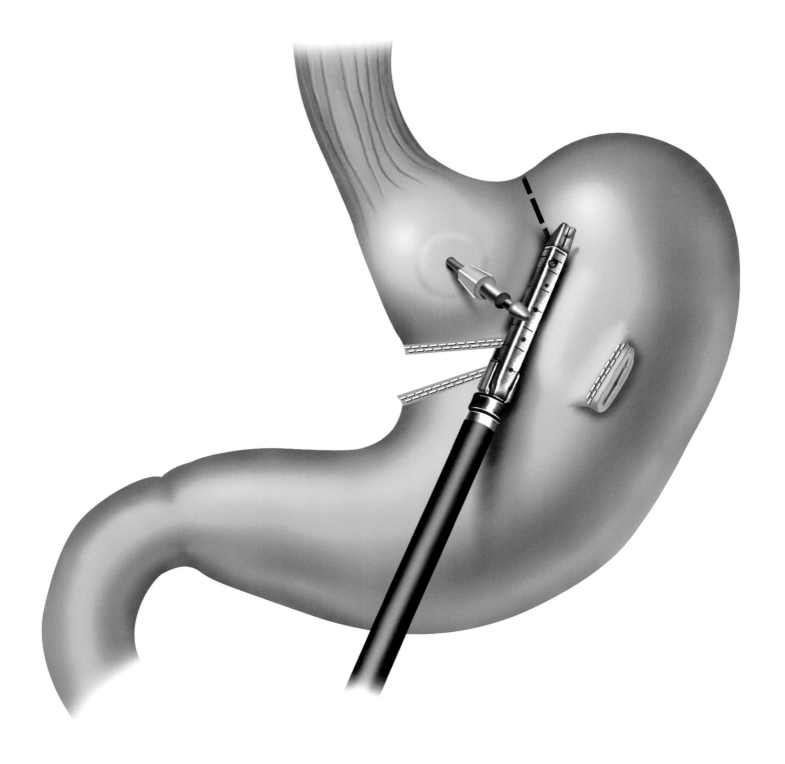

FIGURE I

Transabdominal Circular Anastomosis— Gastrojejunostomy

19. The left inferior port is again removed, and a 21 mm EEA circular stapler is placed through the port site. The staple line of the Roux limb is excised and the EEA stapler is introduced into the lumen of the Roux limb (Figure I).

20. The stapler spike is deployed through the antimesenteric wall of the jejunum and the anvil previously placed in the gastric pouch is held with the Jones anvil holder instrument (Access Surgical) (Figure inset).

21. The anvil and stapler are mated; deployment of the stapler creates the gastrojejunostomy (GJ) anastomosis. The end of the Roux limb is then divided adjacent to the gastric pouch using an endoscopic GIA stapler (3.5 mm staples) and the excised tissue is removed from the abdomen.

22. The anastomosis may then be reinforced with interrupted absorbable sutures. A leak test is performed by instilling 60 mL of saline or dilute methylene blue via a NGT while occluding the Roux limb. Alternatively, the anastomosis may be checked with upper endoscopy or an air bubble test with the GJ anastomosis submerged in saline.

23. A closed suction Jackson-Pratt or Blake drain may be placed (optional) near the GJ anastomosis to identify early leaks and possibly drain subclinical leaks.

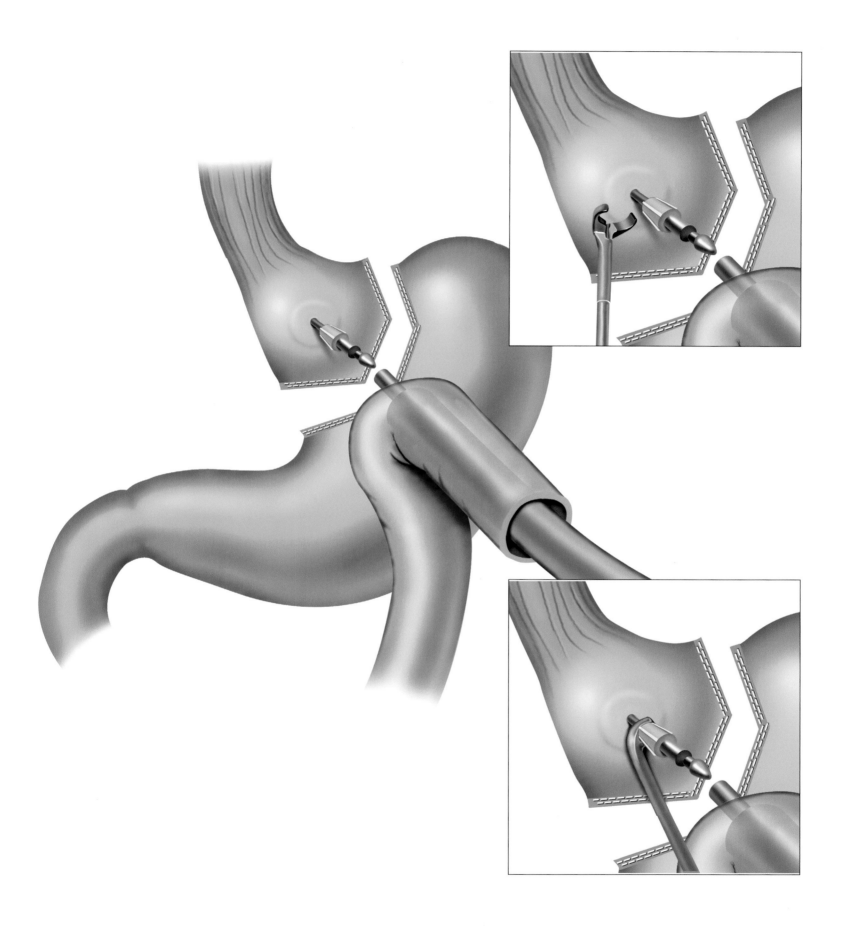

Closure of Mesenteric Defects

24. The window in the transverse mesocolon, the mesenteric defect at the jejunojejunostomy, and the Petersen's defect are closed with silk sutures to prevent internal hernias.

25. Approximately 2 mL of Fibrin glue (Baxter) applied to the gastrojejunostomy and jejunostomy may decrease postoperative leaks (optional).

26. Pneumoperitoneum is evacuated and the fascia at each of the 12 mm port sites is closed with 0 absorbable suture using a fascial closure device. The ports are irrigated with saline. The skin is injected with Marcaine and is closed with 4-0 absorbable subcuticular sutures.

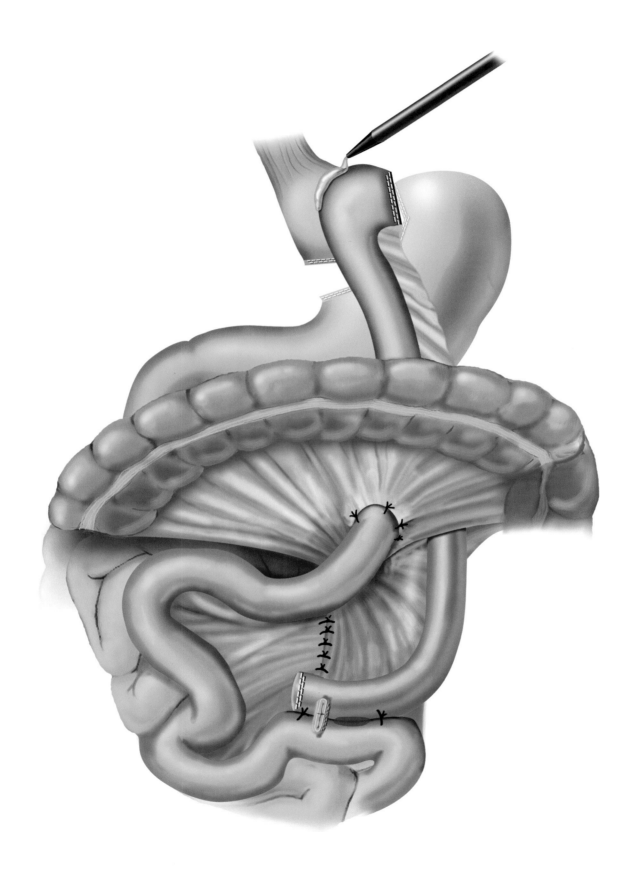

Postoperative Care

Sequential compression devices and subcutaneous heparin are continued postoperatively. If an intra-abdominal drain was placed at operation, oral contrast (methylene blue) may be administered postoperatively to assess for leak. Our practice is to obtain a gastrograffin swallow study routinely on postoperative day 1 prior to beginning a liquid diet. Protein supplements and daily multivitamins are initiated. If the gallbladder is still in place, ursodiol is administered for 6 months.

Suggested Reading

1. National Institutes of Health Consensus Development Conference: G astrointestional surgery for severe obesity. *Ann Intern Med*. 1991;115:956-961.

2. Jones DB, Provost DA, DeMaria EF, Smith CD, Morgenstern L, Schirmer B. Optimal management of the morbidly obese patient. SAGES appropriateness conference statement. *Surg Endosc*. 2004;18:1029-1037

3. Buchwald H, Avidor Y, Braunwald E, et al. Bariatric surgery: a systematic review and meta-analysis. *JAMA*. 2004;292(14):1724-1737.

4. Flum DR, Dellinger EP. Impact of gastric bypass operation on survival: a population-based analysis. *J Am Coll Surg*. 2004;199(4):543-551.

5. Lehman Center Weight Loss Surgery Expert Panel. Commonwealth of Massachusetts Betsy Lehman Center for Patient Safety and Medical Error Reduction Expert Panel on Weight Loss Surgery : Executive report. *Obes Res*. 2005;13(2):205-226.

6. Sjostrom L, Lindroos AK, Peltonen M, et al. Lifestyle, diabetes, and cardiovascular risk factors 10 years after bariatric surgery. *N Engl J Med*. 2004;351(26): 2683-2693.

7. Schumann R, Jones SB, Ortiz VE, et al. Best practice recommendations for anesthetic perioperative care and pain management in weight loss surgery. *Obes Res*. 2005;13:254-266.

8. Jones DB, Blackburn GL, Schneider BE. Patient Safety in Obesity Surgery: Defining Best Practices (DVD). Ciné-Med, Inc., 127 Main Street North, Woodbury, CT 06798.

Commentary

Bruce David Schirmer, M.D.
University of Virginia

The authors described a safe, relatively standardized approach to the performance of laparoscopic Roux-en-Y gastric bypass. The illustrations allow the reader to easily follow the steps of the procedure with alternative choices. Important steps in patient preparation and postoperative care are given.

We use an identical preparation and prophylaxis regimen, with the exception of using low molecular weight heparin instead of standard unfractionated heparin. Our incidence of deep venous thrombosis (DVT) has decreased since making this change and our incidence of transfusion and bleeding has increased. No optimal regimen for DVT prophylaxis has yet been proven by objective data.

Our port placement locates the surgeon's left and right hands on opposite sides of the camera, orienting the camera axis in the plane between the surgeon's hands. The assistant uses a left subcostal (right hand) and a left midlateral abdominal port (left hand). A subxyphoid location of a straight liver retractor (T-bone) is favored by us. One must be careful when having an inexperienced surgeon place a Nathanson retractor that the liver is not damaged.

For the enteroenterostomy, our technique varies only in that we use a double stapling technique to create the anastomosis, with the initial firing being done with a white load of the stapler from the surgeon's left hand (right upper quadrant) port, and the opposite direction stapler being fired through the same enterotomy from the left subcostal (assistant's) port. We also found, through experience, that this anastomosis brought us back to the operating room far more frequently for technical problems than did the gastrojejunostomy. As a result, we adopted the policy of always hand sewing the closure of the enterotomy. A small but definable incidence of stenosis has subsequently been avoided.

We close the enteroenterostomy internal hernia space directly after completing the enteroenterostomy, while the orientation of this area is in the camera view. It is also wise to double check that these mesenteric edges are lying appropriately for closure prior to stapling the enteroenterostomy, to assure the Roux limb is not twisted and the area of anastomosis is not antiperistaltic in its orientation, causing the mesentery to twist under the anastomosis if so created.

In our experience of almost always using a retrogastric retrocolic pathway for the Roux limb, we have found the mesenteric defect is optimally created slightly to the patient's left and above the ligament of Treitz. This places the defect to the patient's left of the middle colic vessels, avoids the proximal jejunum when passing the Roux limb (which is passed to the patient's left of the proximal segment of jejunum), and avoids passage of the Roux limb too low on the stomach, in the antral area, where the lesser curvature vessels limit passage and may be injured. However, the surgeon is urged not to stray too far to the patient's left in making the opening and passage, as we had one splenic injury from such an error. A Penrose drain, sewn to the proximal end of the Roux limb, assists in the passage of the Roux limb into the retrogastric position and assists greatly in the passage of the Roux limb the remainder of the retrogastric distance to lie adjacent to the proximal gastric pouch. In passing the Roux limb into the retrogastric space, care must be taken that the Roux limb is passed with its mesentery oriented downward, and without twists. Failure to ensure this may lead to creation of the gastrojejunostomy incorporating a 180° or 360° twist in the Roux limb mesentery, usually discovered only later when trying to close the mesenteric defects. In our experience, such situations have been met with the expression of great displeasure on the part of the surgeon.

We create the gastric pouch using the second gastric vessel as a landmark, transversely stapling the stomach just below it, then having the anesthesiologist pass a 32 Fr gastric lavage (Ewald) tube, which is positioned along the upper lesser curvature of the stomach, and used to size the gastric pouch. Subsequent firings of the blue load of the stapler are made adjacent to the tube, leading up to the angle of His. The fundus is excluded as much as possible to prevent postoperative pouch dilatation. The lavage tube has added benefit: it is subsequently used as a "backstop" to create the gastrotomy in the proximal pouch prior to stapling, it is used to stent the anastomosis when placing a reinforcing layer of sutures over the enterotomy closure, and it is used to forcefully instill methylene blue dye after the completion of the gastrojejunostomy to test for leaks. In stapling the stomach, one is advised to always be sure tubes are kept out of the path of the stapler.

There are several excellent ways to create the gastrojejunostomy. We formerly used the circular stapler technique as described. However, when the surgeon does not have a highly skilled first assistant, the linear stapling technique is more easily performed by one skilled person. To perform linear stapling, we have had good success with aligning the proximal Roux limb alongside the proximal gastric pouch, using a row of absorbable sutures to hold this position. A single firing of the linear stapler creates an excellent anastomosis. We do NOT limit the size of this anastomosis, but insert over two thirds of the 45 mm stapler. This author remains unconvinced that minimizing anastomotic size produces superior long-term weight loss. It has also been our experience that the linear stapler, so used, produces a lower incidence of anastomotic stenosis postoperatively, with comparable weight loss, to the circular stapling technique.

All mesenteric defects MUST be closed. There is no perfect way to do this. Nonabsorbable sutures incorporating as much structurally sound tissue as possible without injury or obstruction best accomplishes this goal. Suturing to fat will result in large defects once weight is lost, and an appreciable incidence of late hernias. The literature suggests that an antecolic antegastric passage of the Roux limb will decrease the incidence of hernias. However, the distance to pass the Roux limb is longer with this technique and closure of the Petersen's space is more difficult. We have used nonabsorbable suture to incorporate a bite of the Roux limb as it passes through the transverse colon mesentery, two bites of the mesenteric defect at the two and ten o'clock locations, and a bite of the proximal jejunum to simultaneously close the mesenteric defect, prevent the Roux limb from migrating up behind the stomach and becoming kinked and obstructed, and close the Petersen space. A second suture from Roux limb to the four to five o'clock location of the mesenteric defect as well as a third bowel to bowel suture of Roux limb to proximal jejunum about 3 cm below the first suture complete this relatively simple mesenteric closure. It has been associated with a low, but not zero, incidence of internal hernias.

We do not use drains routinely. The nasogastric tube is removed before the gastric pouch division is initiated, and it is not replaced in our practice.

In closing, the technique as described by Dr. Jones et al is a technically sound one which will produce excellent results. Our differences, noted above, give the reader other options to contemplate or try. There are no substantive data to clearly define superiority of any of the differences among these techniques, with the exception that accumulating data may show the creation of a smaller stapled gastrojejunostomy is associated with a higher incidence of stenosis without perhaps an improvement in weight loss or comorbidities.

David R. Flum, M.D., M.P.H.
University of Washington Medical Center

Perioperative prophylaxis to prevent surgical site infection should also include a measurement of fasting bloodglucose and the management of normoglycemia during the procedure with insulin if needed. The appropriate dosing of heparin is still unknown for patients undergoing bariatric surgery. For those with BMI ≤ 40 kg/m^2 we use 5000 units of heparin and make adjustments based on BMI over 40 kg/m^2.

When extending a patient's arms, it is important that appropriate padding be placed in the axillary fold. Patients with significant truncal obesity may be overextended, resulting in a brachial plexopathy and support of the axillae may help avoid this complication.

We place the left subcostal port further toward the axilliary line because we think it provides better access for the EEA stapler later on. We also use a self-retaining retractor for the liver paddle, which will go through the right subcostal port. It is important to get some distance between the working port in the right midquadrant away from the midline port so that when forming the jejunojejunostomy, an appropriate angle between the working ports can be achieved.

Lastly, in super-obese patients, sometimes an additional 5 mm port is required for liver retraction. We have found this to be less important when the patient undergoes a preoperative fast using a very low-calorie diet, which is helpful in reducing the size of the liver.

Our group uses a triple-staple technique to complete the JJ anastomosis. We place the GIA stapler in both the proximal and distal orientation to the biliopancreaticoduodenal (BPD) limb. When we close the jejunotomy defect we avoid narrowing and this leaves a wider JJ anastomosis.

The more the mesentery of the jejunum is divided, the more potential there is for a defect that can cause an internal hernia. We have moved away from a stapled division of the mesentery and it is rarely necessary to open it up to facilitate passage of the Roux limb using the retrocolic/retrograstric approach.

The defect that we place in the transverse mesocolon is usually left of the ligament of Treitz; here it is drawn being to the right. The passing to the left avoids the middle colic artery. We think it is important to close the defects in the mesentery and mesocolon although the evidence to support this is limited. Patients will lose massive amounts of weight after the operation and the resultant defects can be quite significant even when closed. We have also been referred several patients who have had near total loss of the small bowel due to internal hernias. (With both defects closed at the time of initial operation and left open).

We use a ruler to measure the gastric pouch rather than a balloon and are also careful to preserve the nerve of Latarjet as we begin our dissection on the lesser curve. We find that dissecting the phrenoesophageal ligament and mobilizing the angle of His is quite important both to direct the vertical staple line and to avoid bleeding, which can occur when a staple line is placed in this area. After the angle of His is mobilized, the lesser sac dissection extends into the free portion of the posterior stomach. This dissection is complete when a dissector can be placed from the lesser sac up to the angle of His.

The retrogastric membranes that occasionally form between the stomach and the pancreas are important to mobilize at this point if a retrogastric approach is entertained. In the patient with a history of pancreatitis, this space may be obliterated necessitating an antegastric approach.

Although we too place a transgastric anvil, we use an alternative approach in which a single staple line is placed in a transverse fashion 3 cm distal gastroesophageal junction. The central staple is removed from the staple line and we then make a lateral gastrotomy of the type shown here and introduce the 25 EEA stapler into the neogastric pouch space. The stitch attached to the EEA anvil is then brought through to the defect of the staple line on the inferior aspect of the pouch. We then close the lateral gastrotomy and finish the separation of the gastric pouch with a single or sometimes additional vertical fire of a GIA stapler toward the angle of His. The advantages of this inferior orientation are that it directs the anastomosis to the inferior aspect of the gastric pouch, which may facilitate emptying of the gastric pouch and may be easier to complete for retrogastric approaches. The drawn approach may be more appropriate for an antegastric approach. We use a 25 EEA anvil because of the fairly high rate of stricture that we have found to be associated with smaller sizes. When creating the gastric pouch, it is important to first evaluate the width of the stomach in the superior aspect to make sure there is sufficient room laterally to allow the passage of the EEA anvil into the gastric pouch. When in the rare case it is too narrow for that, we do place the anvil using a transesophageal approach.

In patients who weigh more than 450 lbs we have found it helpful to place a tube gastrostomy in the gastric remnant. The infrequent occurrence of gastric remnant bloating can result in serious consequences. This can be alleviated postoperatively by reoperating or by placing a gastrostomy tube in the interventional radiology suites. Once the patients are over a certain weight, the interventional radiology approach is not feasible and the placement of the prophylactic gastrostomy tube has been helpful.

We find it helpful to fasten a Penrose drain on the cut end of the jejunal limb. This drain allows manipulation of the Roux limb as it moves into the retrogastric position with a reticulating grasper. We find that the retrogastric approximation of the small bowel to the gastric pouch reduces tension on the alimentary limb. In placing the EEA stapler through the cut end of the jejunum, we find it helpful to place a traction stitch at the base of the cut end of the jejunum to grasp the jejunum. If the bowel is directly grasped with traction across the EEA, it can occasionally tear. If there is excessive traction on the EEA anvil during its coupling with the EEA stapler the defect in the pouch may widen. This can be avoided by placing a purse-string stitch around the anvil. When closing the defect around the mesocolon it is important to reduce the length of redundant jejunal limb. This may avoid the risk of twisting the Roux limb.

We routinely perform endoscopy at the completion of the anastomosis with a bowel clamp on the Roux limb. This is done to check for hemostasis and to confirm the integrity of the staple line as air is inflated while the anastomosis is submerged in saline.

Stephanie B. Jones, M.D., Beth Israel Deaconess Medical Center Harvard Medical School

Anesthesia for the laparoscopic Roux-en-Y gastric bypass deserves special attention. The incidence of difficult intubation may be increased, and if intubation fails, mask ventilation may be difficult as well. Increased cardiac output and restrictive pulmonary mechanics then lead to a rapid descent in oxygen saturation. Airway adjuncts and assisting personnel must be readily available, and the same cautions apply to emergence from anesthesia. Positioning the table at 25° to 30° reverse Trendelenburg may help maintain adequate oxygen saturation for a longer period of time.

Increased hepatic and renal blood flow results in more rapid metabolism of anesthetic drugs such as neuromuscular blocking agents, impeding the surgical view when muscle relaxation is inadequate. Reverse Trendelenburg positioning may improve ventilation, but cause hypotension. With frequent position changes, the patient must be well secured to the operating table to avoid potential neuropathy. Oro- or nasogastric tubes are often inserted and removed at various points in the procedure, and constant communication must exist between the surgical and anesthetic teams to avoid inadvertent stapling of the tube, or perforation of a fresh gastrojejunal anastamosis.

Intravenous fluid requirements are greater than might be intuitively expected, likely due to extensive bowel manipulation and consequent third-spacing. Adequate fluid resuscitation (approximately 4 liters of lactated Ringer's in our experience) is necessary to avoid postoperative renal compromise. The routine use of antiemetic prophylaxis is important in higher risk patients, especially young women or those with a previous history of postoperative nausea and vomiting, as persistent retching may stress anastamoses. Postoperative narcotics may cause significant respiratory depression in patients with obstructive sleep apnea, and the use of nonopioid adjuncts such as local anesthetics and nonsteroidal anti-inflammatory drugs should be considered when appropriate. Patients using continuous positive airway pressure devices at home should be continued on the therapy in the immediate postoperative period.

Although the number of operations performed per year continues to increase, laporoscopic Roux-en-Y gastric bypass is not a "routine" general surgery procedure. Appreciation of the anesthetic risks and education of the anesthesia team is vital to the success of any bariatric surgery program.

George L. Blackburn, M.D., Ph.D., Beth Israel Deaconess Medical Center
Harvard Medical School

Roux-en-Y gastric bypass (RYGB) is the most common bariatric operation in the United States. The newest developments are in minimally invasive surgery, or laparoscopy. Laparoscopic RYGB has become increasingly common due to advances in technology and surgical skills, along with growing demand from patients. As reported in the Commonwealth of Massachusetts Betsy Lehman Center for Patient Safety and Medical Error Reduction Expert Panel on Weight Loss Surgery Executive Report, the RYGB procedure has acceptably low complications, and is known to produce marked improvement in comorbidities and quality-of-life measures. The laparoscopic approach improves short-term recovery from surgery, and has a lower incidence of incisional hernias than the open RYGB, but it needs to be performed by appropriately trained, qualified, laparoscopic weight-loss surgeon.

Risk of medical errors and complications are most likely to be minimized under the following conditions: 1) rigorous training that puts a strong emphasis on patient safety, and includes close monitoring and supervision of surgeons early in their learning curves, 2) ongoing training and accumulation of experience that takes place in a supportive setting, with extended proctoring by experienced weight-loss surgeons, and 3)high-volume surgeons (50-100 cases per year) operating in properly equipped, high-volume weight loss centers (> 100 cases per year) with integrated and multidisciplinary treatment. High-volume surgeons tend to have better short-term outcomes.

Physiologically, the most important features of Roux-en-Y gastric bypass are the small neogastric pouch and a tight stoma that limit oral intake, making restriction the primary mechanism for weight loss. In addition, the distal stomach and proximal small bowel are bypassed in the Roux-en-Y configuration to result in dumping syndrome and mild malabsorption. A complex series of sequential integrated signals from a synchronized group of hormones secreted by the gut are thought to restore the dysmetabolism of obesity. Studies show return to euglycemia and normal insulin levels within days of surgery, well before any significant weight loss. Increases of PYY and GLP-1 have also been reported as an effect of surgery. A postoperative fall or failure of the ghrelin level to rise after surgery, as it does after weight loss due to food restriction, has also been observed.

The orexigenic foregut hormone ghrelin can exert prodiabetic effects by suppressing insulin secretion, stimulating counter-regulatory hormones, and directly opposing insulin action. Conversely, large (up to 10-fold) and durable (up to 20 years) elevations of GLP-1 or other nutrient-stimulated L-cell hormones, including enteroglucagon, have been documented after Roux-en-Y gastric bypass.

Eric J. DeMaria, M.D.
Duke University Medical Center

Laparoscopic Roux-en-Y gastric bypass to treat severe obesity is a complex and demanding surgical procedure that appears to have one of the steepest learning curves of all laparoscopic surgical procedures. In the current chapter, the authors present an excellent description of the steps involved in performing one technique for laparoscopic gastric bypass surgery. The various steps of the procedure are reviewed in detail with clear drawings to facilitate the reader's understanding.

The authors' technique using the circular stapler for the gastrojejunostomy is only one of the currently available techniques for creating this anastomosis. In contrast, the jejunojejunostomy anastomotic technique they describe is utilized uniformly by the majority of surgeons practicing laparoscopic gastric bypass today. Alternative techniques for the gastrojejunostomy include a completely hand-sewn anastomosis or a linear-stapled technique with closure of the gastrotomy and enterotomy for passage of the stapling device using a hand-sutured closure. Many surgeons prefer the circular stapled technique presented herein because of the resultant uniformity of anastomotic diameter which results. One negative associated with this technique is the need to dilate the abdominal wall to insert the anvil of the stapling device. Although the anvil can be positioned on the end of a nasogastric tube and delivered into the pouch using the transesophageal route, this adds the possibility of the anvil lodging in the esophagus as well as a theoretical concern about intra-abdominal contamination as the nasogastric tube is removed transabdominally.

Our group has found the linear stapled technique to create a reproducible diameter with the additional advantage of avoiding dilatation of the abdominal wall access incision for insertion of the stapling anvil. Cost savings result from using the same stapling device to perform both of the intestinal anastomoses. Finally, we have seen a reduction in the incidence of gastrojejunostomy complications, including acute hemorrhage, leak, and stenosis/stricture compared to other anastomotic techniques, including our previous "open" surgery experience (using a two-layer, hand-suturing technique) and our limited experience with the laparoscopic circular stapled and hand-sewn methods.

The authors also present retrocolic passage of the Roux limb as their technique of choice for the procedure. Many authors today advocate an antecolic orientation of the Roux limb as a method of reducing operative time and eliminating one of the three mesenteric defects of the retrocolic approach, i.e., the mesocolic defect. Unfortunately, time savings with this approach in part results from the general sentiment that closure of the Petersen's defect (between the jejunal mesentery of the Roux limb and the transverse mesocolon) is not necessary. Our group has seen a worrisome increase in the incidence of Petersen's internal hernias when the defect between the Roux limb mesentery and the transverse mesocolon is left open, and we strongly advocate mandatory closure of this defect in every patient undergoing laparoscopic gastric bypass whether the limb is brought up in the retrocolic or antecolic position. We believe the advantages of easier closure and decreased tension on the gastrojejunal anastomosis make the retrocolic approach superior, although admittedly the antecolic approach can also be safely applied in most routine cases as long as Petersen's defect is closed.

In summary, laparoscopic gastric bypass is a complex procedure that requires extensive training and experience to perform safely. Although the myriad technical details of the procedure are not easily described in the abbreviated format of a surgical atlas, the authors have provided sound fundamental information for surgeons and trainees seeking to become familiar with the procedure.

Philip R. Schauer, M.D.
Cleveland Clinic Foundation

Laparoscopic Roux-en-Y gastric bypass (LRYGBP) is one of the most technically challenging laparoscopic procedures requiring advanced suturing, stapling, and exposure skills. Furthermore, the morbidly obese patient presents many anatomic burdens such as a thick abdominal wall, dense intraabdomial fat, and hepatomegaly, which may significantly add to technical difficulties. Careful attention to technical detail, as well as skill development, is essential to mastering this complex operation.

In this chapter, Dr. Jones very precisely describes and skillfully illustrates LRYGBP utilizing a transgastric circular stapler for the gastrojejunostomy and a retrocolic, antegastric Roux limb. This approach is one of many that has been successfully adopted by surgeons worldwide and has yielded very good outcomes in published reports. Surgeons should be knowledgeable of other proven approaches so that he or she can determine which techniques work best in his or her operating environment.

The gastrojejunostomy technique is perhaps the most variable. Three stapling techniques have emerged including the: 1) circular stapler technique with transesophageal insertion as described by Wittgrove and Clark, 2) the circular stapler technique with transabdominal insertion described in this atlas, and 3) the linear stapler technique described by Champion.

No single gastrojejunostomy technique has been proven superior; however, each has relative advantages and disadvantages. The circular stapler creates a consistent stoma diameter and perhaps enables a smaller gastric pouch but appears to have a higher stricture rate (especially with the 21 mm anvil) than the linear stapler technique. The circular stapler approach requires no suturing and thus may be technically easier. Using the circular stapler, however, necessitates two staplers (linear and circular) for each operation, which may increase cost and requires the operating room staff to be skilled with loading and handling two different staplers. The circular stapler requires a larger abdominal access incision, which is vulnerable to wound infection due to contamination from the stapler as it is withdrawn through the incision. A sleeve wound protector or large trocar (20 mm) can reduce port site infections as a result of circular stapler contamination. Transesophageal placement of the anvil affords creation of a very small pouch, but creates the potential of esophageal injury or anvil entrapment as the anvil is passed. Consequently, many surgeons have adopted the transabdominal circular stapler insertion as described in this atlas to avoid potential esophageal injury. Finally, the hand-sewn approach eliminates all of the limitations of the staplers, but requires enhanced suturing skills and may increase operating time compared to the stapling approaches.

Leaks and strictures are the most common complications of the gastrojejunostomy. Avoiding interruption of the gastric pouch vascular supply and excessive tension on the anastomosis are important to avoid leaks and strictures, regardless of anastomotic technique. When using a linear stapler or hand-sewn approach, a stent across the anastomosis (bougie or endoscope) can minimize an excessively tight anastomosis that may lead to stricturing. Intraoperative leak testing as described in this atlas is highly advised since it may uncover an occult leak, allowing operative repair before leaving the operating room. To create another layer of safety, I recommend a two-layer anastomosis using the jejunal serosa as a patch to cover the gastric pouch staple line, as well as the anastomosis. When using a two-layer approach, careful attention must be paid to avoid excess tension on the anastomosis. I also recommend routine placement of a drain posterior to the gastrojejunostomy, which is removed within 7 days of the operation.

The Roux-limb positioning is also highly variable. The retrocolic approach described in this atlas provides the advantage of minimizing tension on the gastrojejunostomy since it follows the shortest route to the gastric pouch. However, the retrocolic tunnel necessitates creation of a mesocolon defect, which can add 15 minutes to the operation, but more importantly adds a potential site of herniation as described in the atlas. For this reason, my preference has been an antecolic, antegastric Roux-limb position that completely eliminates the threat of a mesocolon defect herniation. I have found that even in superobese patients with shortened small bowel mesentery, the antecolic Roux limb can reach the gastric pouch without undue tension.

Laparoscopic Roux-en-Y gastric bypass can be an intimidating procedure, especially to surgeons who are just entering advanced laparoscopic surgery. However, by studying various proven approaches and receiving training supervised by experienced surgeons, many surgeons can master this complex but rewarding operation. Few, if any, other operations provide as much benefit to patients in terms of improving quality of life and longevity.

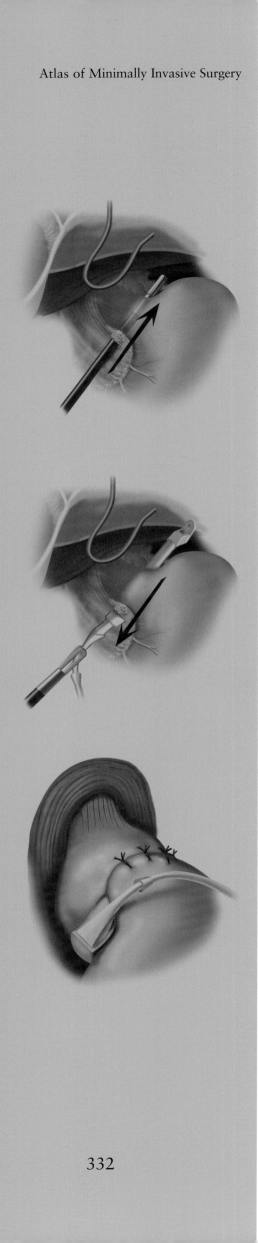

Laparoscopic Adjustable Gastric Banding

Obesity is a major health problem often associated with coronary artery disease, diabetes, hypertension, pulmonary dysfunction, hyperlipidemia, and death. Weight loss surgery remains the best method for attaining significant and lasting weight reduction in the morbidly obese patient. Potential candidates for surgical intervention should have a Body Mass Index (BMI) greater than 40 kg/m^2, or a BMI > 35 kg/m^2 coupled with obesity induced comorbidity. An experienced surgeon in a clinical setting should perform procedures where there exists the capacity for management of these patients, their attendant medical risks, and potential complications. The laparoscopic adjustable gastric band offers an effective means to lose weight with relatively low morbidity and mortality.

Preoperative Preparation

1. Sequential compression devices and subcutaneous heparin are used for prophylaxis against deep venous thrombosis. We administer a first generation cephalosporin for antibiotic prophylaxis. The bladder is emptied preoperatively.

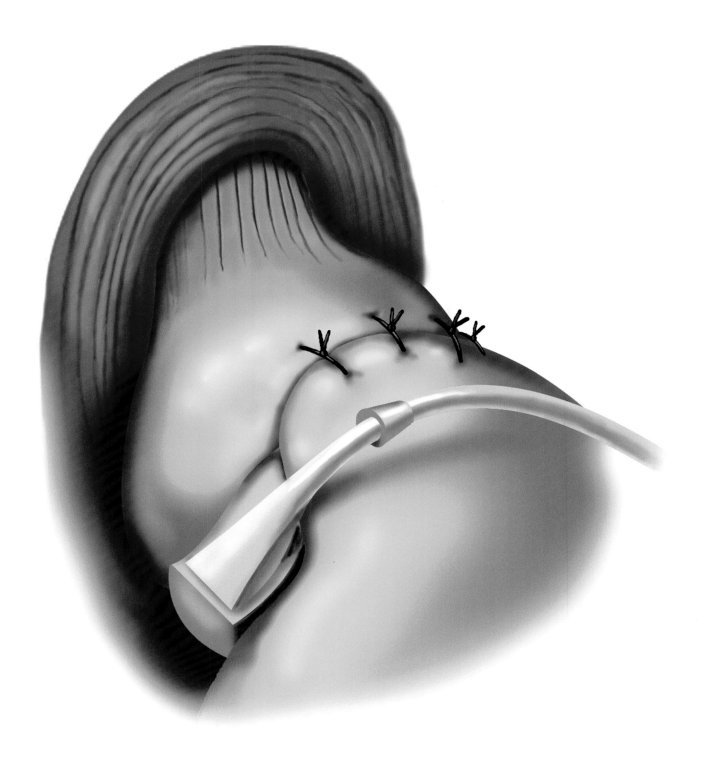

Operating Room Layout

2. The patient is positioned on a padded cushion in the lithotomy position. The arms are secured and padded as shown. The stomach is decompressed with an orogastric tube after induction of general anesthesia.

3. The surgeon is situated between the patient's legs with the assistant/camera operator on the patient's left. The video monitors are placed at the head of the table as shown. Alternatively, many surgeons will prefer to perform this operation with the patient in the supine position, legs together, while standing on the patient's right side.

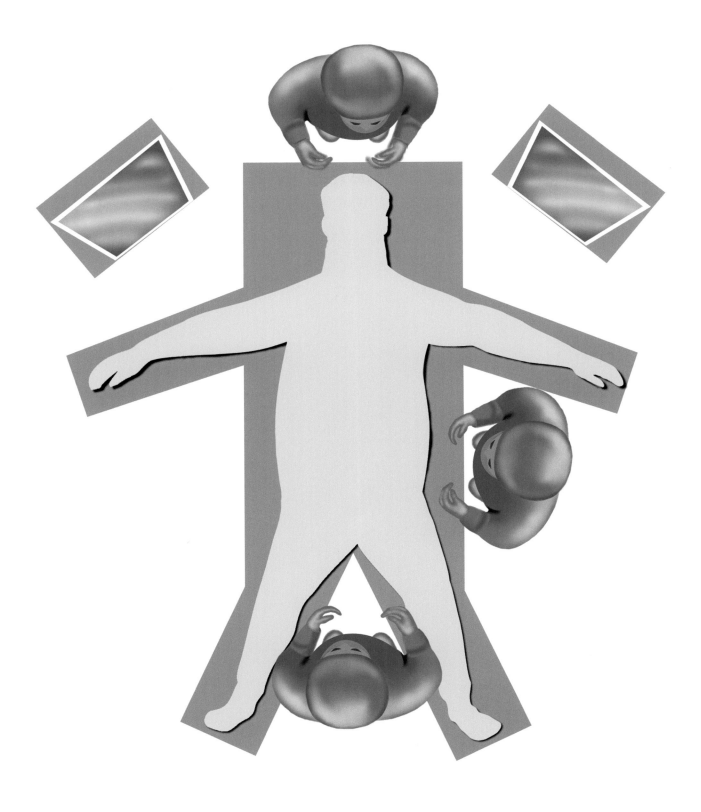

Access and Port Placement

4. Pneumoperitoneum is established using a Veress needle through a small skin nick in the left upper quadrant after a drop test is performed with saline. A 12 mm optical trocar is placed in the left midrectus 15 cm below the xiphoid process using a 0° laparoscope.

5. Port placement varies widely among surgeons. We place a 15 mm subcostal trocar in the left midclavicular line to be used later for band insertion. Three or four additional 5 mm ports are placed as shown. The subxiphoid area (open circle) can be used to insert a Nathanson liver retractor through a 5 mm incision or a standard laparoscopic liver retractor through a 5 mm port.

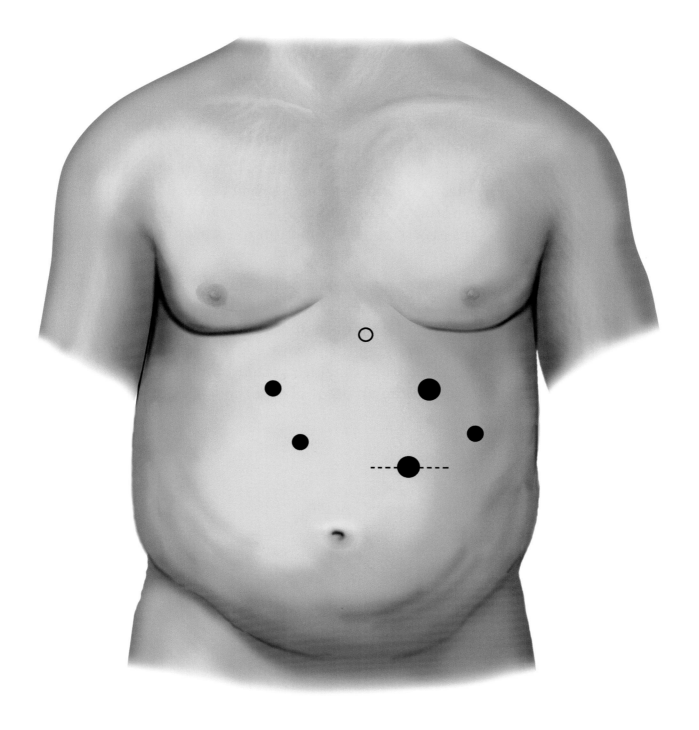

FIGURE C-a,b

Creating a Retrogastric Tunnel

6. Exposure to the hiatus is achieved by retracting the left lateral lobe of the liver anterolaterally.

7. The working space is further exposed by placing the patient in reverse Trendelenburg position, using gravity to drop the bowel and omentum caudally. Retraction on the stomach inferiorly using a Babcock grasper allows for dissection of the angle of His (Figure C-a).

8. The orogastric tube is removed and an intragastric calibration balloon is placed. The anesthesiologist then inflates the balloon with 15 cc of saline. The balloon must be inflated inside the stomach and not the esophagus, otherwise it may cause esophageal rupture. After inflation, the balloon is pulled back to the gastroesophageal junction to approximate the size of the gastric pouch.

9. The avascular space of the pars flaccida (gastrohepatic ligament) is opened, thus exposing the caudate lobe of the liver. Once the right crus of the diaphragm and inferior vena cava are identified, the fat pad overlying the lowest edge of the right crus is scored and a retrogastric tunnel is created bluntly along the posterior gastric wall to the angle of His in the left upper quadrant (Figure C-b).

FIGURE C-a

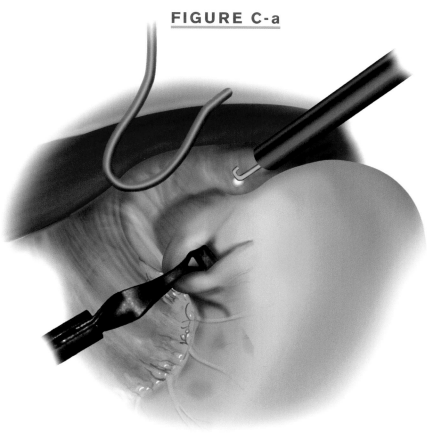

FIGURE C-b

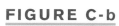

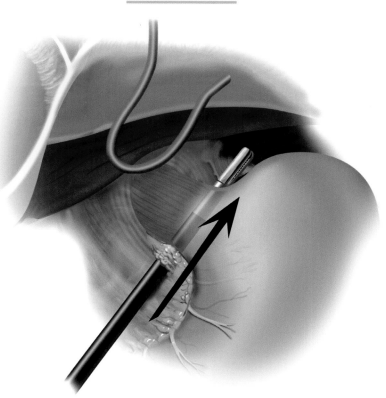

Inserting the Band

10. The band is placed into the abdomen using the Jones inserter device (Access Surgical). The band is attached onto the Jones inserter device (Figure D-a) and fastened into position (Figure D-b). The band/inserter device apparatus is then passed through the 15 mm port (Figure D-c). Alternatively, a previously placed port can be removed and the band/inserter device apparatus can be passed directly through the abdominal wall (Figure D-d).

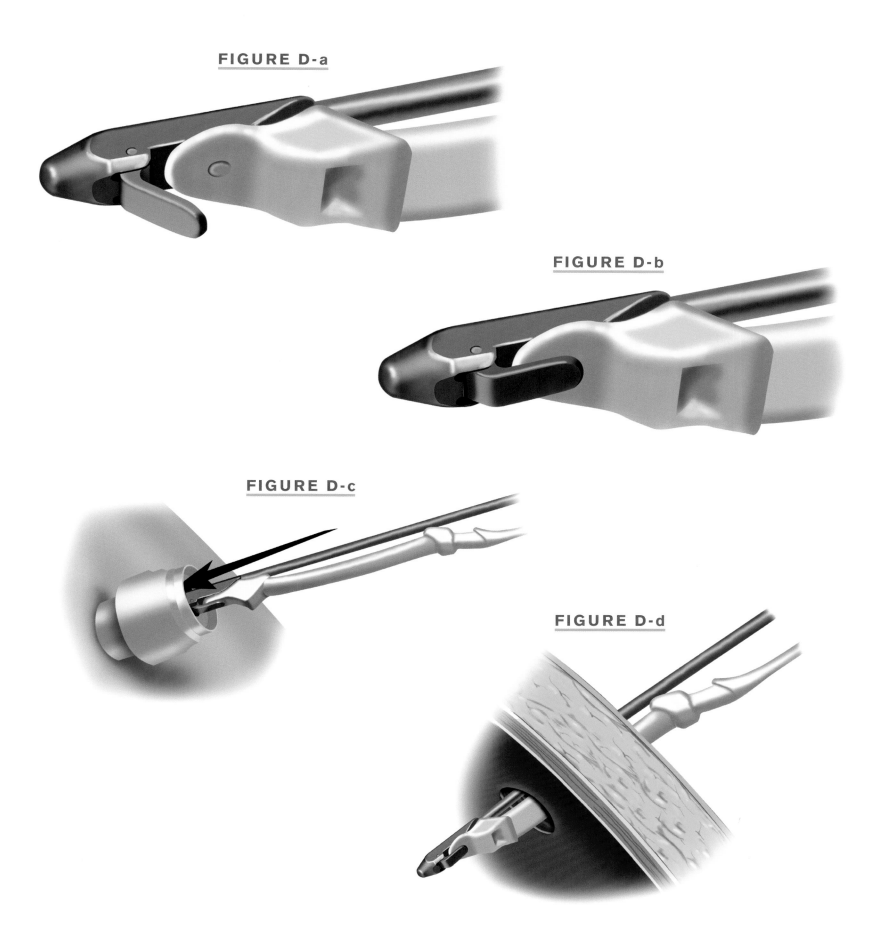

FIGURE D-a

FIGURE D-b

FIGURE D-c

FIGURE D-d

Positioning the Band

11. A grasper passed through the retrogastric tunnel is used to advance the gastric band from the angle of His to the perigastric opening along the lesser curvature.

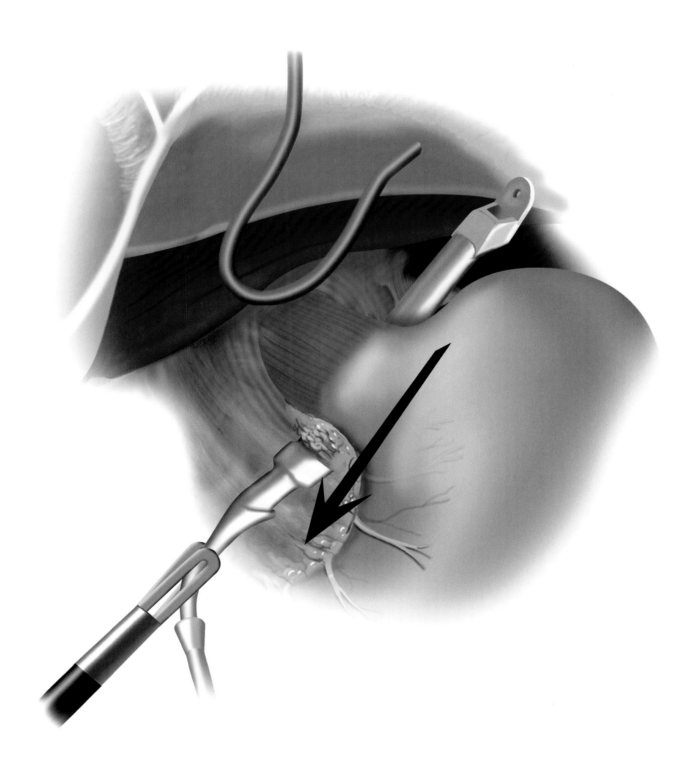

Closing the Band

12. The band is situated around the equator of the intragastric balloon prior to locking. The balloon is deflated prior to the band actually being locked. The band is buckled closed using the Jones hooker and pusher instruments (Access Surgical) (Figure F). These instruments enable one to place adequate traction and countertraction on the buckle necessary for a secure and facile band closure (Figure inset).

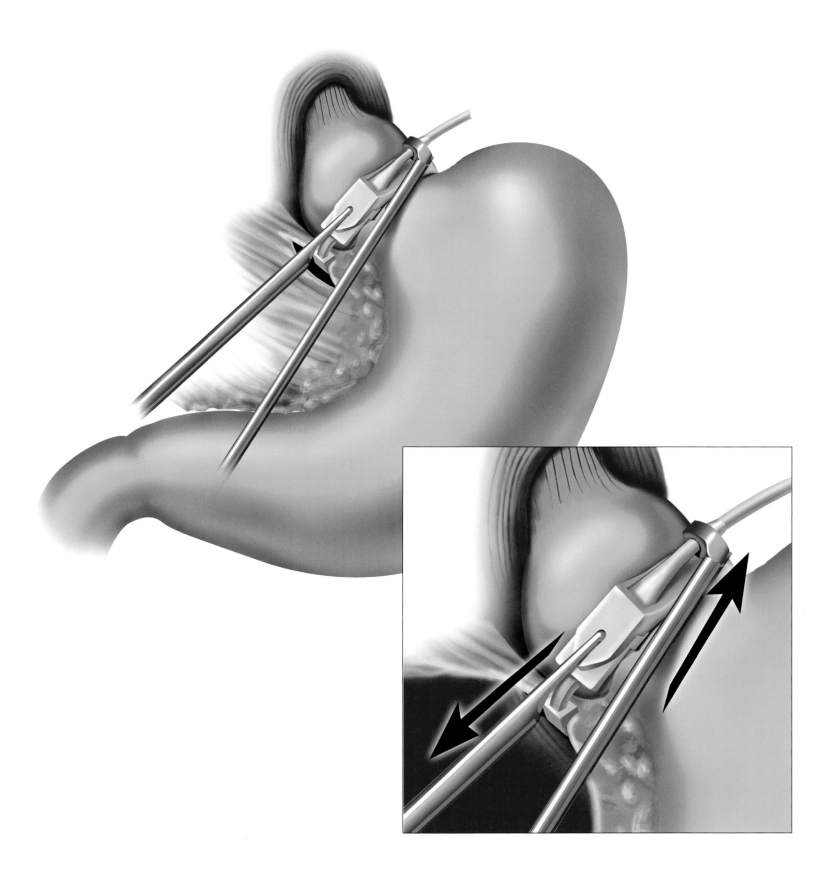

Gastrogastric Imbrication
(Securing the Band in Place)

13. At this point, the orogastric sizing balloon is removed.

14. In order to prevent band slippage or gastric prolapse, four to five interrupted braided nonabsorbable 2-0 sutures complete the gastrogastric imbrication. Alternatively, a running suture can plicate the anterior stomach over the band.

FIGURE G-a

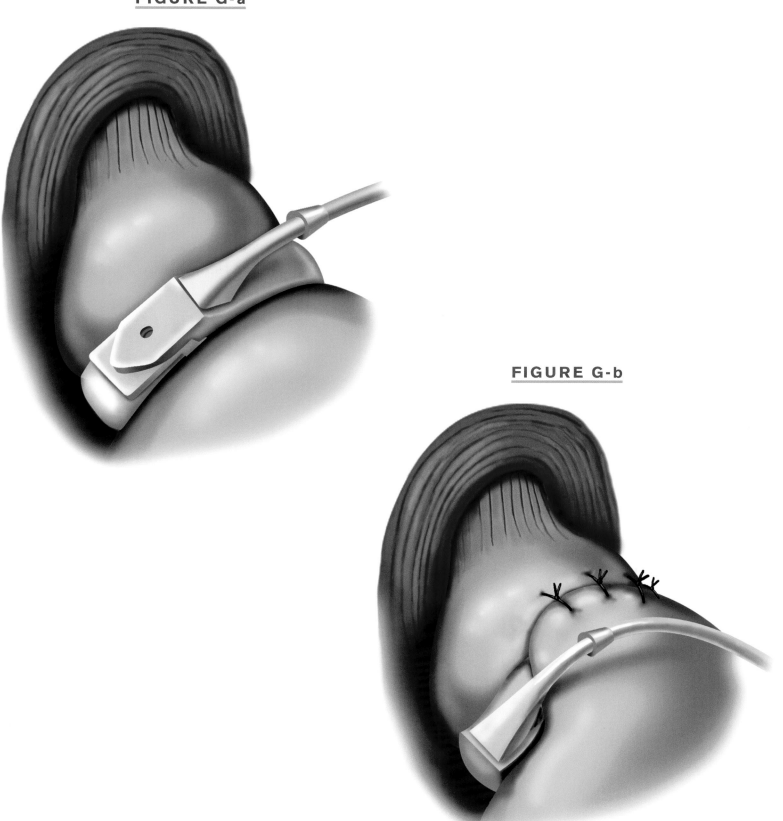

FIGURE G-b

Port Fixation

15. The distal tubing is retrieved through the left paramedian incision (12 mm port site).

16. The 15 mm port site is closed with an absorbable fascial suture; the remaining trocars are removed.

17. In order to facilitate fixation of the access port to the abdominal wall, the skin incision at the 12 mm site is enlarged to afford exposure. The access port and tubing are engaged and excess tubing is placed within the abdomen. The port is then tacked to the anterior rectus sheath with four 0 nonabsorbable sutures.

18. The wounds are irrigated, injected with local anesthetic, and closed with 4-0 absorbable subcuticular sutures. Steri-strips are applied.

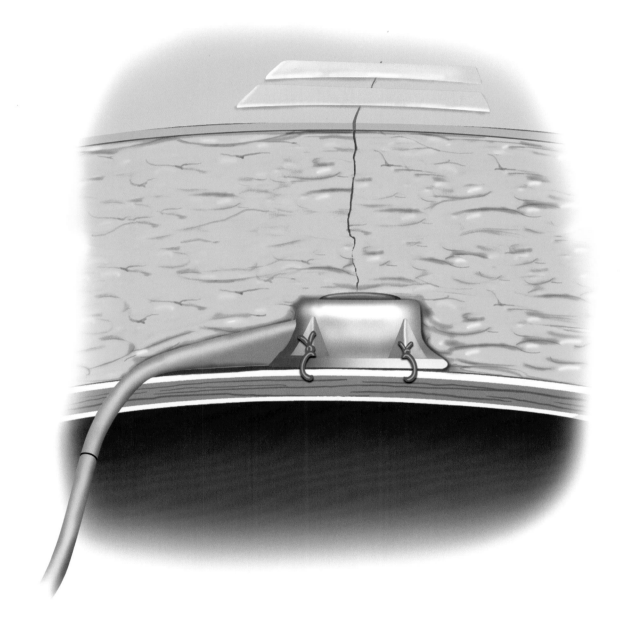

Postoperative Care

Pneumatic compression devices and subcutaneous heparin are continued postoperatively. A gastrograffin swallow is obtained on postoperative day 1 to confirm band position and to rule out leak or obstruction. If the contrast exam is normal, the patient is given a liquid diet. Postoperative adjustment of the band is withheld for 4 to 6 weeks to allow for sufficient encapsulation of the band and resolution of postoperative edema.

Suggested Readings

1. O'Brien PE, Brown WA, et al. Prospective study of laparoscopically placed, adjustable gastric band in the treatment of morbid obesity. *Br J of Surg*. 1999;86:113-118.

2. Chapman AE, Kiroff G, Game P, et al. Laparoscopic adjustable gastric banding in the treatment of obesity. A systematic literature review. *Surgery*. 2004;135(3):326-351.

3. Ponce J, Paynter S, Fromm R. Laparoscopic adjustable gastric banding; 1,014 consecutive cases. *J Am Coll Surg*. 2005; 201(4):529-535.

4. Ogunnaiko BO, Jones SB, Jones DB, Provost D, Whitten CW. Anesthetic considerations for bariatric surgery. *Anesth Analg*. 2002;95:1793-1805.

5. Kelly J, Tarnoff M, Shikora S, et al. Best practice recommendations for surgical care in weight loss surgery. *Obes Res*. 2005;13(2):227-233.

6. Jones DB, Schneider BE, Blackburn GL, Patient Safety in Obesity Surgery: Defining Best Practices (DVD). Ciné-Med, Inc., 127 Main Street North, Woodbury, CT 06798.

Commentary

Jeff W. Allen, M.D.
University of Louisville

The inception of a laparoscopic silicone adjustable gastric band in the 1990s was a quantum leap in bariatric surgery. Commonly abbreviated LAGB, this operation offered a very high rate of laparoscopic completion, a markedly shortened operating time and hospital stay, and perhaps most importantly, the ability to adjust the device postoperatively. Worldwide, surgeons have embraced this technology and this trend is continuing in America in 2005.

This chapter nicely outlines the operative steps in placing a LAGB. On first impression, this technique appears easy and straightforward. While the placement of a LAGB is certainly easier than a laparoscopic Roux-en-Y gastric bypass, it is not an easy operation. Many of the steps have been developed empirically by surgeons who experienced high complication rates initially with LAGB. A good example of this is the retrogastric tunnel, which has evolved from a widely dissected free space including the lesser sac to a blind, blunt tunnel with no dissection essentially "connecting the dots" between the right crus and angle of His.

The modern technique of LAGB is safe and effective and has markedly improved since the early American trials. Improvements in postoperative adjustment strategies have also improved weight loss and decreased postoperative complication. As outlined in this chapter, LAGB is a viable bariatric procedure and is increasing in popularity.

Christine Ren, M.D.
New York University School of Medicine

This chapter is a simple and thorough step-by-step description of how to surgically implant an adjustable gastric band using minimally invasive techniques. The band portrayed in this chapter comes in three different sizes, and can be tailored to the size, gender, and fat distribution of the patient. Many of the techniques can be modified, but in general are adapted for the morbidly obese physique of the patient.

Patient position is important for both patient safety and for surgeon comfort, particularly to maximize ergonomics. The French position with the patient's legs abducted may be helpful for the surgeon, but can be time consuming. The supine position with the surgeon standing on the patient's left is a simple alternative. This would then require a shift of the trocars horizontally across the abdomen in a configuration similar to a laparoscopic Nissen fundoplication, which optimizes angles and decreases instrument torque. The retrogastric placement of the band described represents the greatest evolution in this operation. Specifically termed "pars flaccida," this plane of dissection and band placement has significantly reduced the incidence of gastric prolapse (band slippage) as compared to the earlier "perigastric" dissection.

The gastrogastric imbrication to secure the band is sufficient to maintain band placement. Additional sutures to secure the stomach to the crus is unnecessary and may increase the risk of band erosion. Removal of a hefty anterior fat pad may facilitate suturing by exposing the upper gastric pouch more clearly and ensuring that the suture goes through stomach wall rather than fat.

The most important recent development has been the recognition of small-to-moderate–sized hiatal hernias in this patient population. It is critical to reduce the sliding hernia and primarily repair the crural defect before placing the band. Not only will this prevent future gastroesophageal reflux from developing, but will decrease the risk of gastric perforation during the pars flaccida dissection and the risk of early postoperative obstruction. Repairing the hiatal hernia simultaneously with band placement does not increase the risk of gastric prolapse and should be performed quite liberally. The surgeon who follows the steps of this chapter should be able achieve reproducible results.

David A. Provost, M.D., Parkland Hospital
University of Texas Southwestern Medical Center

Laparoscopic adjustable gastric banding (LAGB) provides the benefits of minimally invasive surgery for the surgical management of morbid obesity, with significantly lower perioperative morbidity and mortality than the Roux-en-Y gastric bypass or the vertical banded gastroplasty. Ease of insertion extends laparoscopic benefits to the extremes of obesity, with rapid recovery and potential reversibility.

Reported outcomes following LAGB vary widely in the literature. Adoption of the "pars flaccida" technique of LAGB placement, instead of the initially described "perigastric" technique, greatly reduced the incidence of posterior prolapse and band erosion. Principles of the pars flaccida technique include creation of a very small proximal pouch, posterior dissection just below the crura above the reflection of the bursa omentalis, improved anterior suture fixation of the fundus and anterior gastric wall over the band, and complete deflation of the band at the time of placement.

As described in the chapter, the pars flaccida technique for band placement utilizes five or six ports, including the liver retactor. Insertion of the band through the abdominal wall, as depicted, obviates the need for a 15 mm port, permitting placement of a 12 mm port in the left subcostal position. Excision of the anterior fat pad overlying the gastroesophageal junction allows improved exposure of the angle of His, dissection of which should stop prior to the most superior short gastric vessels. Initial insertion of the band, prior to creation of the retrogastric tunnel, eliminates the need for the second right-sided 5 mm port for band manipulation. Placing the tail of the band tubing near the angle of His, between the diaphragm and spleen, facilitates grasping of the tubing by the instrument passed behind the gastroesophageal junction as depicted. The band is placed at the "equator" of a 15 mL intragastric balloon pulled back to rest snugly against the crura at the gastroesophageal junction. Deflation of the balloon and retraction of the tube prior to closing the buckle of the band and placing the imbricating gastrogastric sutures ensures creation of a small "virtual" pouch and eliminates the risk of inadvertent suturing of the balloon. The most superior of these sutures must include the fundus near the angle of His to avoid lateral prolapse.

Inflation or adjustment of the band is not performed until a solid diet is initiated at 5 to 6 weeks postoperatively. Successful weight loss with the LAGB is dependent on proper band adjustment. Frequent follow-up evaluations, with adjustments every 4 to 6 weeks as needed for the first year or two provide optimal results.

Paul E. O'Brien, M.D., The Alfred Hospital
Monash University

The key elements to Lap-Band placement are well described in the text. The following comments are to highlight some additional actions or differences in technique which I find can be helpful.

Massive hepatomegaly makes the surgery much harder. The positive predictors of hepatomegaly include male patients, BMI > 50 kg/m^2, high waist circumference, and insulin resistance or clinical diabetes. Preoperative very low calorie diets such as Optifast for 6 weeks is particularly helpful in selected patients.

By far, the best and most cost effective retraction of the liver is achieved with the Nathanson liver retractor. However, you must expect to need time and experience to place it correctly and easily. In retracting the lateral segment of the left lobe, attempt to draw it anteriorly and to the patient's right. Avoid having the vertical component of the retractor in the groove of the falciform ligament.

The precise point for penetrating the peritoneum on the posterior surface of the lesser sac near the right crus is critical for safety and effectiveness. It should be about 0.5 mm in front of the anterior border of the right crus as close as possible to its lower end. The grasper or Lap-Band placer should pass safely and very easily from there to the point of dissection at the angle of His.

I use the calibration tube to determine if the Lap-Band is going to be too tight. Try to anticipate a problem with excess perigastric fat and open a Lap-Band VG for these patients. If you have placed a 10 cm Lap-Band, dissect the lesser curve and anterior gastric fat until the closed band rotates freely while the calibration tube is in place.

I use the balloon on the calibration tube only to identify the esophago-gastric junction by impacting the balloon at the lower esophageal sphincter. The Lap-Band should pass over the highest point of the balloon, not the base of the balloon. If you do the latter, the gastric pouch will be too big and prolapse or symmetrical enlargement may progressively occur. Once the correct line of placement is established and prior to closing the band, the balloon is deflated.

The anterior fixation must commence near (within 1 cm) the greater curve and must continue until the anterior gastric wrap comes close to, but not touching, the buckle. Sometmes four or even five sutures are needed.

I am happy for my patients to start clear oral fluid as soon as they have recovered from the anesthetic. I do a barium meal the following morning to document initial position. I avoid gastrograffin which is unpleasant to take and can lead to vomiting.

Laparoscopic Hepatic Resection

Similar to conventional open techniques, the minimally invasive approach to liver surgery utilizes specialized equipment, including the Nd:YAG laser, ultrasonic dissector, argon beam coagulator, fibrin sealant, endoscopic staplers, and an automatic clip applier. Laparoscopic ultrasound (LUS) proves beneficial in delineating the intraoperative anatomy and identifying lesions contained within the parenchyma.

Laparoscopic techniques are used for diagnostic purposes or for treating benign and/or metastatic disease (wedge resection or segmentectomy), in addition to large/complex hepatic cysts. Primary hepatic tumors may be too large for a safe approach with minimally invasive techniques. A relatively new indication for performing a laparoscopic liver resection is for a living donor left lateral segmentectomy.

FIGURE A-a,b

Surgical Anatomy

One must possess a clear understanding of the difference between the morphologic and functional anatomy of the liver. The liver is functionally divided into a right and left side by Cantlie's line, which is a plane that connects the medial border of the gallbladder to the posterior inferior vena cava (IVC) (Figure A-a). The liver is further divided into eight Couinaud segments based on the portal and hepatic venous circulatory pattern (Figure A-b). The caudate lobe is designated segment I. The left lobe is divided into a lateral section (segments II and III) and a medial segment (IV). The right lobe is divided into an anterior section and a posterior section, each of which has a superior and inferior segment. Segments V, VI, VII, and VIII correspond to the anterior inferior, posterior inferior, posterior superior, and anterior superior segments, respectively. Liver resections are classified as either anatomic or non-anatomic, depending on whether the segmental anatomical classification is observed.

FIGURE A-a

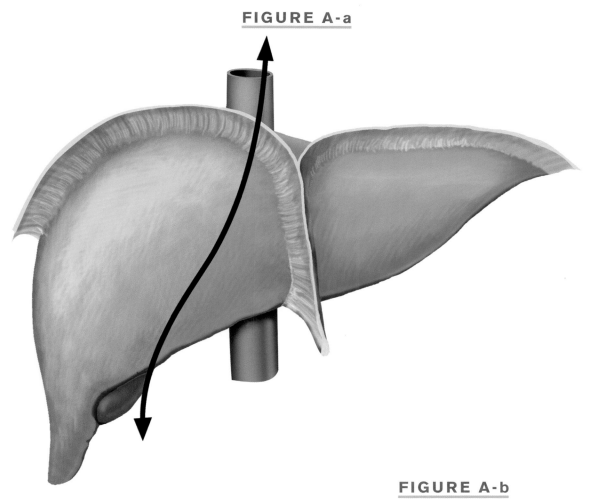

FIGURE A-b

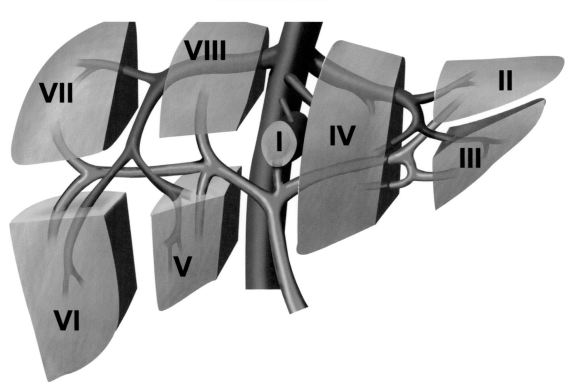

Preoperative Preparation

1. Sequential compression devices and subcutaneously-administered heparin may be used for prophylaxis against deep venous thrombosis. A first-generation cephalosporin is administered for antibiotic prophylaxis. The stomach is decompressed with either an oro- or nasogastric tube and the bladder is emptied with a urinary catheter after induction of general anesthesia. Large bore intravenous access is obtained.

FIGURE B

Operating Room Setup

2. The patient is placed in a modified lithotomy position. All pressure points must be adequately padded.

3. The surgeon stands between the patient's legs. The assistant(s) is situated to the patient's left, while the camera operator stands on the patient's right side.

4. The video monitors are stationed at both sides of the patient's head to facilitate adequate viewing from either side of the table. A laparotomy tray should be available in the event that conversion is necessary.

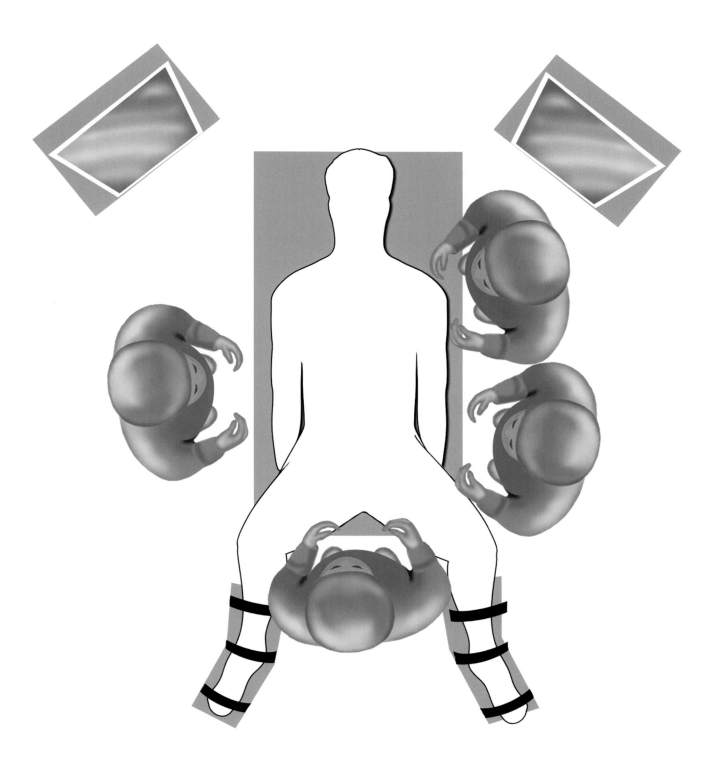

FIGURE C-a,b

Access and Port Placement

5. A supraumbilical incision is used to gain access to the abdomen via an open or closed technique. A 10/11 mm port is placed here and the laparoscope is inserted. Pneumoperitoneal pressure is set to 12 mm Hg to 15 mm Hg. A 30° angled scope facilitates obtaining crucial images. A careful exploration is performed to ensure that no injury occurred during port insertion and that no other abnormalities are present.

6. All subsequently placed ports should be at least 10 mm in size to allow for repositioning the camera during the course of the procedure. A minimum of three more ports are usually necessary (Figure C-a). An irrigation/suction probe is placed through the right subcostal port and the working instruments through the other two.

7. If a more complex procedure is planned and two surgeons are available, the four-hands approach can be utilized, which requires placing five working ports (Figure C-b). Using this technique, one surgeon operates the ultrasonic dissector and grasper, and the other controls the scissors and clip applier. Alternatively, a hand port can be placed (dashed line) to aid in the dissection and specimen retrieval.

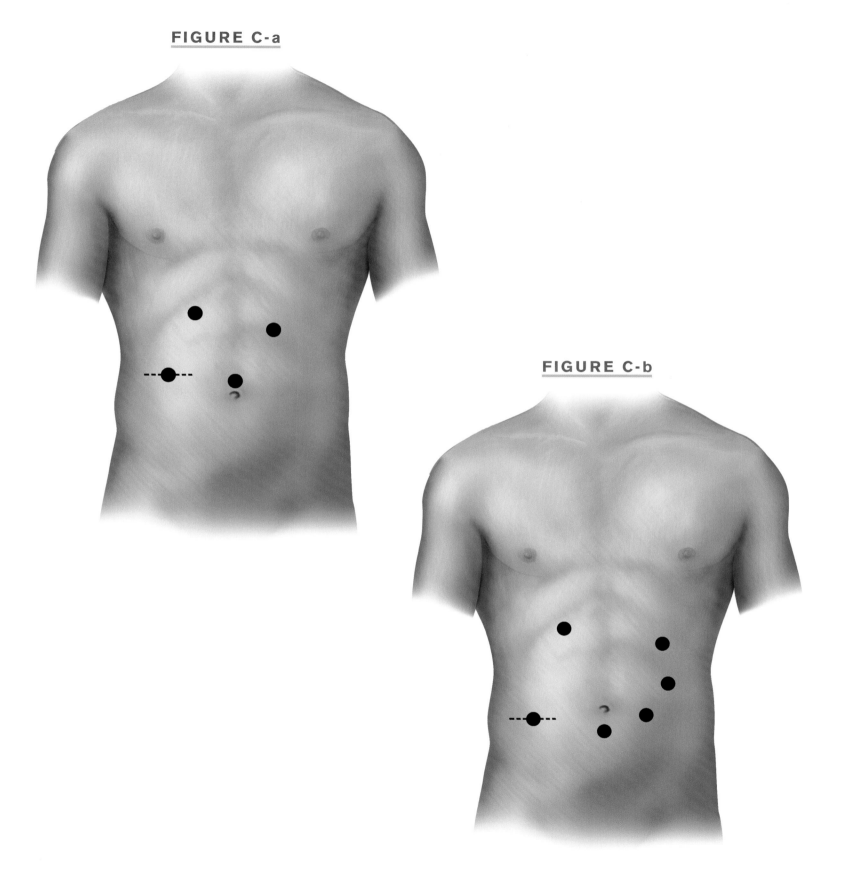

FIGURE C-a

FIGURE C-b

Mobilizing the Liver

8. The hepatic ligaments are divided in a similar manner as with open surgery. The round ligament and falciform ligament are divided between surgical clips or with an endoscopic stapling device to allow the liver to be mobilized from the abdominal wall. Next, depending on where the area of interest is located, the right and/or left triangular ligament is divided to further mobilize each lobe.

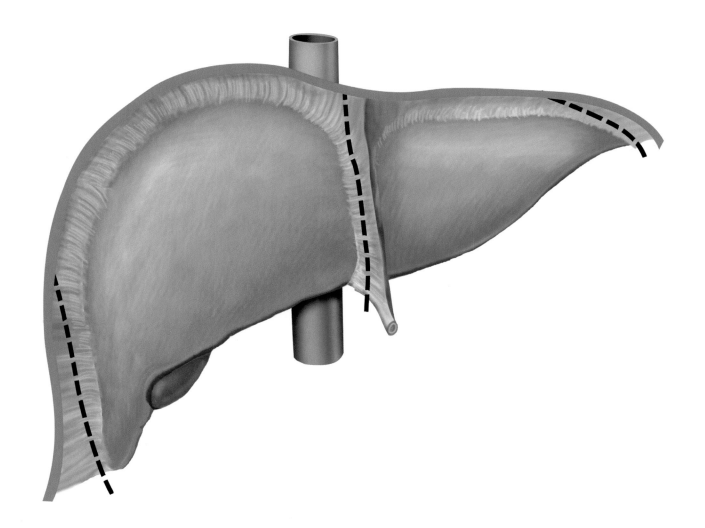

Laparoscopic Treatment of Simple Liver Cysts

Simple cysts of the liver contain clear, serous fluid and usually remain asymptomatic. However, as cysts enlarge in size and increase in number, they can become symptomatic by compressing adjacent structures and can cause abdominal discomfort, gastric or duodenal obstruction, jaundice, or even portal hypertension. They can also become secondarily infected, bleed, or rupture into the peritoneal cavity.

FIGURE E-a,b

Draining and Excising the Cyst Wall

1. Liver cysts usually appear as a bluish-colored, convex-shaped protrusion from the liver surface. Once the dome of the cyst is clearly identified, curved scissors or a cauterized hook are used to puncture the anterior cyst wall (Figure E-a). The cyst fluid is aspirated and sent for Gram's stain and culture. The cyst usually collapses as the fluid is removed. The opening in the cyst wall is then enlarged and any remaining fluid is drained.

2. Next, the exposed part of the cyst wall is excised. The portion of the wall that is protruding above the surface of the liver is grasped and circumferentially excised with a harmonic scalpel, cautery, or scissors to within 2 mm of the junction between the cyst wall and liver parenchyma (Figure E-b). The specimen is sent for pathologic review. Excision of the cyst wall is important to assess for the presence of malignancy and to prevent fluid reaccumulation.

FIGURE E-a

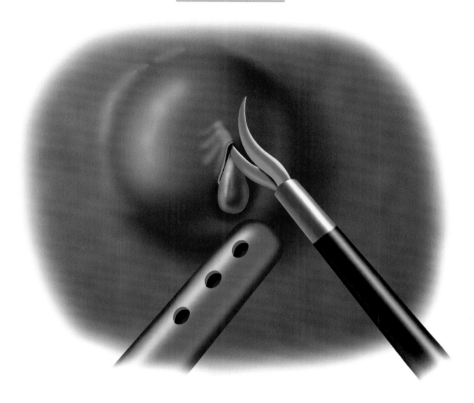

FIGURE E-b

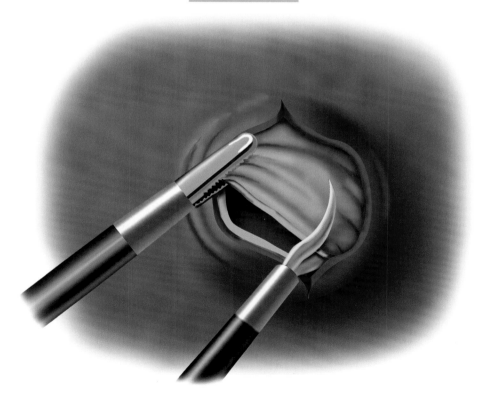

Laparoscopic Treatment of Hydatid Cysts

Hydatid cysts form secondary to a parasite infection from the tapeworm *Echinococcus granulosus*. Hydatid cysts can become secondarily infected by bacteria, and can lead to cholangitis by rupturing into the bile ducts. Anteriorly located cysts should undergo complete cyst excision, while cysts located posteriorly or near the IVC should be "unroofed" using a similar technique as that described for treating a simple cyst. Prior to draining the cyst, it should first be injected with alcohol or hypertonic saline to kill the indwelling parasites. Its contents are then aspirated, being careful to prevent peritoneal spillage, and the dome of the cyst wall is removed.

FIGURE F-a,b

Excising a Hydatid Cyst

1. For hydatid cysts located on the anterior surface of the liver, total pericystectomy is the preferred procedure. The cyst need not be injected or aspirated dry if it is to be removed entirely. Hydatid cystic disease often produces perihepatic inflammatory adhesions; these are divided with electrocautery to clearly expose the cyst. Once exposed, the liver capsule (Glisson's capsule) surrounding the cyst is circumferentially scored using an Nd:YAG laser set at 50 W (Figure F-a).

2. Slow, meticulous dissection is then continued circumferentially around the lesion (Figure F-b). An electrocautery spatula or an ultrasonic dissector (set to low power) can be used to perform the dissection. Blood vessels and bile ducts larger than 1 mm to 2 mm in diameter should be individually ligated with surgical clips or a stapling device in order to maintain hemostasis and prevent postoperative bile leaks. A double-clipping technique should be employed to avoid inadvertent avulsion of a single clip during the dissection. Selective use of arteriography and cholangiography (via a cholecystectomy and transcystic approach) can be helpful in delineating the anatomy of large cysts.

3. Once the entire cyst is excised en bloc, it is extracted through the periumbilical incision in an entrapment sac, being careful not to spill any contents in the peritoneal cavity. The fascial incision may need to be enlarged in order to remove the specimen, which can also be morselized inside the bag in order to facilitate extraction. Fibrin sealant can be injected into the cyst cavity to assist with hemostasis and help prevent a bile leak.

FIGURE F-a

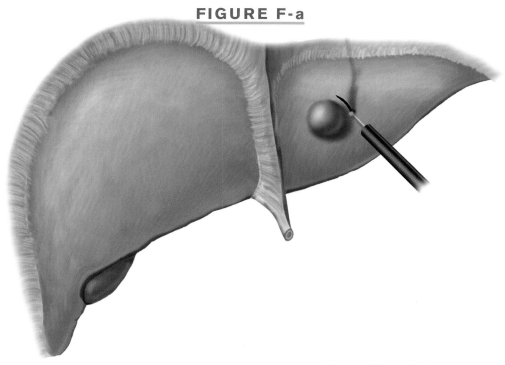

FIGURE F-b

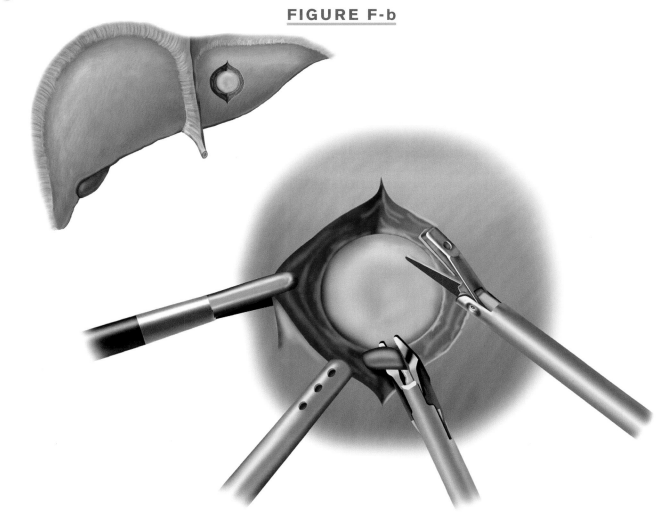

Laparoscopic Wedge Resection or Enucleation

Laparoscopic techniques can be used to resect focal liver lesions. A 2 cm circumferential margin should be obtained. Patients with a solitary liver metastasis are ideal candidates for the minimally invasive approach. The technique for enucleating these lesions is similar to that as described for excising a hydatid cyst.

FIGURE G

Performing a Wedge Resection

1. Using the Nd:YAG laser, Glisson's capsule is circumferentially incised 2 cm from the lesion. An irrigation and suction catheter is used to clear the smoke and keep the operating field dry during the course of the dissection. Electrocautery, an endoscopic stapling device (2.5 mm staples), and/or an ultrasonic dissector are used to continue the circumferential dissection around the lesion, being careful to maintain an adequate margin of resection. Atraumatic graspers are used to expose the dissection plane. A double-clipping technique can be used to control and ligate the larger blood vessels and bile ducts.

2. An extraction bag is used to extract the specimen through the umbilical fascial incision. The resected specimen should not be morselized, as this will interfere with an appropriate pathologic examination. Fibrin sealant is applied to the cavity or cut surface of the liver. For large resections, a cholangiogram should be obtained via a cholecystectomy and transcystic approach to assess for evidence of a bile leak.

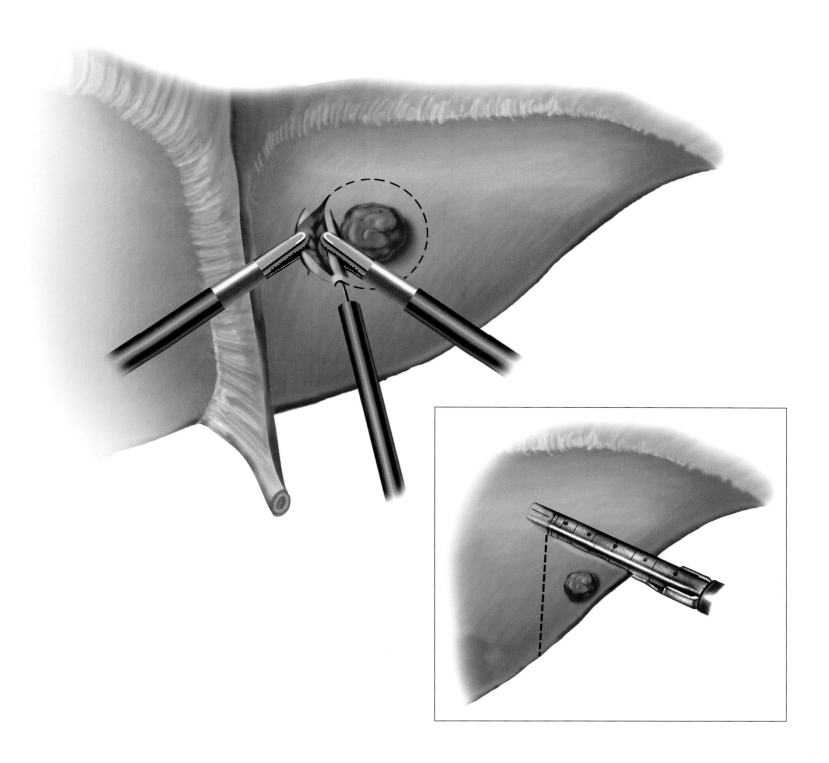

Laparoscopic Left Lateral Segmentectomy

For larger lesions that are not amenable to a wedge resection, a laparoscopic segmentectomy can be performed. This technique adheres to functional anatomic divisions. Lesions located in the left lateral lobe can also be resected laparoscopically, but should only be performed by surgeons with expertise in open liver surgery and advanced laparoscopic techniques. The use of a hand port greatly assists in the exposure and dissection. The principles for performing a left lateral segmentectomy (segments II and III) can be applied to other segmentectomies. Although some surgeons choose not to obtain control of the porta hepatis, we have described this technique below.

FIGURE H-a,b

Controlling the Porta Hepatis

1. The lesser omentum is opened to expose the portal triad. Careful dissection is used to clear the surrounding tissue from the portal triad. A right-angled dissector is gently passed posterior to the portal vein (Figure H-a).

2. Using this dissector, umbilical tape is doubly passed around the portal triad, thus forming a circumferential loop. The two ends of the umbilical tape are exteriorized through a lateral port site. These two ends are then passed through a section of rubber tubing, which is cut long enough to allow for one end to be in close proximity to the portal triad and the other to remain outside the patient. This configuration creates a tourniquet that can be tightened, should it be necessary, around the portal triad by sliding the rubber tubing toward the patient (Figure H-b). Tourniquet occlusion of the portal triad, or the Pringle maneuver, should not be applied for more than 30 minutes at a time.

FIGURE H-a

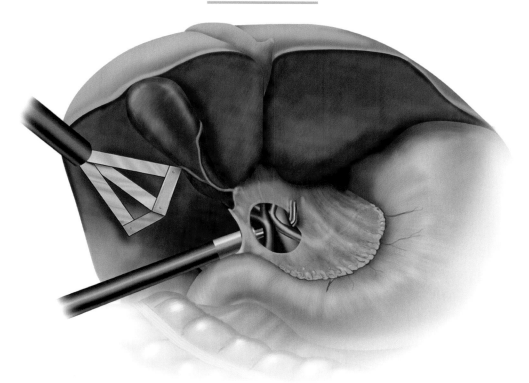

FIGURE H-b

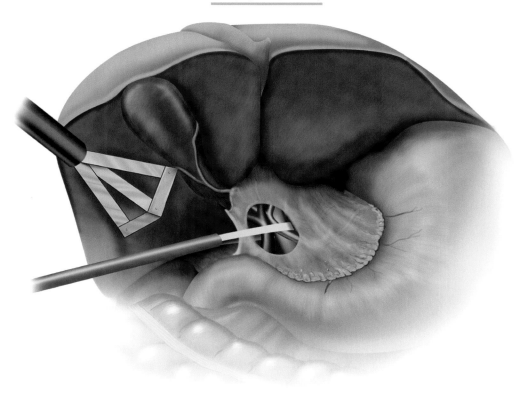

FIGURE I

Ligating the Left Hepatic Vein and Resecting the Specimen

3. The falciform ligament and left triangular ligament are completely divided in order to expose the suprahepatic IVC and root of the left hepatic vein. The section of the left hepatic vein outside the liver is clearly exposed, bluntly dissected free of surrounding tissue, and carefully encircled with a right-angled dissector. If the left hepatic vein is not amenable to extrahepatic exposure and ligation, the procedure may be converted to a laparotomy or pursued laparoscopically, as some surgeons routinely do not control the hepatic vein.

4. Once isolated, the left hepatic vein is ligated with a 0 silk suture. Intracorporeal knot-tying techniques should be used in order to avoid tension on the vein, and the ends of the suture should be cut long to prevent knot slippage.

5. Once the left hepatic vein is ligated, Glisson's capsule is incised with a Nd:YAG laser or electrocautery along a line that is to the left and parallel to the falciform ligament. Deeper dissection through the liver parenchyma is continued with a combination of electrocautery, ultrasonic dissection, laparoscopic Kelly fracture technique, and/or hydrodissection (high velocity, high pressure water). The dissection should be carried out in an inferior to superior direction, thus dividing segment III prior to segment II. The field must be kept clean and dry with an irrigation/suction device. The double-clip technique should be used to ligate all vascular and biliary pedicles. As the dissection proceeds superiorly, the last major structure to be encountered will be the intrahepatic left hepatic vein.

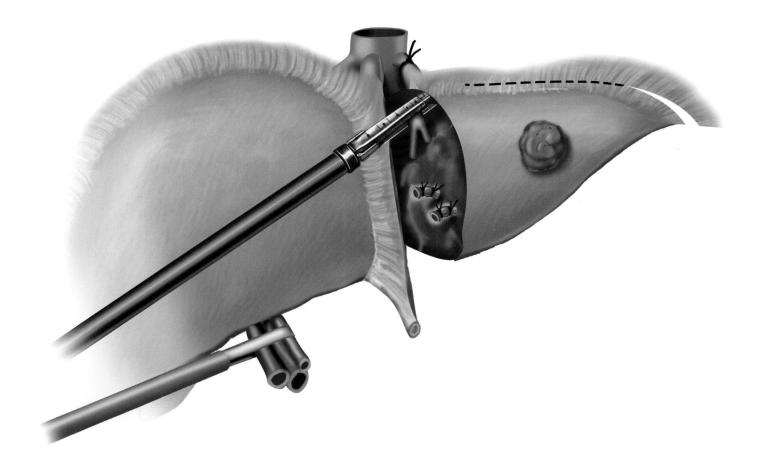

Ligating the Left Hepatic Vein and Resecting the Specimen, Continued

6. The left hepatic vein is divided with a single firing of an endoscopic linear stapler (2.5-2.8 mm staples). Any remaining parenchymal attachments are divided to completely separate the left lateral lobe from the liver. Any bleeding from the raw surface of the cut liver may be controlled with a combination of electrocautery, argon beam coagulation, and application of fibrin sealant to the entire surface. Furthermore, a greater omental flap can be used to cover the cut edge.

7. The specimen is placed in an extraction bag and removed through the umbilical incision. Due to the large specimen size, the umbilical incision is enlarged and part of the specimen (away from the lesion) can be morselized, if necessary, to facilitate extraction. If bile leak is a concern, a cholangiogram can be obtained (via a cholecystectomy and transcystic approach).

8. The right upper quadrant is observed for adequate hemostasis and/or any evidence of a bile leak. One or two closed suction drains are left in place through the lateral port sites. The trocars are removed under direct vision and the fascia and skin incisions are closed in the usual manner.

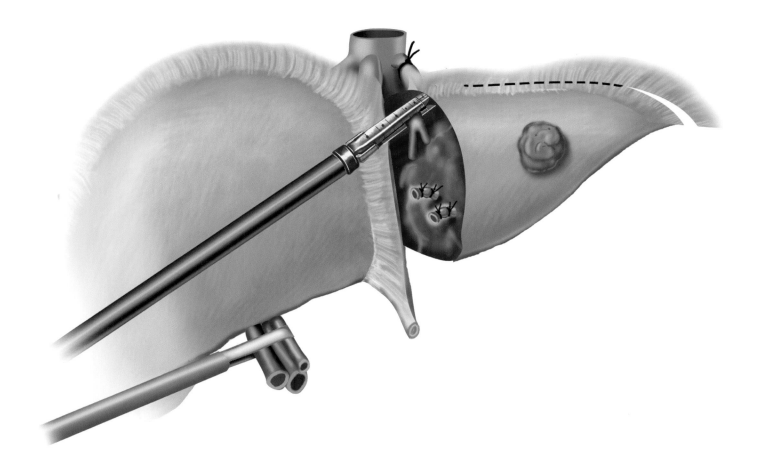

Postoperative Care

Pneumatic compression devices and/or subcutaneous heparin are continued postoperatively. Antibiotics are usually continued for 24 hours postoperatively. Patients are usually able to tolerate liquids and solid food within 24 to 48 hours after the operation. Closed suction drains can be removed by postoperative day 2 or 3 if there is no evidence of a bile leak. Liver function tests, coagulation profile, serum electrolytes, and complete blood counts are monitored as necessary.

Suggested Readings

1. Blumgart LH, ed. *Surgery of the Liver and Biliary Tract*. 2nd ed. New York: Churchill Livingstone; 1994.

2. Katkhouda N, Mavor E, Gugenheim J, Mouiel J. Laparoscopic management of benign cystic lesions of the liver. *J Hepatobiliary Pancreat Surg*. 2000;7:212-217.

3. Cherqui D, Husson E, Hammoud R, et al. Laparoscopic liver resections: a feasibility study in 30 patients. *Ann Surg*. 2000;232(6):753-762.

Commentary

Morris E. Franklin, Jr., M.D.
Texas Endosurgery Institute

Preparation of the patient for laparoscopic liver surgery should include preoperative imaging. In addition to having radiographic images available, preparation should be made for intraoperative ultrasound should the need arise. In the operating room, I prefer to stand on the patient's left side. The camera operator also stands on the left while the assistant stands on the patient's right side. The monitors are placed at the head so as to facilitate moving of equipment and personnel about the table.

Large hepatic cysts (6-7 cm) as well as those that are enlarging or symptomatic, may be drained surgically. Drainage of hepatic cysts may be performed sharply with scissors or, preferably, an ultrasonic scalpel may be used to drain the cyst and obtain hemostasis. In wedge resection of hepatic lesions, surgical staplers and a bipolar device should be readily available in the event that a deep resection might be required. Peripherally located lesions may be resected by merely stapling across the send-out portion of the left lobe of the liver. We have recently begun to use staple line buttress material (SeamGuard) to help control bleeding. We rarely utilize the outlined method for controlling the porta hepatis. Instead, we control bleeding as it is encountered. When control is necessary, a laparoscopic bulldog Glassman clamp is preferable to a tourniquet as it frees up a hand and provides a convenient way for occlusion of the porta hepatis.

Justin S. Wu, M.D., Kaiser Permanente Medical Center
University of California, San Diego

The authors have carried laparoscopic surgery to a higher level of achievement with this chapter. Most laparoscopic hepatic procedures have been limited to diagnostic procedures such as laparoscopic-guided liver biopsies and small peripheral wedge resections. With the recent advent of laparoscopic ultrasound, laparoscopic biopsies of intrahepatic lesions are feasible and more accurate. In addition, one can detect tumors that are often missed by CT scans.

Recently, therapeutic laparoscopic liver operations have been performed with treatment of biliary cysts (excisions, evacuation, and marsupialization), hydatid cysts, and wedge resections of small primary or metastatic neoplasms. With the innovations of laparoscopic cavitron ultrasonic surgical aspirator (CUSA), the argon beam coagulator (ABC), Nd:YAG laser, and fibrin sealant, formal laparoscopic hepatic segmentectomies are now feasible.

This chapter succinctly describes the fundamentals of preoperative preparation, operating room setup, access and port placements, and mobilization of the liver. Specific laparoscopic treatment of simple liver cysts, hydatid cysts, wedge resection and enucleation, and a formal left lateral segmentectomy are shown with clear explanations and vivid illustrations. The latter procedure is certainly revolutionary, and with mastering these basic principles, one can apply these techniques to other anatomic or nonanatomic liver resections.

Scott R. Johnson, M.D., Beth Israel Deaconess Medical Center Harvard Medical School

Laparoscopic hepatobiliary surgery has primarily included cholecystectomy, common bile duct exploration, and cyst fenestration. In the last several years, a number of authors have published data describing techniques for resectional procedures. This includes techniques for nonanatomic, segmental, and, more recently, formal lateral segmentectomy, right and left hepatectomy, and even right trisegmentectomy. The development of these procedures is the natural progression of minimally invasive techniques that are made possible by improved understanding of hepatic anatomy, as well as improved equipment.

Hilar dissection to include isolation of the porta hepatis, for a Pringle maneuver or for isolation of lobar vessels and bile ducts, can be accomplished readily with use of the harmonic scalpel. Parenchymal dissection is generally achieved using any or all of a number of devices, including the harmonic scalpel, tissue link, or endovascular staplers. While each has its proponents, it is likely that all should be given consideration during performance of resectional procedures. The importance of using a hand-assisted technique cannot be overemphasized for all but the most easily accessible lesions. Hand assistance greatly facilitates parenchymal dissection by allowing the assistant to open the dissection plane and also aid in hemostasis when larger vessels are encountered. Tactile reinforcement during non-anatomic resections is paramount to achieving adequate tumor margins and can only be obtained with hand-assisted techniques. Judicious use of laparoscopic ultrasound should also be considered an essential component of minimal invasive hepatobiliary surgical armamentarium. The frequent use of ultrasound not only will aid in determining resection planes, but will also facilitate identification of major portal pedicles or hepatic venous tributaries that will require meticulous technique for identification and control. Ultrasound will also prove itself during nonanatomic resections to ensure adequate tissue margins are preserved.

Steven M. Rudich, M.D., Ph.D.
University of Cincinnati College of Medicine

In preparing the patient for surgery, we often place a central line to ensure our ability to infuse large volumes of fluid, as well as to measure the central venous pressure. Our technique is to perform most hepatic procedures with two surgeons (and sometimes one assistant). The patient is placed supine. If a right-sided liver lesion is encountered, we place the patient in a left-lateral decubitus position. Furthermore, for patients with cirrhosis, we monitor the coagulation function, as well as platelet counts. We tolerate an INR greater than 2.0, but we try to infuse fresh platelets if the count is less than 50,000 if the INR is elevated. Prior upper abdominal surgery, including cholecystectomy, should not preclude a try at laparoscopic liver surgery. The same applies for patients with ascites.

For access and port placement, we use a 10/12 mm balloon trocar. The balloon trocar allows us to pull up (water-ski) and as such, gives us more maneuverability during laparoscopy. There is wide variability in port size. We try to use 5 mm ports as much as possible, as the trocar size decreases risks of postoperative ascites becoming a significant issue—in terms of ascites leakage.

Instead of the technique outlined by the authors, we often use a hand-assist port to help in large or complex resections. To do this, a 7 cm to 8 cm skin incision is made (usually on the right side), slightly above the umbilicus. The rectus muscle is cauterized prior to entering the abdominal cavity. The Geldisc is placed. This allows you to use one hand to assist in dissection, as well as placement of instrument.

We use reticulating staplers liberally during laparoscopic liver surgery and have found them quite effective. We routinely staple across the round ligament and use the harmonic scalpel to "take down" the right and left triangular ligaments. This is especially helpful and safe when the patient has cirrhosis.

Excising the cyst wall can also be accomplished with the use of a harmonic scalpel. For large, complex cysts, the use of endoreticulating staplers may make the resection safer and simpler. I would note that we have found few instances to operate on simple hepatic cysts, as illustrated here. When cysts become complex, multiple, or if there is a suspicion of carcinoma, then sometimes there is cause to explore, sample and remove.

For the treatment of hydatid cysts, the operation can be performed using the laparoscope; for larger cysts, wedge resection may be easier and safer. Our bias has been to use as few clips as possible during laparoscopic hepatic surgery. The clips interfere with the use of staplers, as well as the harmonic scalpel. Both of these tools we rely on quite liberally. In such a large cyst, one should consider use of a hand port to ease dissection, as well as recovery of the specimen.

For wedge resection, most practitioners would consider a 1 cm margin as oncologically acceptable. Depending upon the presence of liver disease (i.e., cirrhosis), as well as placement of secondary lesions, we often treat patients with greater than one lesion. We have found the argon beam coagulator invaluable for marking the liver, as well as to achieve hemostasis. Depending upon the location of the lesion, we often use reticulating staplers to do most of the heavy lifting for wedge resections, especially for more peripherally based lesions. If the lesion is larger, we do not hesitate to place in a hand port to assist in surgery, as well as removal. We also rely quite heavily on intraoperative ultrasound. Using this device allows us to evaluate for other lesions, as well as to show us where major (and minor) hepatic veins and portal venous structures lay in relation to the lesion(s). Besides using fibrin sealant, there are a host of other hemostatic agents (Flo-Seal, Knu-Knot Surgical, fibrin glue), which should be available to assist the surgeon performing laparoscopic liver surgery.

For left lateral segmentectomy, with proper patient positioning, lesions in the right posterior segments (including segments VI and VII) are amenable to a laparoscopic approach. For a simple left lateral segmentectomy (or most other laparoscopic liver surgery), we have not had the need to control the porta in the same manner described by the authors, and do not. In many cases, it will be very difficult and unnecessary to obtain such control. We would advocate the use of a hand-assist port for all "major" hepatic resections, including a left lateral segmentectomy.

In performing a routine left lateral segmentectomy, we do not find that control of the left hepatic vein is warranted. After scoring the resection plane with the hot cautery, we would start paryenchymal dissection with the harmonic scalpel and use reticulating staplers liberally, especially in areas in which vascular/biliary structures are apparent. Most laparoscopic left lateral segmentectomies, with a hand-assist port can be performed in well under 2 hours. During the parenchymal dissection, we keep careful attention to the central venous pressure. We try to maintain these in the 5 mm Hg to 8 mm Hg range and will use vasodilators to achieve such. We believe this decreases intraoperative bleeding.

Patients tolerate these laparoscopic resections (whether wedge or partial lobectomies) quite well. We start oral intake the day following surgery and most patients are discharged home within 48 hours. For a routine exploration and radiofrequency ablation, many patients are discharged within 24 hours, if not the same day.

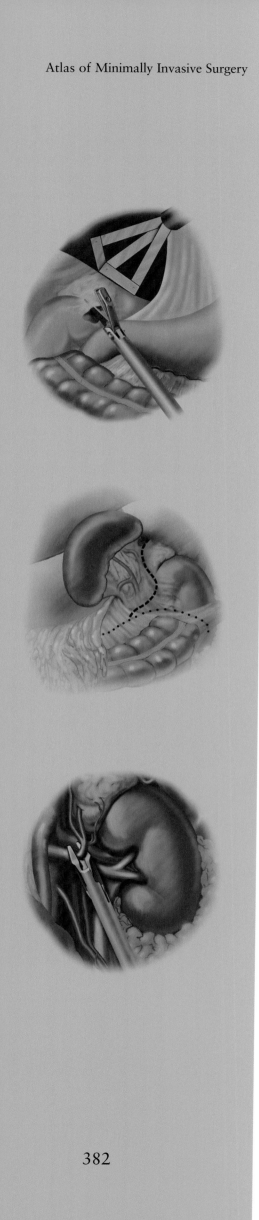

Laparoscopic Adrenalectomy

Laparoscopic adrenalectomy has become the procedure of choice in appropriately selected patients with pheochromocytoma, Cushing's syndrome, aldosteronoma (Conn's syndrome), adrenal metastases, and carcinoma and/or incidentaloma measuring less than 6 cm. While many surgeons will tackle large tumors as well, many believe that these tumors (> 6 cm) may be better approached through an open technique due to the high propensity for carcinoma and local invasiveness. The preoperative preparation of patients with hormonally active tumors is crucial for the overall success of adrenalectomies.

Anatomic differences between the right and left adrenal glands necessitate a slight variation in technique owing to differences in venous drainage and surrounding structures. Three different approaches have been described and utilized for performing a laparoscopic adrenalectomy: 1) transabdominal lateral flank approach, 2) anterior transabdominal approach, and 3) retroperitoneal approach. Most surgeons favor the transabdominal lateral flank approach for several reasons, including a large working space, gravity retraction of surrounding structures, and easy access high in the retroperitoneum. This technique shall be described in detail.

Preoperative Preparation

1. Patients with hormonally active tumors (e.g. pheochromocytoma) should be adequately treated and controlled prior to undergoing operation (e.g. with hydration and alpha blockade with phenoxybenzamine and if persistent tachycadia, followed by beta blockade). Sequential compression stockings and subcutaneous heparin may be used for prophylaxis against deep venous thrombosis. Intravenous antibiotics, usually a first-generation cephalosporin, are administered prophylactically. After induction of general anesthesia, the bladder is emptied with a urinary catheter and the stomach is decompressed with an orogastric tube. Laparoscopic ultrasonography may be helpful to identify the adrenal gland and adjacent structures in obese patients.

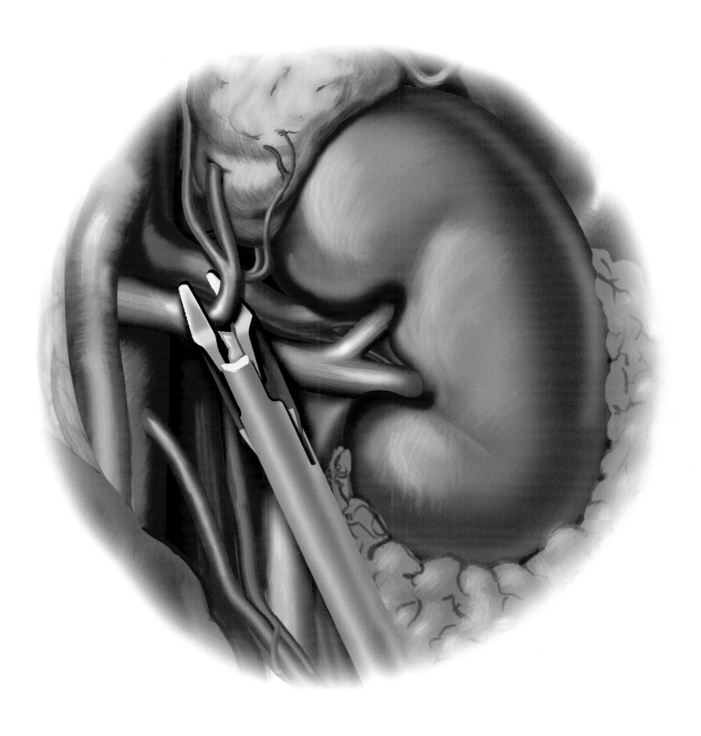

Right Adrenalectomy

Operating Room Setup

2. The patient is positioned in the lateral decubitus position with the right side rotated upward and the table flexed 30° at the waist. A pillow may be placed between the knees. Placing the patient in reverse Trendelenburg position further facilitates subsequent port placement and gravity retraction of adjacent organs.

3. All pressure points must be adequately padded and a bean-bag device is used to secure the patient's position when rotating the table to facilitate exposure and viewing during the procedure.

4. The surgeon and camera operator usually stand to the left or anterior to the patient, while the assistant stands on the opposite side of the table. The video monitors are stationed at both sides of the patient's head to facilitate adequate viewing from either side of the table. A laparotomy set should be readily available should emergent conversion be necessary secondary to uncontrolled bleeding.

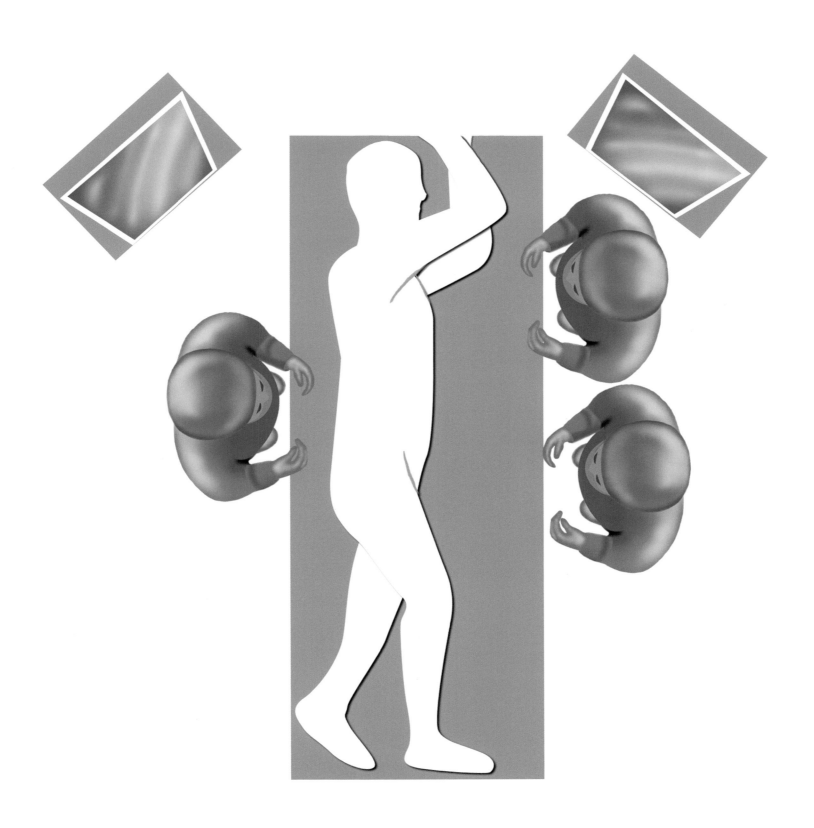

Access and Port Placement

5. The optimal configuration of port placement follows the subcostal margin. Initial access is obtained just medial to the anterior axillary line about two fingerbreadths below the costal margin. Pneumoperitoneum can be obtained with either an open or closed technique via a Veress needle.

6. A direct-view optical trocar can be utilized for placing the first port to minimize the incidence of intra-abdominal injury during this step.

7. The remaining three ports are placed under direct vision, in an anterior to posterior direction. One port should be a 11 mm-sized port to allow for insertion of a surgical clip applier; the other two are 5 mm in size.

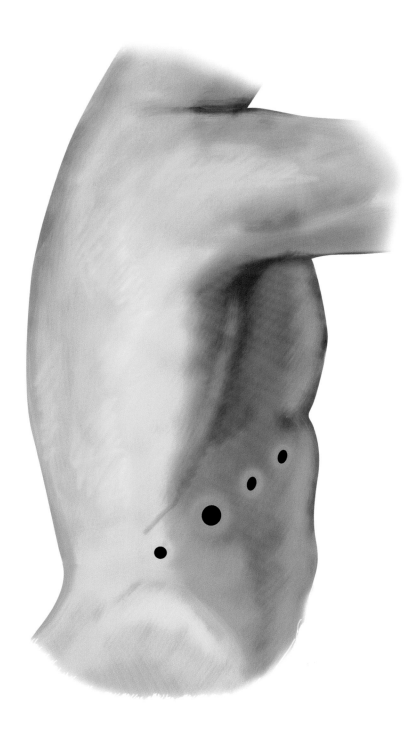

FIGURE C

Exposing the Right Adrenal Gland

8. Exploratory laparoscopy must first be performed to assess for any evidence of liver metastasis or other upper abdominal pathology.

9. The right lobe of the liver is mobilized anteriorly and medially by incising the triangular ligament to the level of the diaphragm. A liver retractor placed through the most medial port will adequately retract the right lobe once it has been mobilized. It is usually not necessary to mobilize the hepatic flexure of the colon. The right adrenal gland is situated in the perinephric fat at the superior pole of the right kidney and posterolateral to the inferior vena cava (IVC).

10. The adrenal gland is exposed from the overlying retroperitoneal and perinephric fat using a combination of ultrasonic coagulation and blunt dissection.

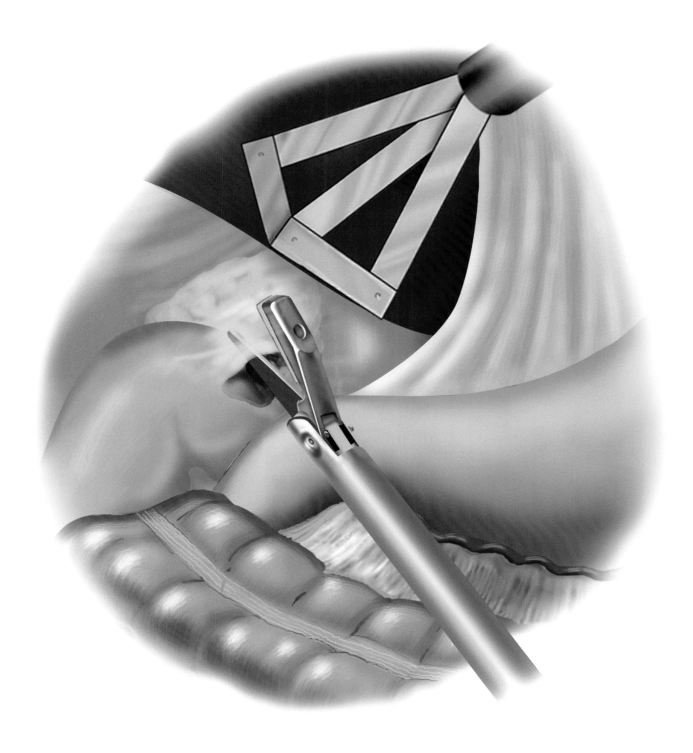

Dissecting the Right Adrenal Gland and Dividing the Right Adrenal Vein

11. The adrenal gland itself is manipulated by grasping the periadrenal fat or by gently pushing the gland with the instrument; care is taken not to violate the adrenal capsule in order to avoid spillage of tumor cells.

12. Dissection with an ultrasonic coagulator begins at the medial margin and is carried both superiorly and inferiorly to mobilize the adrenal gland off the IVC. It is crucial to maintain exposure and orientation of the IVC at all times to avoid injury. In this manner the adrenal gland is reflected laterally.

13. The right adrenal vein is exposed as the gland is mobilized off the IVC. The right adrenal vein is short and empties directly into the IVC. The adrenal vein is circumferentially mobilized with a right angle dissector and divided between surgical clips (two clips are placed on the IVC side).

14. The adrenal gland is then dissected free from its surrounding tissue and attachments using an ultrasonic coagulator. The numerous small arterial branches that supply the adrenal gland are usually adequately controlled with ultrasonic coagulation.

15. Once completely freed, the gland is placed in an impermeable entrapment sac and retrieved through the 11 mm port site. The specimen should be evaluated to confirm that the lesion lies within the resected specimen. The operative field is inspected for adequate hemostasis and secure positioning of the surgical clips. The ports are removed under direct vision and the fascia and skin incisions are closed in the usual manner.

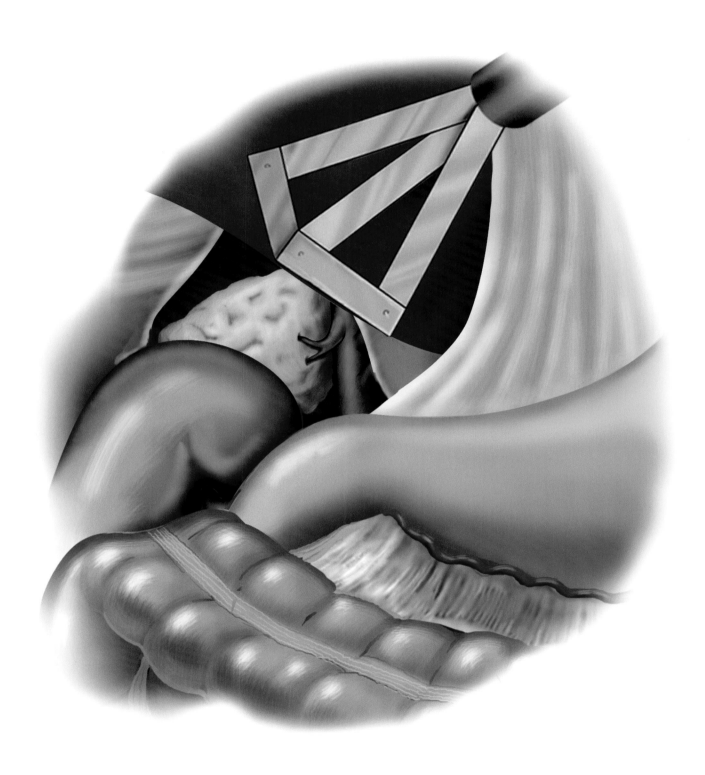

Left Adrenalectomy

FIGURE E

Operating Room Setup

1. The patient is positioned in the lateral decubitus position with the left side rotated upward and the table flexed 30° at the waist. A pillow may be placed between the knees. Placing the patient in reverse Trendelenburg position further facilitates subsequent port placement and gravity retraction of adjacent organs.

2. All pressure points must be adequately padded and a bean-bag device is used to secure the patient's position when rotating the table to facilitate exposure and viewing during the procedure.

3. The surgeon and camera operator usually stand to the right or anterior to the patient, while the assistant stands on the opposite side of the table. The video monitors are stationed at both sides of the patient's head to facilitate adequate viewing from either side of the table. A laparotomy set should be readily available should emergent conversion be necessary secondary to uncontrolled bleeding.

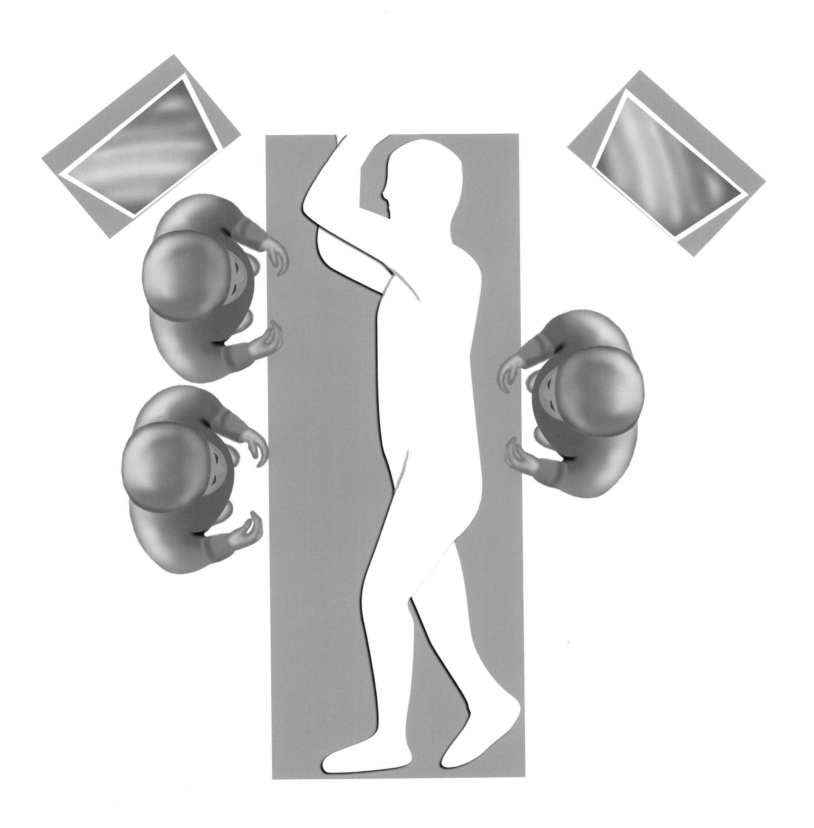

Access and Port Placement

4. The optimal configuration of port placement follows the subcostal margin. Initial access is obtained just medial to the anterior axillary line about two fingerbreadths below the costal margin. Pneumoperitoneum can be obtained with either an open or closed technique via a Veress needle.

5. A direct view optical trocar can be utilized for placing the first port to minimize the incidence of intra-abdominal injury during this step.

6. The remaining three ports are placed under direct vision, in an anterior to posterior direction. One port should be a 11 mm-sized port to allow for insertion of a surgical clip applier; the other two are 5 mm in size. The lateral most port is usually placed after mobilizing the splenic flexure of the colon to avoid injury.

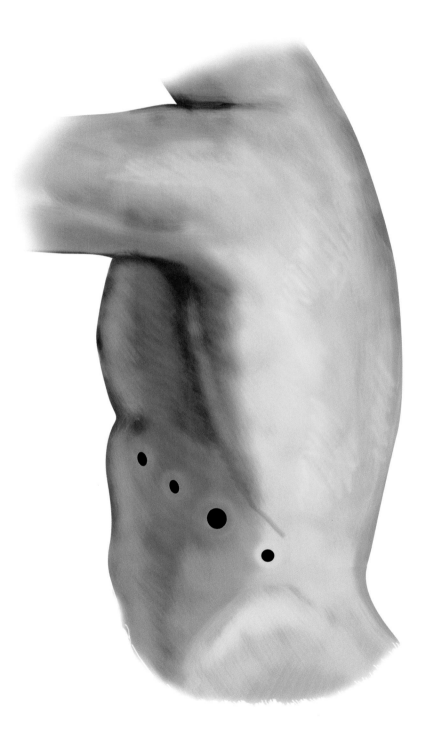

Exposing the Left Adrenal Gland

7. The splenic flexure of the colon is mobilized away from the inferior pole of the spleen by dividing the splenocolic ligament. Gravity retraction allows the colon to fall away from the operative field.

8. Next, the lateral attachments of the spleen and the splenorenal ligament are divided up to the level of the diaphragm. This mobilization is facilitated by gravity allowing the spleen to fall anteriorly and medially away from the retroperitoneum. The lateral and posterior attachments of the left kidney should not be divided as this will cause the kidney to fall forward and obstruct exposure of the adrenal gland.

9. The left adrenal gland is contained in the perinephric fat at the superomedial pole of the left kidney. The tail of the pancreas often needs to be somewhat mobilized as well in order to clearly visualize the renal hilum, inferior aspect of the adrenal gland, and left adrenal vein.

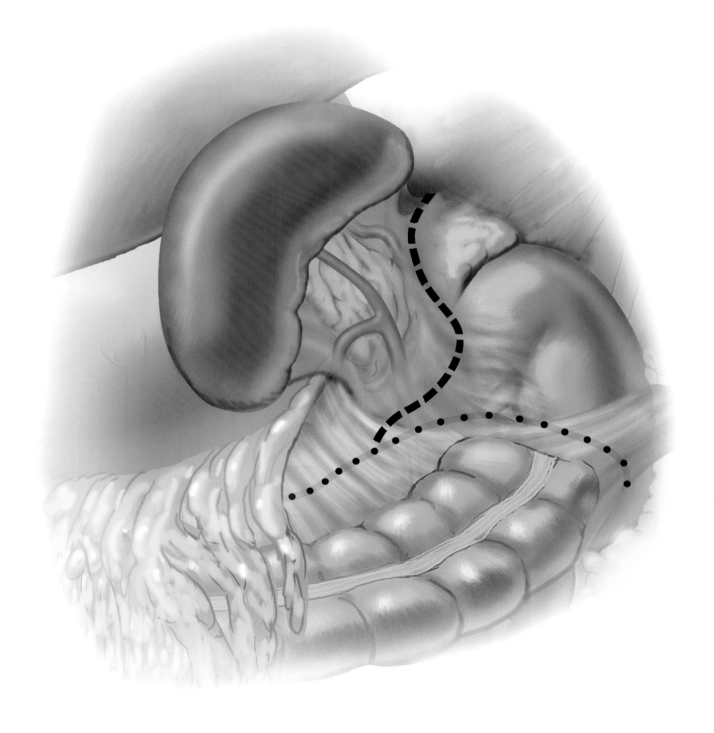

Dissecting the Left Adrenal Gland and Dividing the Left Adrenal Vein

10. The left adrenal vein courses from the inferomedial aspect of the adrenal gland and empties into the left renal vein. The adrenal vein should be localized, circumferentially dissected free, and divided between surgical clips (two clips are placed on the renal vein side). The inferior phrenic vein usually drains into the left adrenal vein proximal to its junction with the left renal vein. Depending on where the left adrenal vein is divided and the exact anatomy of the inferior phrenic vein, the latter may need to be separately divided between surgical clips as well.

11. Next, the left adrenal gland is circumferentially dissected free using an ultrasonic coagulator to control its numerous arterial branches. Specimen retrieval and closure are identical to that as previously described for a right adrenalectomy.

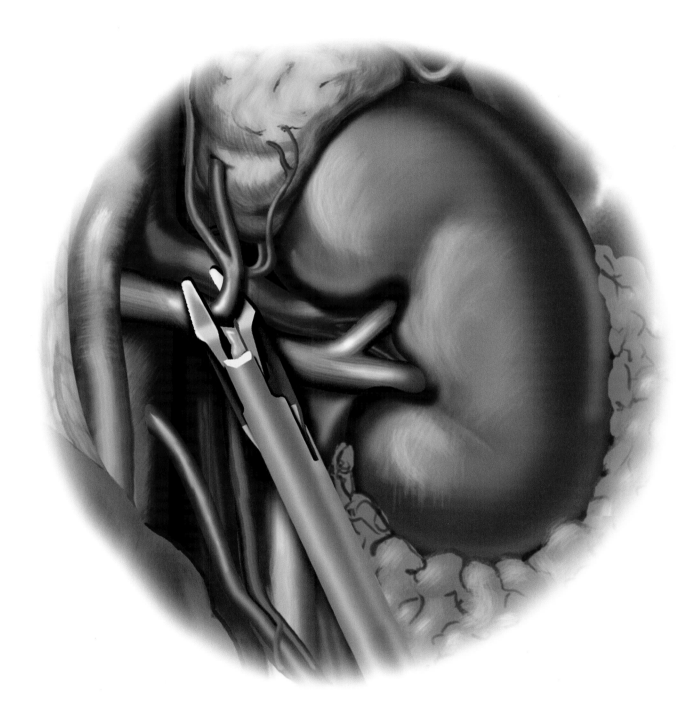

Postoperative Care

Sequential compression devices and/or subcutaneous heparin are continued postoperatively. Provided there was no colonic injury during splenic mobilization, postoperative antibiotics are usually not necessary. Oral intake is advanced as tolerated. If needed, appropriate steroid replacement therapy should be instituted.

Suggested Reading

1. Brunt LM, Moley JF, Doherty, GM, Lairmore TC, DeBenedetti MK, Quasebarth MA. Outcomes analysis in patients undergoing laparoscopic adrenalectomy for hormonally active adrenal tumors. *Surgery* 2001;130:629-635.

2. Brunt LM. Laparoscopic adrenalectomy In: Jones DB, Wu JS, Soper NJ, eds. *Laparoscopic Surgery: Principles and Procedures*. 2nd ed. New York: Marcel Dekker. 2004;379-394.

3. Gagner M, Lacroix A, Bolte E, Pomp A. Laparoscopic adrenalectomy: the importance of a flank approach in the lateral decubitus position. *Surg Endosc*. 1994;8:135-138.

Commentary

Michael S. Nussbaum, M.D., The University Hospital
University of Cincinnati

Laparoscopic adrenalectomy has become the gold standard for the majority of adrenal lesions. The overall benefits to patients are multiple. It is tempting to have more liberal indications for "incidentalomas" when a procedure is easier and safer to perform. However, it is important to recognize that the indications for adrenalectomy have not changed. The direct benefits of the laparoscopic approach over open adrenalectomy include: less blood loss, decreased analgesic requirement, shorter hospital stay, earlier return to work and normal activities, and a lower risk of wound complications such as infection and incisional hernia. All of these benefits lead to a lower overall cost of the procedure.

While the majority of adrenal lesions can be approached laparoscopically, there are clear contraindications to the laparoscopic approach. These include: lesions that a larger than 8 cm, malignant lesions, extra-adrenal pheochromocytoma, patients with an uncorrectable coagulopathy, prior abdominal surgery that prevents safe laparoscopic access (a rare occurrence), and any contraindication to general anesthesia or pneumoperitoneum.

The lateral transabdominal flank approach that is described in this atlas is clearly the best approach for the majority of situations. The advantages that this positioning provides are clearly outlined. When positioning the patient on the operating table, it is essential to prepare, drape, and secure the patient to allow access to the opposite side of the midline so that the patient can be rotated from an almost 90° lateral position to an almost supine position. Such rotation will allow for safer abdominal access, as well as manipulation of the surrounding structures by the use of gravity.

When dissecting the adrenal gland, it is very important not to disrupt or damage the adrenal capsule. This is especially important when dealing with a pheochromocytoma or a potentially malignant neoplasm. The gland itself should rarely be grasped, rather the periadrenal fat can be grasped or the gland can be retracted with a blunt probe or gauze dissector. A useful concept to keep in mind when performing a laparoscopic adrenalectomy is to dissect the surrounding structures away from the gland (i.e., dissect the patient off of the adrenal gland). In the process of dissection, if there is significant bleeding or an obvious vascular injury, the first step should be to apply direct pressure with a gauze dissector to the area that is bleeding. This is not a time to panic! Frequently, application of pressure for 5 minutes is enough to slow the bleeding to allow laparoscopic control. If bleeding persists, direct pressure can be maintained until the patient has been opened and the bleeding addressed in an open fashion. Other complications to be aware of and vigilant to avoid include pancreatic injury, bowel injury (hepatic and splenic flexure of colon), and diaphragm injury.

Identification of the adrenal gland can be difficult at times, particularly in obese patients with a large amount of retroperitoneal fat. On the left side, a useful technique is to find the phrenic vein on the left diaphragm and to follow the inferior phrenic vein down to the left adrenal vein. Intraoperative laparoscopic ultrasonography utilizing a 10 mm, 7.5 MHz laparoscopic probe can also be very useful in situations where the adrenal lesion is difficult to find. This is particularly helpful in localizing small adenomas in obese patients. Ultrasound is also useful in identifying anatomy such as localizing the adrenal vein, assessing for invasion of malignancies, and identifying extra-adrenal pheochromocytomas.

The postoperative management of most patients following a laparoscopic adrenalectomy is very straightforward and most patients should be ready for discharge by the first or second postoperative day. A liquid diet can be started immediately and advanced as tolerated. Hydrocortisone replacement should be administered for Cushing's patients, mineralocorticoid replacement following bilateral adrenalectomy, and oral potassium replacement should be continued after aldosteronoma resection. The patient can be discharged when ambulating and tolerating a regular diet and oral medications.

L. Michael Brunt, M.D., Barnes- Jewish Hospital
Washington University School of Medicine

Laparoscopic adrenalectomy has become the preferred method for removal of the vast majority of adrenal tumors and Dr. Jones et al have done a nice job illustrating the essential steps in carrying out this operation. The color drawings capture the key relationships in adrenal anatomy and the text highlights the important technical details involved in each step for both the right and left sides. Surgeons who attempt this operation should be prepared with a thorough knowledge of adrenal anatomy and the atlas succeeds in this regard. Like the authors, I prefer the transabdominal lateral approach to adrenalectomy. For the right side, the three key components to the operation in my experience are: 1) thorough mobilization of the liver by dividing the right triangular ligament, 2) meticulous dissection of the adrenal/IVC border and isolation of the adrenal vein, and 3) dissection of the inferior-lateral border where the adrenal sits on top of the right kidney. Care should be taken in this last step in the dissection to not extend it too inferiorly where a superior pole renal artery branch could be injured. My preference is to use the L-hook electrocautery for the entire dissection on the right side, whereas an ultrasonic coagulator greatly facilitates the dissection on the left.

For left adrenalectomy, the three key steps as illustrated in the atlas are: 1) dividing the splenocolic and splenorenal ligaments, 2) development of the plane between the tail of pancreas and kidney to expose the renal hilum and adrenal, and 3) dissection of the left adrenal vein. The operation can be carried out with only three ports if the surgeon is experienced. As the tail of the pancreas is reflected medially, both the splenic artery and vein are usually visible. Care should be taken retracting the pancreas as it can be easily injured and bleed or leak pancreatic fluid postoperatively. My approach to the left adrenal vein is to first define the medial and lateral borders of the adrenal gland and to then proceed caudally to its inferior-medial border where the vein lies. I use the hook cautery to define the inferior margin of the gland, but, like the authors, prefer the ultrasonic coagulator for division of the remaining attachments. In some cases, the left adrenal gland can be difficult to locate, especially if the patient is obese or has Cushing's syndrome. Laparoscopic ultrasound can be very useful in such patients to locate the adrenal and define its relationship to the left kidney and other adjacent structures.

Postoperatively, most patients can be discharged the day following surgery unless additional monitoring is needed for hormone replacement or blood pressure management. Since bleeding is the most common complication of laparoscopic adrenalectomy, our practice has been to obtain a complete blood count the morning after surgery and to assess electrolytes and serum creatinine in patients with hormonally active tumors. By properly selecting patients for operation and using a careful and meticulous dissection technique that follows the sequence outlined in this atlas, a high degree of success can be expected.

Michel Gagner, M.D., New York-Presbyterian Hospital
Weill Medical College of Cornell University

Since its first description in 1992, laparoscopic adrenalectomy has proven to be the procedure of choice for the surgical treatment of benign adrenal disease. Multiple reports have consistently demonstrated the well-known benefits of minimally invasive surgery, including a decreased hospital stay, analgesic needs, blood loss, and recovery time, over the conventional approach.

Although some authors advocate the retroperitoneal approach, the technique of choice by most surgeons performing laparoscopic adrenalectomy is the transabdominal lateral approach, originally described by me in 1992. Positioning of the patient in lateral decubitus uses the force of gravity to help retract the surrounding organs (including the bowel), and effectively exposes either adrenal gland for laparoscopic intervention. As a result, there is reduced dissection and minimal retraction of the vena cava and other adjacent structures.

On the left side, a laparoscope is then inserted in the most anterior trocar and the surgeon will work laterally with a two-hand technique through the other two trocars. Working with the laparoscopic scissors with cautery or the ultrasonic scalpel, in the right hand, and a curved dissector in the left hand, the splenic flexure is mobilized medially to move the colon from the inferior pole of the adrenal and expose the lineorenal ligament. Mobilization allows instruments to be inserted more easily and helps prevent inadvertent trauma to the colon or spleen during instrument insertion. Then, the lineorenal ligament is incised inferosuperiorly approximately 1 cm from the spleen. The dissection is carried up to the diaphragm and stopped when the short gastric vessels are encountered posteriorly behind the stomach. This maneuver allows the spleen to fall medially, thus exposing the retroperitoneal space. The lateral edge and anterior portion of the adrenal gland will become visible in the perinephric fat superiorly and medially. Laparoscopic ultrasound may be used as an adjunct to identify the adrenal gland, the mass within the gland, and the adrenal vein. Grasping the perinephric fat, dissection of the lateral and anterior part of the adrenal gland is carried out. Hook elecrocautery or ultrasonic scalpel is a useful instrument for this phase of dissection.

Most left adrenal veins are about 10 mm in diameter and can be clipped with medium to large titanium clips placed with clip applier. With a right-angle dissector, the adrenal vein is dissected from its insertion into the left adrenal gland. It's not necessary to identify and dissect the origin of the vein from the left renal vein.

On the right side, the liver often must be mobilized to obtain the best exposure of the junction between the adrenal gland and the inferior vena cava. This is the key for providing adequate exposure of the right adrenal vein and its entry into the vena cava. The right lateral hepatic attachments and the triangular ligament are, therefore, dissected from the diaphragm using laparoscopic scissors or ultrasonic scalpel

The inferolateral edge is then mobilized, and dissection is continued afterwards medially and upward, along the lateral edge of the vena cava. The adrenal vein should be visualized at this stage. This vein is often short and sometimes broad. Usually the vein can be clipped with medium to large titanium clips, and at least two should be applied at the vena cava side. If there is not enough space for clips, then a vascular cartridge of a 30 mm or 45-mm laparoscopic stapler is used for secure division of the right adrenal vein. Smaller veins may be encountered superiorly; these should be clipped or cauterized to prevent bleeding.

Additional reported complications may result from injury to structures in the area of dissection, adjacent to the adrenals, including the kidney, colon, tail of the pancreas, and the stomach on the left side. On the right side, the liver and the duodenum are at risk.

Because both adrenals are located in close proximity to major blood vessels (the hilum of kidneys and the vena cava), massive bleeding is a potentially disastrous complication.

Furthermore, dissection high in the abdomen could result in diaphragmatic injury, leading to potential tension pneumothorax.

Pheochromocytoma constituted for 25% of the pathologies in our series. These tumors were larger than in patients with other diseases: 6.3 cm versus 3.9 cm ($P<.05$). In addition, operative time was longer: 2.5 hours versus 1.8 hours ($P<.05$). During the removal of these tumors, hypertension occurred in 56% of patients and hypotension in 52%. Moreover, almost 60% (7/12) of our postoperative complications were in pheochromocytomas.

The accumulated data suggest that there are very few absolute contraindications for laparoscopic adrenalectomy. At the present time, we consider invasive adrenal carcinoma to be the only absolute contraindication for the laparoscopic approach, due to the possible extent and complexity of the operation required. An open technique also may be more desirable for patients with malignant pheochromocytoma when metastatic nodes are present in the periaortic chain or close to the bladder. Several authors differentiate between the biologic behavior of adrenal metastasis and primary adrenal cancer as to their suitability for the laparoscopic technique.

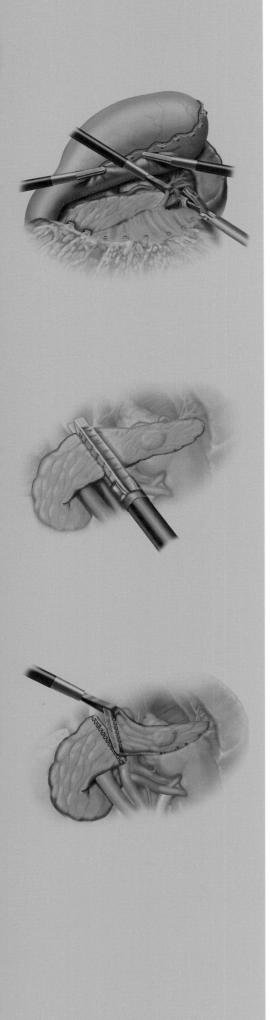

Laparoscopic Distal Pancreatectomy

Laparoscopic pancreatic surgery is employed for oncologic staging, resections of neuroendocrine or cystic tumors, and treating complications of pancreatitis, including pseudocyst drainage procedures and necrosectomies. When planning a distal pancreatectomy, even if a spleen-preserving operation is intended, the patient should be preoperatively prepared for a splenectomy in the event that intraoperative bleeding, adherence, or invasion into other organs mandate such a procedure. Thus, the patient should receive vaccinations for encapsulated bacteria (Pneumovax, HIB, *Neisseria meningitidis*) 2 to 3 weeks prior to the procedure. Otherwise, the vaccinations should be administered 1 to 2 weeks postoperatively.

Preoperative Preparation

1. A mechanical bowel preparation may be administered at the surgeon's discretion. Sequential compression stockings and subcutaneous heparin may be used for prophylaxis against deep venous thrombosis. Intravenous antibiotics, usually a first-generation cephalosporin, are administered prophylactically. After induction of general anesthesia, the bladder is emptied with a urinary catheter and the stomach is decompressed with a nasogastric tube.

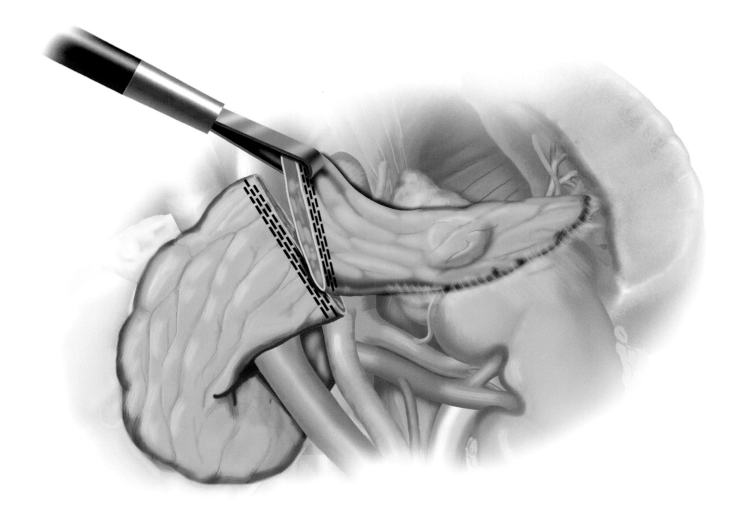

Operating Room Setup

2. The patient is placed in a modified lithotomy position on a cushioned bean bag with the surgeon standing between the legs. The patient's thighs should not be excessively flexed so as to impede any instrument's range of motion. All pressure points must be adequately padded and the bean-bag device is used to secure the patient's position when rotating the table to facilitate exposure and viewing during the procedure.

3. The assistant is situated to the patient's right, while the camera operator stands on the patient's left side (or vice versa).

4. Alternatively, the patient can be placed supine with the surgeon standing to the patient's right, and the assistant on the left.

5. The video monitors are stationed at both sides of the patient's head to facilitate adequate viewing from either side of the table. A laparotomy set should be available on the back table should emergent conversion be necessary. Additionally, laparoscopic ultrasound may be invaluable as a tool to identify liver lesions and anatomy.

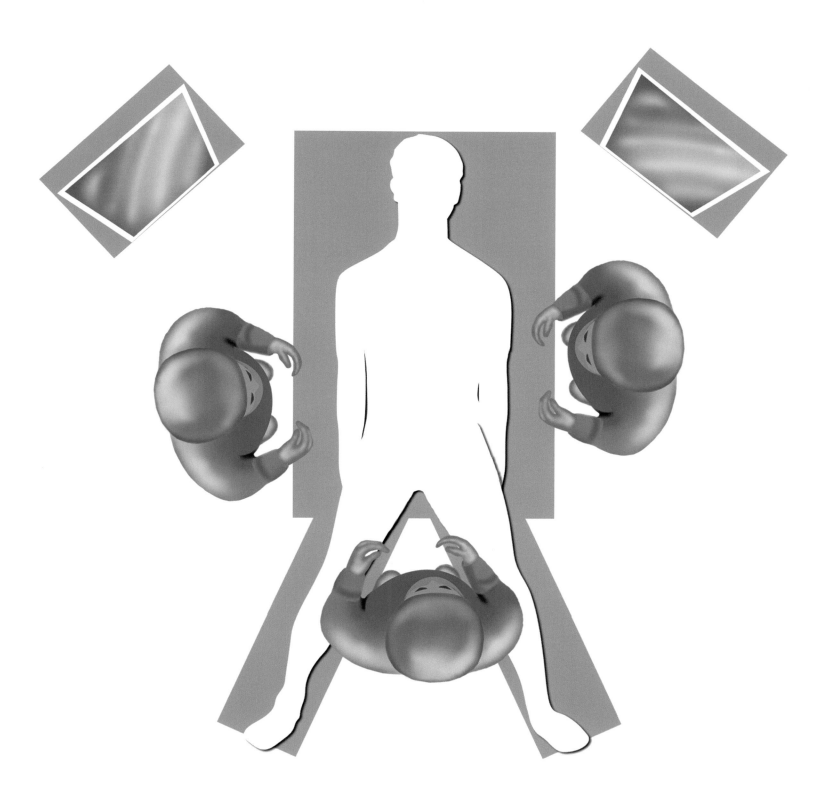

Access and Port Placement

6. The optimal configuration of port placement varies depending on the indications for the procedure. The camera is usually best positioned at the umbilicus and the working ports are at adequate distances to allow appropriate manipulation of the instruments and proper exposure of the pancreas. An angled laparoscope is used to facilitate better visualization of structures.

7. Pneumoperitoneum is obtained through an infraumbilical incision with either an open or closed technique. One 12 mm port is required to introduce an endoscopic linear stapler, while the remaining ports can be 5 mm in size. In order to perform a splenectomy, a left subcostal port in the midclavicular line will be required. The ports can be arranged as shown, with the 12 mm port placed at an appropriate distance to facilitate stapling across the pancreas. Surgeons may wish to employ a hand port in order to regain tactile sense, aid in dissection, and retrieve specimens.

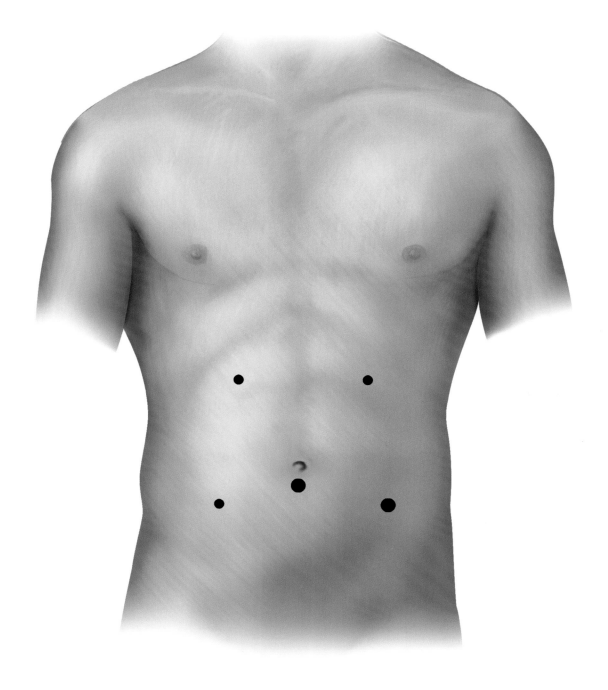

Distal Pancreatectomy With Splenectomy

FIGURE C

Exposing the Pancreas

1. Exploratory laparoscopy must first be performed to assess for any evidence of carcinomatosis and/or liver metastasis.

2. Next, the lesser sac is entered by creating a window in an avascular area of the gastrocolic omentum. This dissection is extended along the greater curve of the stomach using an ultrasonic coagulator or surgical clips to include ligation of all the short gastric vessels. This wide mobilization allows for better visualization of the pancreas. The splenic flexure of the colon is also dissected free from the inferior pole of the spleen in a medial to lateral direction, thus dividing the splenocolic ligament.

3. The stomach is retracted cephalad by grasping the posterior aspect with atraumatic graspers. This plane between the posterior stomach and the anterior surface of the pancreas should be relatively easy to develop. Dense adhesions here can be secondary to malignancy and/or previous episodes of pancreatitis and conversion to an open procedure may become necessary. Laparoscopic ultrasonography may better assess the extent of and resectability of a pancreatic tumor.

4. The posterior peritoneum overlying the superior and inferior borders of the pancreas is carefully incised. Gentle blunt dissection and anterior retraction of the pancreas develops the plane between the pancreas and the underlying retroperitoneal fat. Dissection should be performed medial to the inferior mesenteric vein (IMV), while recognizing the variable anatomy of the IMV, as it can drain into the splenic vein, superior mesenteric vein, or the confluence of the two. An ultrasonic coagulator is used to ligate any small vessels encountered in this posterior plane.

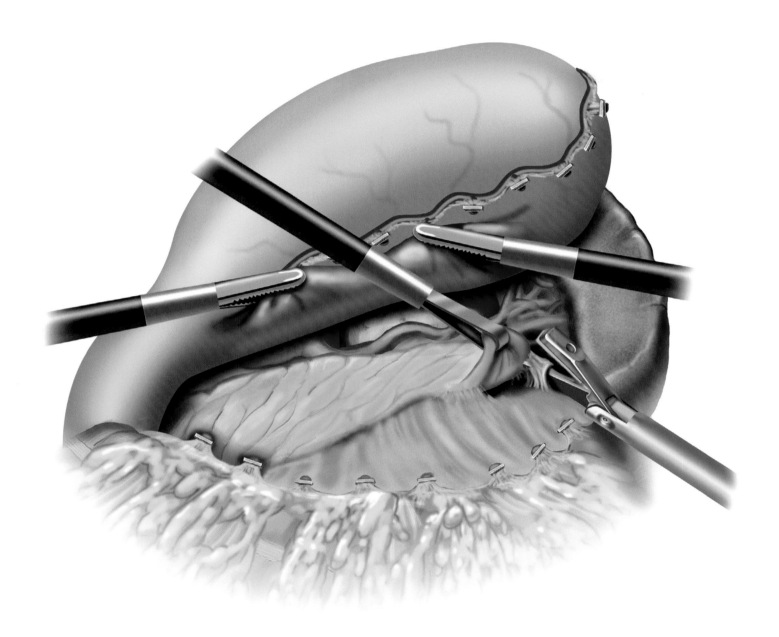

FIGURE D

Dividing the Pancreas and Splenic Vessels

5. The splenic artery coursing along the superior border of the pancreas is then identified, isolated at the point of intended pancreatic transection, and ligated with either surgical clips, suture ligatures, or an endoscopic vascular stapler (2.5 mm staples).

6. Careful blunt dissection of the pancreas from the underlying retroperitoneum allows identification of the splenic vein. With great care to avoid hemorrhage, the splenic vein is similarly isolated and can be divided using an endoscopic stapler with a vascular load (2.5 mm staples).

7. The pancreas itself can be divided using an endoscopic linear stapler, ultrasonic shears, or electrocautery, of which we prefer the former. The posterior jaw of the stapler must be inserted very carefully as to not injure any underlying vascular structures. Depending on the thickness of the gland, 2.5 mm to 3.5 mm staples should be employed in order to achieve an adequate seal of the parenchyma and more importantly, the pancreatic duct. The proximal remnant staple line can be oversewn and/or a fibrin sealant applied. The pancreatic duct may be directly ligated with sutures.

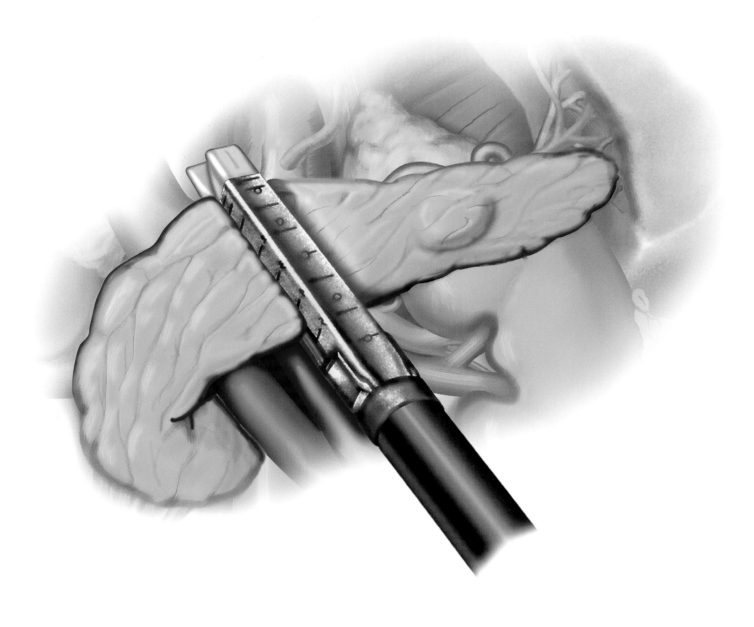

Removing the Specimen

8. Once the splenic vessels have been ligated, the posterior plane of the pancreas is developed in a medial to lateral direction, ultimately freeing the most distal aspect of the pancreatic tail from the underlying retroperitoneal fat. Gentle upward retraction of the pancreas facilitates exposing any vessels in this plane, which can be ligated with an ultrasonic coagulator.

9. After the pancreatic specimen is completely mobilized, the splenorenal and splenophrenic ligaments are divided, thus freeing the entire specimen. Once the operative field is inspected for hemostasis, the 12 mm port is exchanged for an 18 mm port. A specimen retrieval bag is inserted and the specimen is placed completely inside. The 18 mm port is removed while retaining control of the bag-pursestring suture. Digital fracture technique or ringed forceps can assist in removal of the spleen. The pancreatic specimen should be left intact for pathologic investigation.

10. Once the operative field is reinspected for satisfactory hemostasis, a closed suction drain is placed near the pancreatic stump to facilitate drainage of a postoperative leak, should one occur. The fascial and skin incisions are closed in the usual manner.

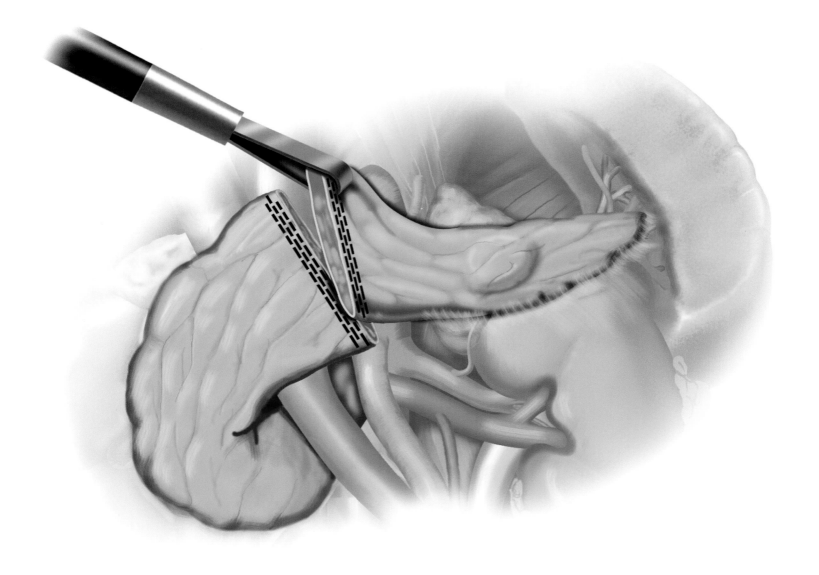

Distal Pancreatectomy With Splenic Preservation

FIGURE F

Lateral to Medial Dissection

The general exposure and dissection are similar to that as previously described. However, some important differences need to be highlighted.

1. Some surgeons advocate leaving the short gastric vessels intact when planning splenic preservation. Although this is the ideal situation, this can compromise exposure and visibility of the pancreas.

2. The splenic artery and vein should be localized and isolated as before should significant bleeding during the pancreatic dissection mandate ligation and splenic resection.

3. The pancreatic dissection usually begins laterally. The tail of the gland is gently retracted anteriorly and medially, while any branches from the splenic vessels to the pancreas are ligated with an ultrasonic coagulator. Dissection is carried medially until the point of intended pancreatic transection. An endoscopic linear stapler is used as previously described to transect the pancreas.

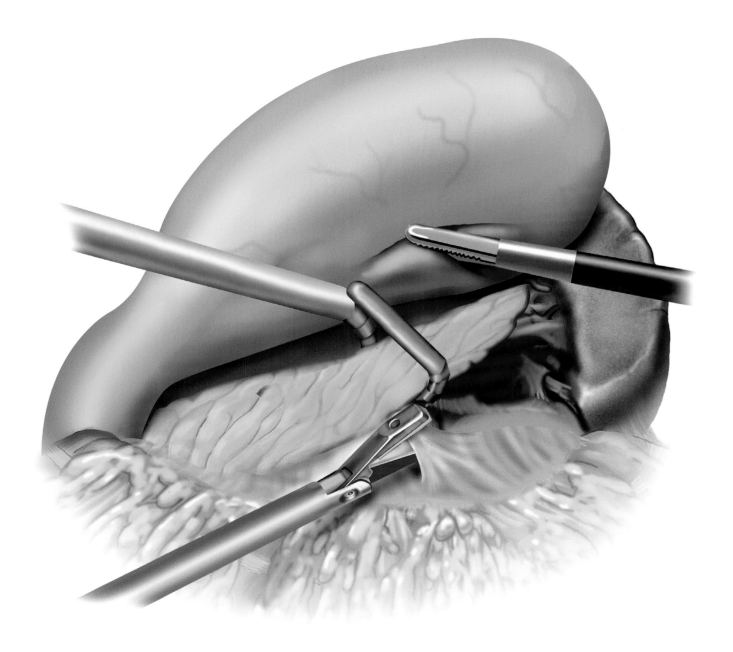

Postoperative Care

Sequential compression devices and/or subcutaneous heparin are continued postoperatively. Provided there was no colonic injury during splenic mobilization, postoperative antibiotics are usually not necessary. A nasogastric tube may be left in place until return of bowel function. The output and character of the drainage, including the amylase content, from the closed suction drain should be monitored to assess for a pancreatic duct leak. Somatostatin is not routinely administered. Serum glucose levels should also be monitored closely as some patients may require insulin.

Suggested Reading

1. Cushieri A, Jakimowicz JJ. Laparoscopic pancreatic resections. *Semin Laparosc Surg.* 1998; 5:168-179.

2. Patterson EJ, Gagner M, Salky B, et al. Laparoscopic pancreatic resection: single institution experience in 19 patients. *J Am Coll Surg.* 2001;193:281-287.

3. Vezakis A, Davides D, Larvin M, McMahon MJ. Laparoscopic surgery combined with preservation of the spleen for distal pancreatic tumors. *Surg Endosc.* 1999;13:26-29.

Commentary

Stanley W. Ashley, M.D., Brigham and Women's Hospital
Harvard Medical School

Despite scattered reports of small experiences with minimally invasive pancreaticoduodenectomy, most surgeons remain skeptical that this technical tour de force, particularly the complex reconstruction, can be truly of benefit. In contrast, distal pancreatectomy is a laparoscopic procedure that makes sense. Although no randomized trials have been performed, several series suggest that this procedure is accompanied by a more rapid recovery, less pain, and improved cosmesis than open operation. Unfortunately, distal pancreatectomy, with or without splenectomy, remains a relatively infrequent operation. Indications include benign and malignant neoplasms and the complications of pancreatitis, including pseudocyst, organized necrosis, and fistula.

Resectable adenocarcinomas of the pancreatic tail are extremely rare and, unless discovered incidentally at a very small size, would not usually be appropriately managed with the laparoscope. The best lesions for this approach are small and, particularly if the spleen is to be spared, unaccompanied by significant pancreatic inflammation. If there is significant suspicion of malignancy, it is inappropriate to attempt to spare the spleen. The benign islet cell tumor, particularly the insulinoma, is perhaps most ideal for this approach, although this can be more complicated if the lesion is not completely localized preoperatively. In the patient who has had only venous sampling that suggests a tail lesion, we have found that laparoscopic ultrasound can be useful in identifying these tumors intraoperatively and in identifying an appropriate site for pancreatic transection. This technology may be useful in determining the extent of resection for other lesions as well. If this is not revealing, it is usually necessary to palpate the pancreas to identify these tumors, rather than proceeding with a blind resection. Under these circumstances, a hand port may prove useful. Mucinous cystic tumors represent another appropriate indication; in this case, the index of suspicion for malignancy should determine the need for accompanying splenectomy. The suspected intraductal papillary mucinous tumor (IPMT) is a somewhat more complicated situation because of the not-infrequent necessity for removing additional pancreas based on dysplasia of the ductal epithelium on frozen section of the initial specimen—despite this, it seems reasonable to proceed with a laparoscopic resection when preoperative imaging suggests that the disease is confined to the tail,

421

recognizing that it may be necessary to convert to an open procedure if intraoperative sections prove suspicious.

Although minimally invasive approaches to the complications of pancreatitis have been employed, distal pancreatectomy, as described here, is seldom the appropriate procedure. Occasionally, a small, asymptomatic pseudocyst, where the distinction from a cystic neoplasm is an indication, may be approached using these techniques. In contrast, most symptomatic cysts are more appropriately drained internally. The lesions are large, interfering with exposure, and the accompanying adhesions often preclude a successful laparoscopic approach; the splenic vein is typically thrombosed, producing left-sided portal hypertension that may be difficult to maneuver. A preoperative evaluation of ductal anatomy, usually by endoscopic retrograde cholangiopancreatography (ERCP) is indicated to rule out the presence of a more proximal ductal stricture, precluding simple distal resection. Necrosis of the pancreatic tail may be debrided using minimally invasive techniques—typically a catheter is placed from the flank preoperatively and the tract dilated, permitting insertion of the scope and piecemeal necrosectomy. Pancreatic fistulas likewise are often accompanied by an intense inflammatory fibrosis along the tract, making minimally invasive approaches less feasible.

With regard to the technical aspects of the operation, we have tended, except for more central lesions, to position the patient in nearly full right lateral decubitus with the option to airplane the patient back to the left when necessary. Our port placements are similar to those described although we would emphasize that, particularly in larger patients, one cannot be too cephalad with the position of the working ports. Even when we are attempting to preserve the spleen, we like to begin laterally—we have found dissection more proximally may be unnecessary and separation of the splenic veins more difficult. However, occasionally, when we know we will be taking the spleen, we have isolated and divided the splenic artery before beginning our dissection. We usually proceed initially by taking down the splenic flexure. We leave some omental tissue on the inferior pole of the spleen to use as a handle for gentle elevation and then dissect medially onto the anterior surface of the pancreatic tail. Attachments along the inferior border of the pancreas are divided. Although some surgeons have reported being able to salvage the spleen based on preservation of the short gastrics alone, we have not found this to be the case and take these vessels relatively early to facilitate exposure. Once the inferior pancreatic border is defined, we grasp this with an atraumatic grasper and, if we are attempting to preserve the spleen, elevate this gently off the splenic vessels using a combination of blunt dissection with a peanut and the harmonic scalpel. In contrast, if the spleen is to be sacrificed, we divide its phrenic attachments relatively early and then enter the plane posteriorly, reflecting the spleen and tail to the right to the point of division. We have occasionally found that a hand port, placed in a subcostal position to permit extension with conversion, can considerably enhance the exposure.

Particularly when there is accompanying inflammation, the pancreas may be too thickened to divide with the laparoscopic staplers and, in this situation, we have been satisfied with the use of the harmonic scalpel. Although we have not oversewn pancreatic staple lines, we do place a running absorbable suture when we have divided the pancreas with the harmonic scalpel. We always leave a closed suction drain.

If splenectomy has been performed, once the specimen has been freed, we typically divide the splenic attachments to the pancreas and remove the pancreas first. We have worried about disrupting the pancreatic architecture when the spleen is morcellated in the same bag. After separation, the pancreas is placed in a bag first and removed; typically this is possible with minimal extension of the 12 mm port incision. The 12 mm port is then replaced with the 18 mm and a larger bag used for morcellation of the spleen itself.

Mark P. Callery, M.D., Beth Israel Deaconess Medical Center Harvard Medical School

Pancreatic resections, all agree, are among the most technically demanding operations general surgeons will perform. The pancreas is a formidable adversary because of its inherent diseases, and because of the vascular and locoregional anatomy it straddles. This chapter nicely provides the basics of preoperative preparation, operating room setup, and one suggestion for trocar placement. It only scratches the surface, I believe, of what you really need to know to attempt a laparoscopic distal pancreatectomy.

Is the disease process and location amenable to a laparoscopic approach? Indeed, this is a rewarding technique for resecting focal cystic lesions or possible neuroendocrine tumors well out in the left pancreas. For bulky neoplasms, and especially potential carcinomas anywhere in the gland, I still select open pancreatectomy. This is because there exists no evidence-based consensus that laparoscopic pancreatectomy is equivalent oncologically. If chronic or acute pancreatitis is present, tissue planes will disappear, the pancreas will be very difficult to manipulate, and the risks for sudden fierce hemorrhage will increase.

Is it safe to try this procedure? Only if you are experienced in open distal pancreatectomy. After all, the procedure as described departs little from descriptions of the open procedure other than to apply laparoscopic techniques. If you can get through these steps safely, and the anatomy is clear and manageable, then access and technique should not really matter. It is the regional vascular anatomy, however, that makes pancreatic surgery perilous. Any injury to the portal venous system will bleed profusely, often be hidden by the pancreas, and will extend further if recovery maneuvers fail. Your only option will be emergency laparotomy, but the damage will be done.

Here are a few technical caveats I have learned. Don't tie up assistant instruments holding up the stomach. Once you have entered the lesser sac, and exposed the anterior pancreas (Figure C), simply suture the greater curve of the stomach as necessary up to the anterior abdominal wall. Consider pancreatic mobilization medial to lateral (tail), and not always vice versa. Use laparoscopic ultrasound so you know where the vessels, and the lesions, are, as you will lack palpation and at times visualization. Avoid dividing the splenic vein within the pancreatic parenchyma. The autostaplers do not always perform as flawlessly as Figure D would suggest. Oversew the pancreatic duct in the remnant staple line, and even secure neighboring omentum or fat to it. For larger specimens, consider using hand-assist devices early in the operation for ease and later retrieval.

If everything goes absolutely perfectly with this approach as summarized, and if the anatomy is as straightforward as the illustrations depict, you may be able to do this safely. But if any trouble is encountered, it will be your experience with open pancreatic surgery, and not advanced laparoscopy, that will determine your success.

Horacio J. Asbun, M.D.
John Muir Health

Minimal access surgery techniques have rapidly evolved to include a variety of complex surgical procedures. Even though laparoscopic pancreatic surgery is still not universally practiced, laparoscopic distal pancreatectomy is safe and readily feasible. In experienced hands, the procedure has striking advantages over its open counterpart. The minimal access approach suits distal pancreatectomy well because of the advantages in visual magnification, the inherent delicate manipulation of tissues, the decreased blood loss, the enhanced access to the pancreas and the absence of need for reconstruction. These advantages however are present only when the operator is an experienced laparoscopic surgeon with extensive expertise in open pancreatic surgery and a clear understanding of pancreatic diseases.

Indications for the procedure are, in general, similar to an open distal pancreatectomy. In selected cases, however, there could be a more liberal indication to do the procedure with a palliative intent in patients with malignancies of the body and tail. This is based on the lesser negative impact that the minimal access approach has on the patient's quality of life.

In the presence of a small lesion, the laparoscopic approach is limited by the inability to palpate the lesion. Nevertheless, the use of intraoperative ultrasound markedly enhances the laparoscopic approach and surgeons dealing with the procedure must have experience in its use. Even though not commonly needed, the operation can also be performed in a hand-assisted manner. As it is well described by the author in this chapter, the surgery can be done either with spleen preservation or with a splenectomy. The indications to include or not to include a splenectomy should not be affected by the fact that the procedure is being done using the minimal access method. Robotic-assisted laparoscopic distal pancreatectomy has been described and may have a role in the splenic-preserving procedure. However, its advantages over the traditional laparoscopic technique done by an experienced surgeon are still to be proven.

A contraindication to the laparoscopic approach is the presence of portal hypertension, either generalized, or limited to the splenic circulation. Relative contraindications include: the presence of a very large solid lesion, severe prior episodes of pancreatitis with residual scarring, or prior pancreatic surgery that would preclude clear identification of the anatomy. The greater extent of medial dissection occasionally needed during a distal pancreatectomy is not a limitation to the laparoscopic approach. Distal resection of the neck, body, and tail of the pancreas can be safely done. In fact, in experienced hands, the laparoscopic approach to the area of the neck of the pancreas may be even safer than its open counterpart.

The technical steps of the procedure are well described and illustrated by the author in this chapter. The principles of the technique are thoroughly depicted. Our approach to the procedure is similar to the one described with the following variants:

Patient position: The patient is placed in a modified right lateral decubitus position that would allow for rotation to the left or right during the procedure. In our experience, this facilitates the exposure of the operative area by allowing gravity do a significant portion of the retraction of the neighboring organs. Care is taken to secure the patient in the position, as well as to avoid any points of significant pressure, hyperextension, or hyperflexion. The surgeon stands to the right of the operating table.

Exposing, dissecting and dividing the pancreas: We start the dissection by performing a wide mobilization of the splenic flexure, as well as the descending colon. Given the lateral position of the patient, this dissection allows for displacement of the colon and omentum medially by gravity. The lesser sac is entered from its lateral aspect, and the gastrocolic omentum is divided and ligated from lateral to medial. This maneuver readily exposes the distal pancreas and avoids losing time in the dissection of the different layers of fibroadipose adhesions that surround the splenocolic ligament. Once the distal pancreas has been exposed, the dissection is continued in a clockwise manner, starting at the lower edge of the pancreas from lateral to medial. When in the right plane, this dissection is readily done with ultrasonic energy in a relatively avascular plane. The first named vascular structure that is found is the inferior mesenteric vein. Depending on the indications for the procedure, the dissection is stopped here and attention paid to the division of the pancreas or the dissection continued further medially. When needed, the inferior mesenteric vein is ligated. If more of a subtotal pancreatectomy is necessary, the dissection is continued medially along the lower edge of the pancreas. The area of the ligament of Treitz and the fourth portion of the duodenum are now exposed and care is taken to avoid injury. Following the lower edge of the pancreas, the next vascular structure that is evident is the superior mesenteric vein heading cephalad to travel under the neck of the pancreas. The posterior aspect of the tail and body of pancreas has been exposed during the dissection of the lower edge of the pancreas and partially separated of its posterior attachments by gentle blunt dissection. This aids in further facilitating the dissection and exposure of the inferior edge when going from lateral to medial. At the chosen site of pancreatic division, additional posterior dissection is now performed from caudad to cephalad up to the superior edge of the pancreas. As described in the chapter, the splenic vein is exposed and if needed isolated. Passing a Penrose drain to encircle the pancreas aids in its retraction when a splenic preserving procedure is planned.

Pancreatic division: In some cases, the pancreatic parenchyma is too thick at the division site and the use of a stapler is not advised. In that situation, our preference is to divide the pancreas with ultrasonic shears in a fish-mouth fashion. The proximal divided edge is then sutured with a running nonabsorbable monofilament suture. Particular care is taken to suture shut the pancreatic duct opening. This is done in similar manner as in an open procedure.

After the posterior dissection and ligation of the vessels is completed, attention is paid to the dissection of the superior edge of the pancreas that is now done from medial to lateral, continuing in a clockwise manner. Up to this stage, the superior attachments of the body and tail of the pancreas lateral to the division site had been kept intact. The dissection of the superior edge is continued reaching the end of the tail of the pancreas laterally. The pancreatic mobilization is then completed.

If a splenectomy is performed, a small serosal band between the upper pole of the spleen and the diaphragm can be left undivided until the specimen is within the retrieval bag. This facilitates the manipulation and placement of the specimen in the bag by keeping the specimen anchored superiorly. As described by the author, when retrieving the specimen, care should be taken to preserve the pancreatic specimen intact for pathologic examination.

Even though unusual, the procedure can always be converted to an open procedure if felt needed. As in any other advanced laparoscopic procedure, and experienced operator will not hesitate to do so when he/she feels that the quality or safety of the operation can be compromised by continuing with the minimal access approach.

Michel Gagner, M.D., New York-Presbyterian Hospital Weill Medical College of Cornell University

Given its anatomic relationships and location, laparoscopic access to the pancreas is reserved for well-trained surgeons in advanced laparoscopic surgery and they must have access to the required technology to perform these kinds of procedures.

Few surgeons have expertise in these techniques. Available data suggest that it is feasible, safe, and beneficial for the patient in terms of reduced hospital stay, reduced postoperative pain, faster return to normal activities, and better scar scores. However, morbidity and mortality rates and operative times have not been significantly different than the traditional open approach.

Distal pancreatectomy can be done either with or without splenic preservation. The spleen-sparing techniques are particularly indicated for patients with benign diseases, since extended lymphadenectomy needed for malignancy is still controversial and considered inadequate by laparoscopy.

Splenic salvage can be done by either dissecting the superior edge of the pancreas from the vessels emerging from the splenic vein and artery or by transecting these vessels at the level of the pancreatic section and resectioning them between the tail of the pancreas and the splenic hilum. In the latter procedure, similar to Warshaw's technique, short gastric vessels are needed for splenic perfusion.

These techniques require a longer operative time and laparoscopic surgical expertise; vascular damage and hemorrhage may occur due to the delicate maneuvers needed to dissect the upper margin of the pancreas. In such cases, the only way to preserve the spleen is to leave the short gastric vessels intact. The surgeon must keep this in mind at the beginning of the procedure and avoid transection of these vessels, as they might be needed for unexpected splenic salvage.

Since Warshaw's technique carries a risk of splenic infarction and abscess, I recommend looking at the spleen before terminating the procedure to evaluate the need for splenectomy if major ischemia exists.

Some surgeon transect the pancreas alone with staplers, while others divide it along with cautery or ultrasonic shears. In some situations with a fibrotic gland, and if an increased risk of important bleeding when dissecting the main splenic vessels exists, ligation of the splenic artery close to its origin maybe the best strategy. This maneuver will reduce the risk of major bleeding and could also be used as an attempt to reduce the size of the spleen, facilitating subsequent steps of the operation.

In order to prevent fistula formation, some authors favor the application of fibrin glue, even if there is no statistically significant study supporting this addition. Others suture the anterior and posterior capsule with a running suture, and even fine suture the pancreatic duct itself. Drainage routinely used, may increase fistula formation, paradoxically.

Hand-assisted laparoscopic surgery may bear some advantages in difficult cases involving large tumors, intraoperative bleeding, dense adhesions, in possible vascular involvement or malignancy, and obesity.

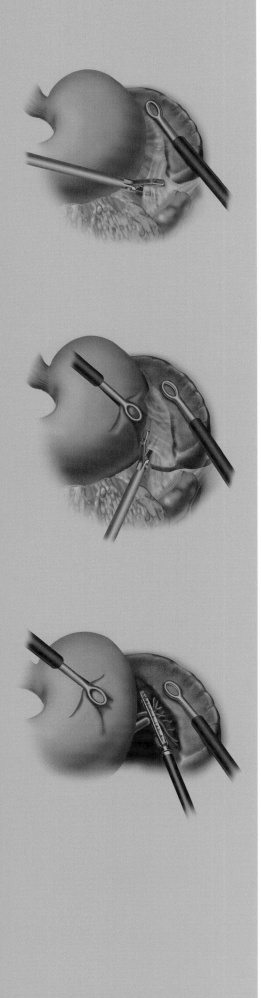

Laparoscopic Splenectomy

Splenectomy can relieve symptomatic splenomegaly (an anatomical problem), and treat hypersplenism (a functional problem), and provide diagnosis (e.g., Hodgkins). The laparoscopic approach has gained favor for normal-sized spleens. However, large spleens can also be safely resected with the laparoscopic approach as one gains sufficient experience. A hand-port can be of assistance in such cases. Rarely, diagnostic laparoscopy is indicated for blunt or penetrating trauma. If an elective splenectomy is planned, the patient should receive vaccinations for encapsulated bacteria (Pneumovax, HIB, *Neisseria meningitidis*) 2 to 3 weeks prior to the procedure. Otherwise, the vaccinations should be administered 1 to 2 weeks postoperatively.

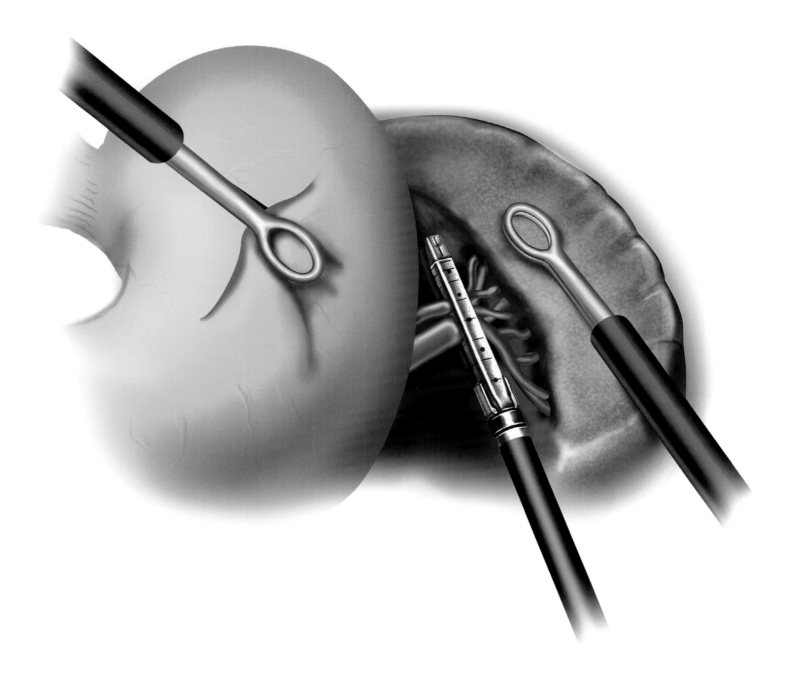

Review of the Anatomy

The spleen is suspended in its anatomical location by way of peritoneal-based ligamentous attachments. Adjacent structures include the splenic flexure of the colon, tail of the pancreas, left kidney, left adrenal gland, stomach, and diaphragm. The ligamentous attachments are sequentially divided to mobilize the spleen and obtain adequate exposure of the splenic hilum. The tail of the pancreas is directly adjacent to the splenic hilum and the splenic artery and vein course along the superior border of the pancreas, with the vein lying posterior to the artery.

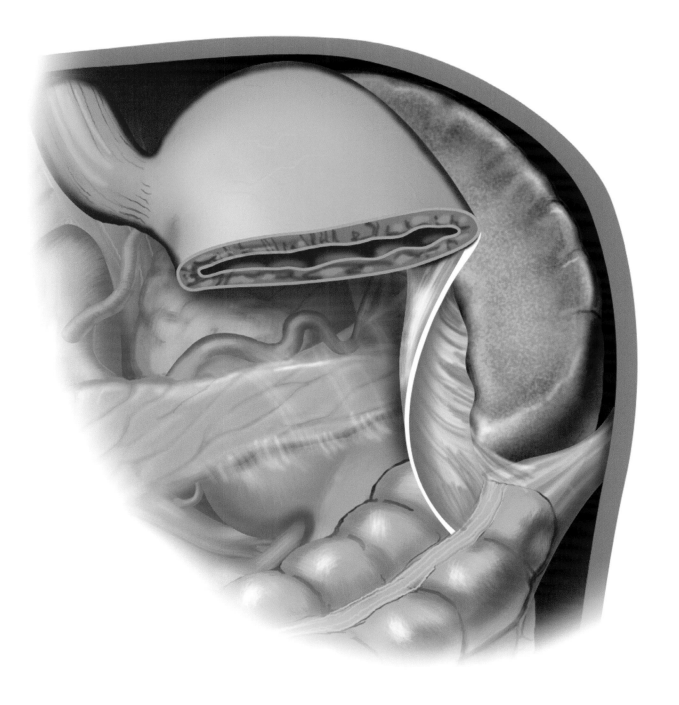

Recognizing Accessory Spleens

Accessory spleens are found in 10% to 20% of patients and should be resected. It is important to locate accessory spleens even if resection is not planned. The most common locations are depicted in Figure B, including hilar, omental, mesocolic, and mesentery.

Preoperative Preparation

1. Sequential compression stockings are nearly always used and subcutaneous heparin may be added for prophylaxis against deep venous thrombosis. Intravenous antibiotics, usually a first-generation cephalosporin, are administered prophylactically. After induction of general anesthesia, the bladder is emptied with a urinary catheter and the stomach is decompressed with a nasogastric tube or orogastric tube.

2. A blood type and screen should be obtained preoperatively in the event that hemorrhage would necessitate urgent transfusion. Patients with severe thrombocytopenia should have a preoperative hematology consult and possible treatment with intravenous steroids and/or immune globulin. Rarely will patients require a blood and/or platelet transfusion intraoperatively. In patients with severe thrombocytopenia, it can be useful to angio-embolize the splenic artery on the morning of the planned splenectomy.

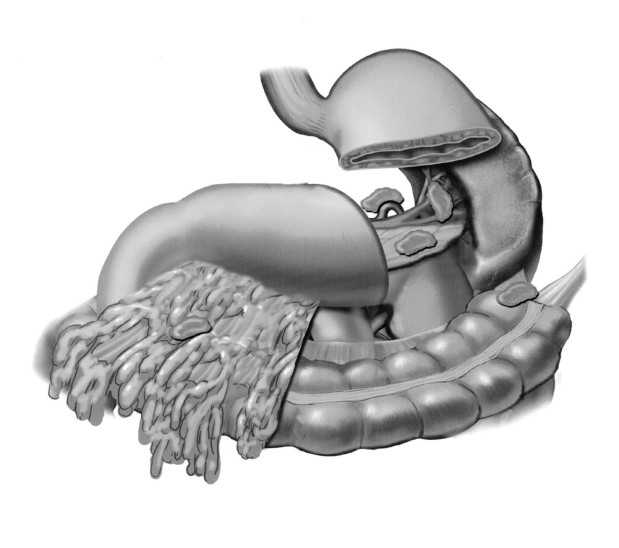

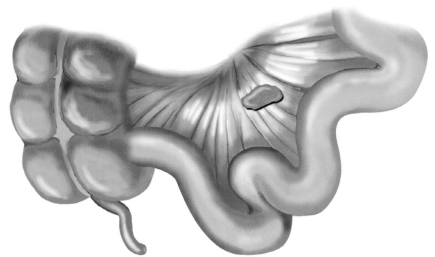

FIGURE C

Operating Room Setup for the Lateral Approach to Splenectomy

3. A right semilateral decubitus position with the operating table flexed approximately 30° is recommended. Variations from this setup are considered for surgeon preference and patient body habitus. All pressure points must be adequately padded and a bean-bag device is used to secure the patient's position. Elevating the kidney rest will additionally help to increase the space between the costal margin and iliac crest.

4. The surgeon and camera operator stand on the patient's right side while the assistant is on the left. The video monitors are stationed at both sides of the patient's head to facilitate adequate viewing from either side of the table.

5. When preparing and draping the patient, it can be helpful to mark the site for a left subcostal incision in case an emergent conversion to open should occur. The umbilicus should remain visible to serve as a landmark during the procedure. A laparotomy set should be open on the back table as well.

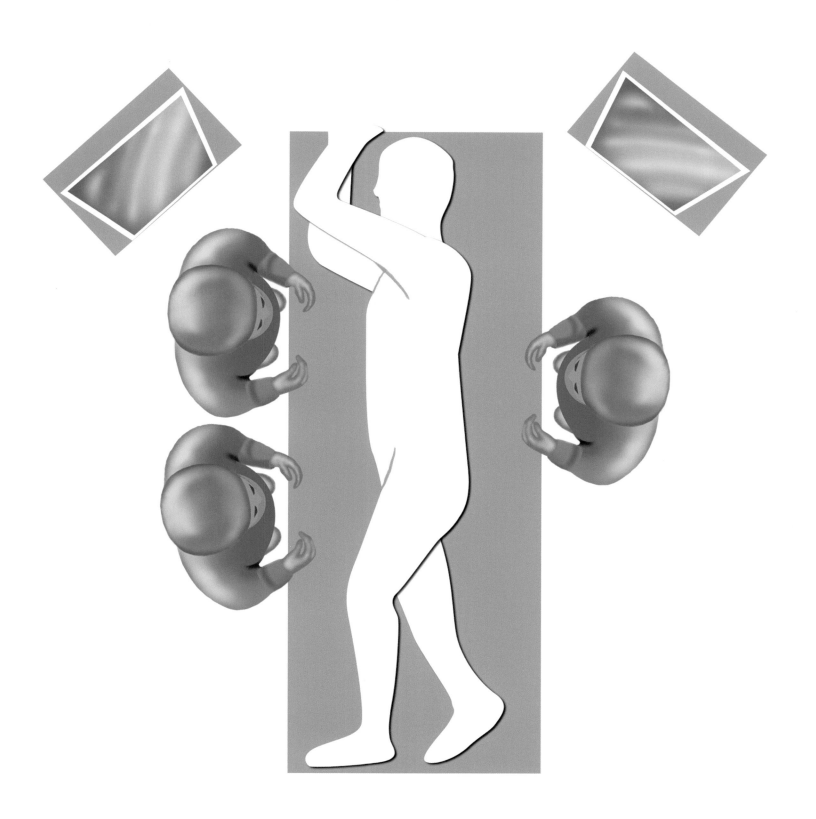

Access and Port Placement

6. A Veress needle can be used to obtain initial access just medial to the anterior axillary line and inferior to the left costal margin.

7. The first port is placed commonly in the left midclavicular line approximately 6 cm below the costal margin with an optical trocar. Exact port position varies by patient and spleen size. All subsequent ports are placed after initial visual survey to assess optimal port positions. For most patients, the optimal configuration of port placement parallels the costal margin, with the most medial port being just left of the midline and the most lateral port in the midaxillary line. A 12 mm port is placed inferior to an imaginary line connecting the other three 5 mm ports, as depicted in Figure D.

8. Alternatively, in patients with a small body habitus or a large spleen, it may be preferred to obtain pneumoperitoneum via an infraumbilical incision and an open approach.

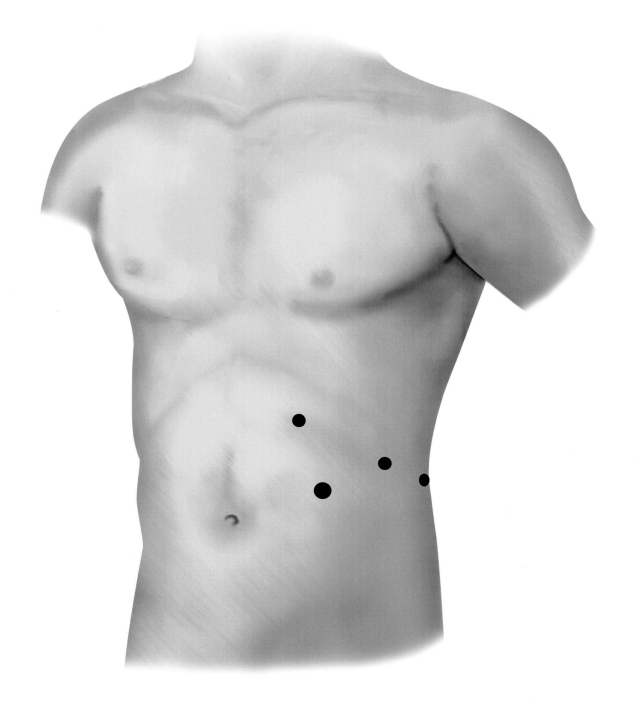

Dividing the Splenocolic Ligament

9. The patient is placed in steep reverse Trendelenburg position to facilitate inferior retraction of the colon. The inferior pole of the spleen is mobilized by dividing the attachments to the colon and the lateral abdominal wall. Extreme care must be taken to not injure the colon or the spleen during retraction. The dissection is carried out in a medial to lateral direction. These ligaments are relatively avascular and any vessels encountered can usually be controlled with ultrasonic shears or similiar tools.

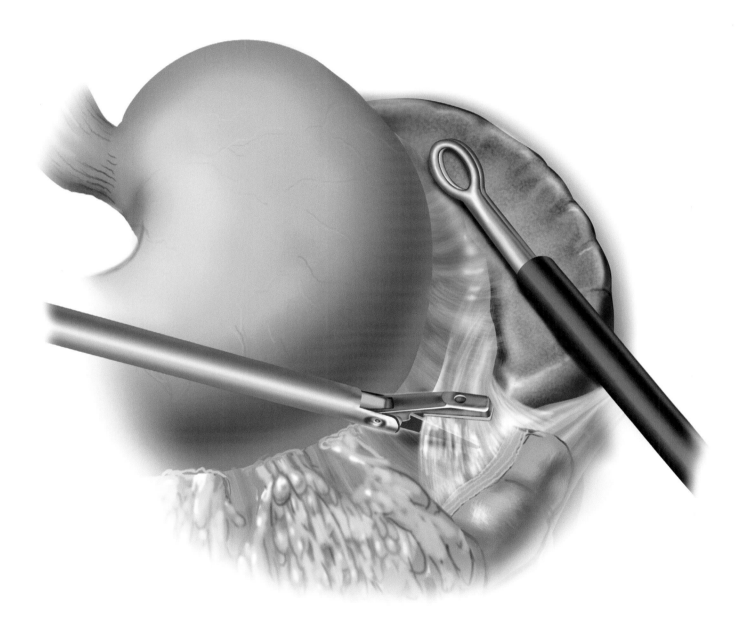

Dividing the Splenorenal Ligament

10. The splenorenal ligament is divided along the entire craniocaudal length of the spleen, being careful to not violate Gerota's fascia. This maneuver will facilitate medial retraction of the spleen for subsequent hilar dissection. Alternatively, the gastrosplenic ligament can be divided before the splenorenal ligament.

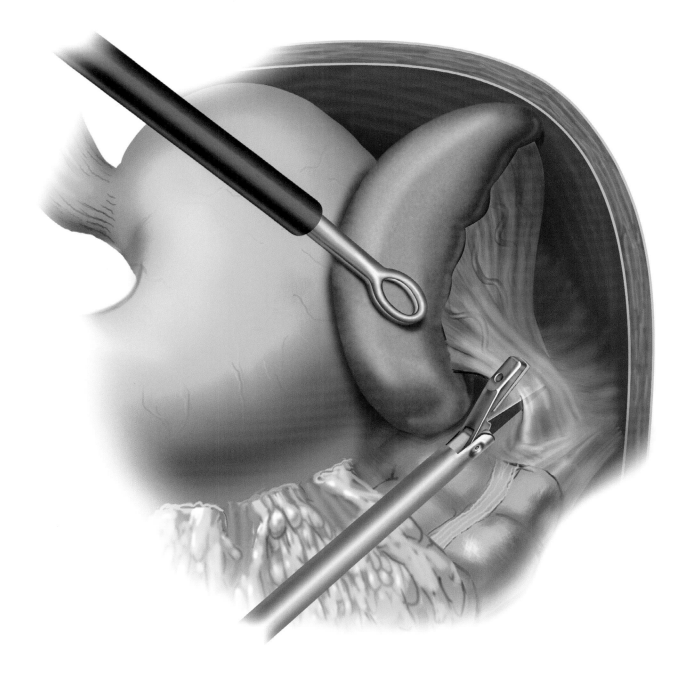

Dividing the Gastrosplenic Ligament and Short Gastrics

11. The ultrasonic coagulator is used to divide the gastrosplenic ligament, containing the short gastric vessels. Extreme care must be taken to not avulse these vessels during the dissection. The entire ligament is divided along the greater curve of the stomach, and, finally, the splenophrenic ligament is divided at the superior pole of the spleen, making sure to completely mobilize the upper pole of the spleen.

12. Dividing the gastrosplenic ligament exposes the lesser sac. If the hilar dissection is anticipated to be difficult, the splenic artery can be localized and ligated with a single clip or suture proximal to the hilum along its course at the superior border of the pancreas. Judicious use of clips is important, as use of the endoscopic stapler may be prohibited if clips are used in proximity to the splenic hilum. Remember that the splenic artery is quite tortuous throughout its course and that it is easily injured.

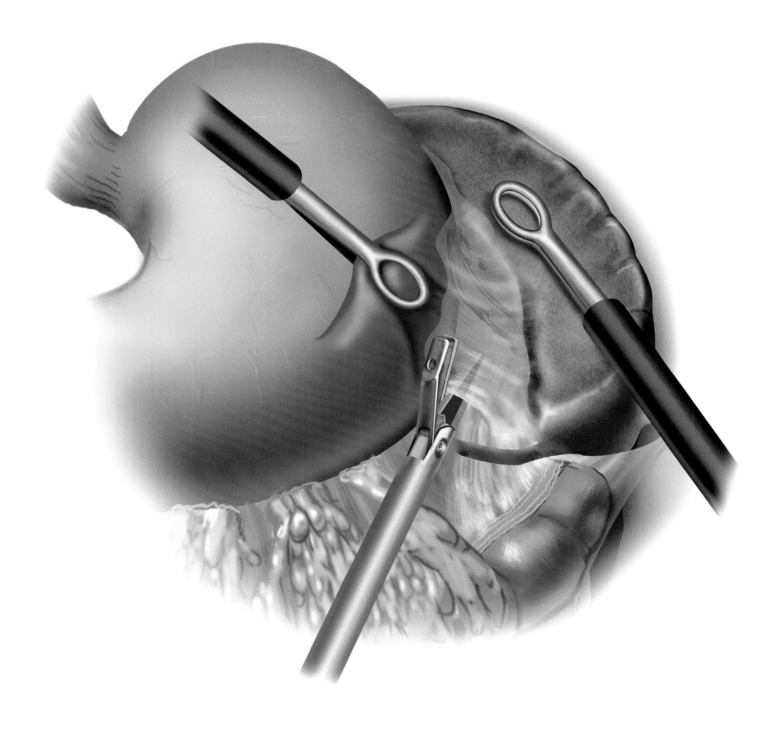

Dividing the Splenic Hilum

13. With the spleen circumferentially mobilized, the hilar dissection can be carried out from either the anterior or posterior aspect, depending on the position of the hilar vessels. The assistant gently elevates and retracts the spleen to expose the hilum, which facilitates determining the relationship of the pancreatic tail to the hilar vessels. The vessels are divided using an endoscopic linear cutting stapler with a vascular load (2.5 mm staples). After firing each staple load and opening the instrument jaws, be prepared to immediately close the instrument jaws to pressure occlude any troublesome bleeders.

14. Alternatively, each hilar branch can be separately dissected and controlled with surgical clips. It is noteworthy to recognize that the use of clips prevents the subsequent use of a stapling device. The linear stapler does not fire and cut through clips—substantial hemmorhage can result!

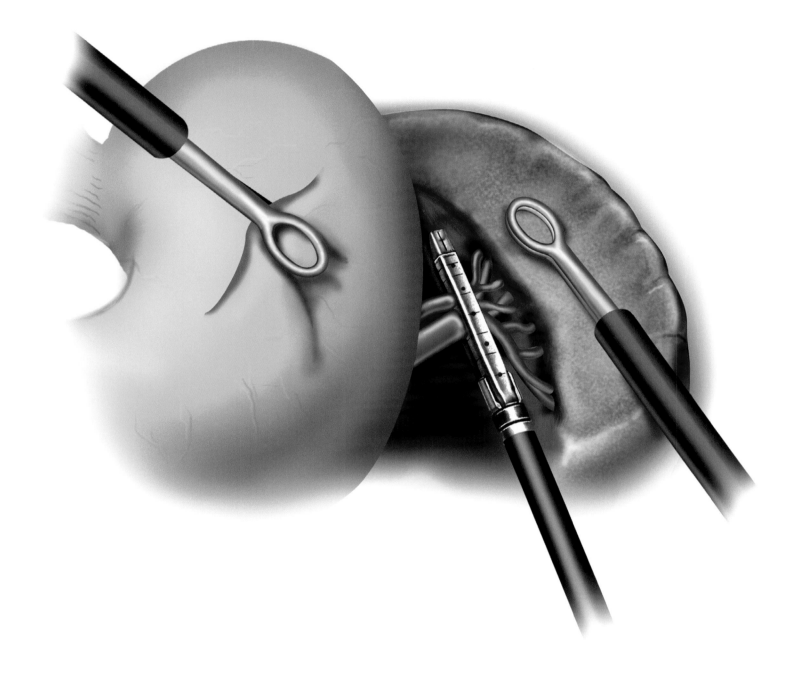

FIGURE I

Preparing for Extraction

15. Once the operative field is inspected for hemostasis, the 12 mm port is exchanged for an 18 mm port. A specimen retrieval bag is inserted and the spleen is placed completely inside. The bag should be of adequate strength to prevent rupture and subsequent intra-abdominal dissemination of splenic tissue (resulting in splenosis). The bag is closed at its apex with a pursestring suture.

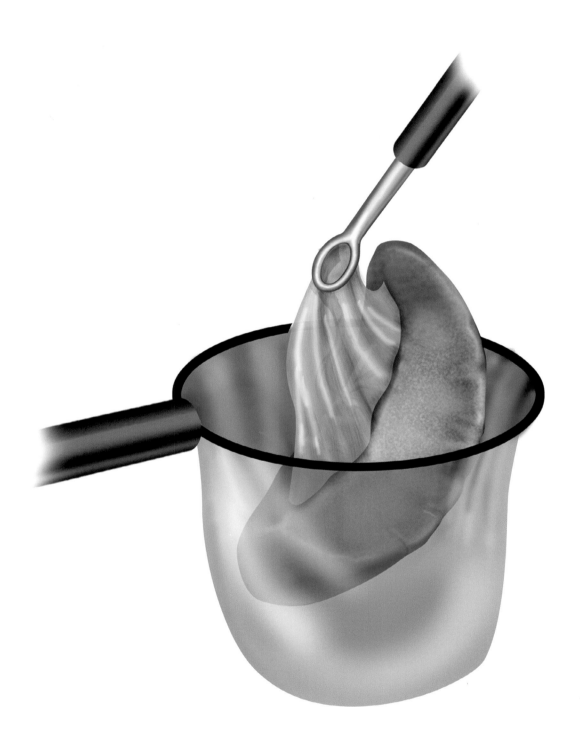

Removing the Specimen

16. The 18 mm trocar is removed while retaining control of the pursestring suture. The spleen is removed through this fascial incision in a piecemeal fashion, unless it is being resected for a solid tumor. Digital fracture technique and/or ringed forceps can assist in removal of the splenic fragments. The incision may need to be extended to remove the specimen. Care must be taken to not contaminate the wound with splenic tissue.

17. Penetrating towel clips can be used to temporarily close the fascia and/or skin for leak-free insufflation. Once the left upper quadrant is reinspected for satisfactory hemostasis, the fascial and skin incisions are closed in the usual manner. A closed suction drain can be left in place at the surgeon's discretion.

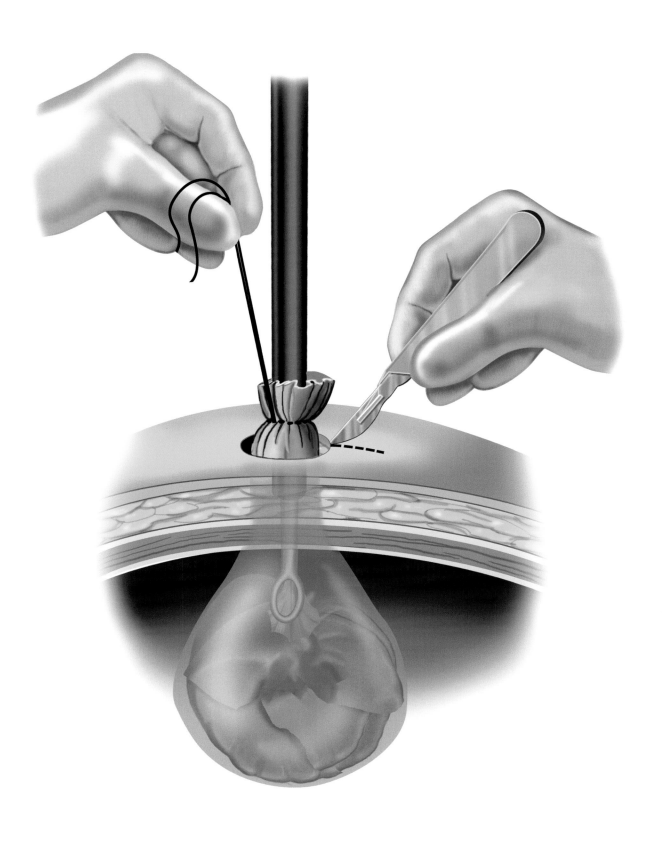

Postoperative Care

Sequential compression devices and/or subcutaneous heparin are continued postoperatively. Provided there was no enteric injury, postoperative antibiotics are usually not necessary. A nasogastric tube is optional, but may be left in place until return of bowel function, at which time it is removed and oral intake is advanced as tolerated.

Suggested Reading

1. Park A, Birgisson G, Mastrangelo MJ, Marcaccio MJ, Witzke D. Laparoscopic splenectomy: outcomes and lessons learned from over 200 cases. *Surgery*. 2000;128:660-667.

2. Brodsky JA, Brody FJ, Walsh RM, Malm JA, Ponsky JL. Laparoscopic splenectomy: experience with 100 cases. *Surg Endosc* 2002;16:851-854.

3. Katkhouda N, Mavor E. Laparoscopic splenectomy. *Surg Clin North Am*. 2000;80:1285-1297.

Commentary

**James Ellsmere, M.D., Beth Israel Deaconess Medical Center
Harvard Medical School**

Most centers consider laparoscopic splenectomy the approach of choice for elective patients requiring splenectomy. The only absolute contraindication to a laparoscopic approach is cirrhosis with portal hypertension. The relative contraindication remains massive splenomegaly. What constitutes massive splenomegaly is debatable. A spleen greater than 30 cm should be removed with an open or alternatively, a hand-assisted technique. Smaller spleens in patients with inadequate room between their costal margin and their iliac crest can be difficult to remove laparosopically. The most important consideration is whether there is adequate working space to establish pneumoperitoneum. This must be determined on a case-by-case basis.

The dissection involves five stages, including: 1) division of the short gastric vessels, 2) division of the splenocolic ligament, 3) ligation of the inferior pole vessels, 4) division of phrenic attachments of the spleen, and 5) hilar control. Direct grasping of the spleen may lead to capsular tear so it should be avoided. When manipulating the spleen, the operator should grasp the remnants of the ligamentous attachments or, preferably, use a blunt retractor. Noting the color changes in the spleen as the segmental vessels are divided is helpful to understanding the patient's specific vascular anatomy. Hilar control can be accomplished with a single or multiple firings of a vascular load on laparoscopic linear stapler. Alternatively, clips can be used, but the surgeon must be aware that they may interfere with further stapler firings.

Removing the spleen is an often underappreciated stage of the operation. Care must be taken not to damage the capsule prior to placing the spleen into the retrieval bag. Morcellating the spleen can be a tedious process, but care must also be taken not to inadvertently damage the retrieval bag, or worse, the surrounding viscera.

Antonio Garcia-Ruiz, M.D., Hospital Central Militar

Laparoscopic splenectomy has been mostly for treatment of idiopathic thrombocytopenia purpura patients. In these cases, the relatively normal size of the spleen allows me to work perfectly with only three trocars (one 12 mm and two 5 mm). Regarding accessory spleens, I routinely order a nuclear scan on these patients to rule out accessory spleens in the lower right quadrant where they may be out of my laparoscopic sight. Trocar site planning is a key factor for laparoscopic splenectomy and is totally related to the size of the spleen. In a normal-sized spleen, I start making a 15- mm transverse skin incision immediately below the left subcostal margin, from the midclavicular line to the lateral border of the rectus abdominis muscle. With blunt dissection, assisted by a pair of "S-shaped" retractors, I access the peritoneal cavity and insert a 12-mm Hasson trocar. However, in a splenomegaly case, I would have to lower my trocar sites accordingly. In all my cases, but one, I've been able to work them out adding only two more 5-mm trocars (one under the xyphoid process and the other over the midaxillary line, avoiding the splenic flexure attachments of the colon). I use a 5-mm angled scope to be able to change the position of my camera and improve my surgical view.

Different than the beautifully illustrated technique in this chapter, I divide the gastrosplenic ligament first, and then the splenocolic and splenorenal ligaments, leaving the splenic hilum for last. The reason for this order is that the splenorenal ligament holds the spleen in a convenient position for taking down the gastrosplenic ligament and the short gastric vessels, diminishing the potential for bleeding at this point. To divide the splenic hilum, in my early cases I used laparoscopic vascular staplers. In my last 10 cases I have used laparoscopic vessel sealing-cutting technology (Ligasure, Tyco Healthcare, Boulder, Colo) with excellent results. The advantages I have found with this instrument are a higher vessel sealing power and the ability to use it as many times as needed. Once the specimen is free inside the abdominal cavity, bagging it may be very cumbersome. One trick is to use gravity to your advantage and a very durable bag for extraction. At this time, the surgical bed has a 20° head-up tilt. After dividing the hilum, I flip the spleen over to have the hilum, facing up and place it under the transverse colon. I insert the bag and unroll it very carefully over the liver, directing its opening to my camera. Then, with my left hand grasping the lower edge of the bag opening and my right hand grasping the perihilar tissue on the specimen, I ask the anesthesiologist to tilt the surgical bed head-down and slowly slide the specimen inside the bag. Remember, the larger the specimen, the more difficulties you may find bagging it. Unfortunately, there is no efficient solution yet to morcellate the specimen for extraction. My choice still is to aspirate as much as possible with the aspiration cannula and then to use the ring forceps to extract what remains in the bag. I have found the reinforced nylon-polyurethane bag (Lap-Sac, Cook, Spencer, Ind) to be the best choice.

John F. Sweeney, M.D.
Baylor College of Medicine

When performing laparoscopic splenectomy, we prefer to place patients in a partial right lateral decubitus position after induction of general anesthesia as the authors have described. The operating table is flexed to expose the area between the left costal margin and iliac crest. With the patient secured to the operating room table, we then place the patient in steep reverse Trendelenburg position and role the operating table to the patient's right, thereby providing a near right lateral decubitus position. If however conversion to an open splenectomy is required, the operating table can be easily rolled to the patient's left, providing a near supine position.

Intra-abdominal access is then obtained per the surgeon's preference. We feel it is important to place this first camera trocar midway between the umbilicus and the left costal margin in the midclavicular line. Two 5 mm trocars are then placed in the upper midline or to the left of midline along the costal margin. Before beginning the laparoscopic splenectomy, a careful search for an accessory spleen(s) must be undertaken. Accessory spleens, found in 5% to 15% of the population, are most commonly located in the splenic hilum, along the route of the splenic vessels, in the greater omentum and along the left gonadal vein. The splenic flexure of the colon is then mobilized and an additional 12 mm trocar is placed in the left anterior axillary line, below the costal margin. This trocar will ultimately be used for dividing the splenic hilum using an endoscopic stapler with a vascular staple cartridge. The spleen is then mobilized and the splenic hilum divided as the authors have described. Another option that will limit blood loss is to identify and divide the splenic artery before proceeding with mobilization of the spleen.

Hand-assisted laparoscopic splenectomy (HALS) should be considered in patients who have significant splenomegaly or patients who require intact removal of the spleen. When HALS is indicated, a 7 cm incision is made in a left paramedian position, and the surgeon's left hand is placed into the abdomen. A hand-port device is utilized by some surgeons in this setting although we do not routinely use this device. We find that gas leakage can be contained by tightening the incision with a towel clamp. The conversion rate to open splenectomy in the setting of splenomegaly is significant. HALS decreases the conversion rate, while preserving the benefits of laparoscopy (e.g., less post-operative ileus, shorter length of stay, earlier return to work).

Matthew M. Hutter, M.D., M.P.H., Massachusetts General Hospital Harvard Medical School

Laparoscopic splenectomy has quickly become the preferred approach for removing the spleen for almost any indication, except trauma, active hemorrhage, or the truly massive spleen. This chapter does an excellent job of illustrating and highlighting many of the important technical aspects of safely removing the spleen laparoscopically.

Removal of the spleen should always be approached with a healthy respect for the robust blood supply coursing through this organ. It is imperative to have proper control, and sufficient dissection and visualization, to adequately characterize the hilar structures before proceeding with transection. One must quickly convert to an open procedure when things are not going well, or exposure or visualization is inadequate. Conversion should be done before frank, uncontrollable hemorrhage develops and a life-threatening situation ensues.

Removing massive spleens has been safely described, but this should only be tackled by the experienced laparoscopic surgeon, with a low threshold for conversion to an open procedure. Adjuncts such as a hand port may prove to be useful in the setting of massive splenomegaly, or early in one's experience in spleens of moderate size.

I like the way the authors highlight the perils of using clips before staples—a practice that is dangerous and can lead to staple misfirings and hemorrhage. This point is not always appreciated by the novice or infrequent laparoscopist and is worth emphasizing again.

The key aspect to laparoscopic splenectomy is finding the right balance between adequate mobilization of the splenic attachments to allow you to fully characterize the splenic hilum, without taking too many of these splenic suspensory ligaments, which compromises exposure. It is best not to circumferentially mobilize the spleen, but to leave the superior pole attachments (when they exist) so that the spleen hangs from the sidewall. This technique allows gravity to work for you as a retractor, not against you. This concept must be foremost in your mind during the dissection and the problem must be anticipated, because once the wrong ligaments are released and the spleen flops in your way, it is too late. Should this happen, a fan retractor or a flexible liver retractor can be useful.

The other key technical point is to fully characterize the hilar vessels before transecting them. They do not have to be completely skeletonized, but the relationship of the vessels to the pancreas and to the concavity of the spleen must be visualized so that a clear transection line is determined. This proposed transection line must be in line with the trocar through which the stapler passes, and must be delineated in this 3-D space from start to finish, and anteriorly and posteriorly, before the transection begins. By fully characterizing the optimal path of the stapler, one is less likely to damage the pancreas, hemitransect a vessel, or jam the stapler into the superior pole of the spleen before the hilar vessels are controlled. If there is some bleeding, and the proposed path has been clearly characterized, then a stapler can be quickly reapplied to achieve control before visualization is lost. If there is any concern of damage to the tail of the pancreas, a drain should be left and checked later for amylase content.

David W. Easter, M.D.
University of California, San Diego

Laparoscopy is considered whenever splenectomy is indicated. Splenic trauma is not excepted from this list, though appropriate cases are rare with current imaging capabilities. Common indications for splenectomy include ITP (immune thrombocytopenia purpura) and CML (chronic myelogenous leukemia.) One diagnostic theme helps determine which patients are suitable for surgical intervention, i.e., the "battleground" concept. If one considers that the circulating levels of platelets and/or red cells are a balance between production and destruction, then it becomes clear that altering the balance is the surgeon's goal. A bone marrow aspiration is required in situations when this balance is not completely clear, to assure the surgeon (and patient!) that cellular production is adequate.

The laparoscopic approach does not make sense when: 1) production of cellular elements is significantly impaired, 2) the entire organ's architecture must be inspected intact, or 3) other concurrent procedures diminish the value of the minimal access approach. Patients with very large spleens, or with severe thrombocytopenia, are considered for preoperative embolization of the splenic artery. Even in situations of severe thrombocytopenia, platelet infusions are given only after control of the splenic artery, as ongoing consumption often precludes any hope of significantly improving platelet counts prior to such control.

We prefer the right lateral decubitus position, with the table rolled slightly to the left. The skin is superstitiously marked prior to insufflation at two fingers distance below the left costal margin in case an emergency open incision is required. Our first port is usually placed in the midclavicular line just superior to the level of the umbilicus, but this varies by patient and spleen size. Subsequent ports are placed after initial laparoscopic inspection.

One favorite technique of ours is to mobilize all splenic attachments, in no particular order, such that the spleen is held primarily by its hilar vessels. Next, the "anaconda" flexible retractor is placed through a lateral port and engaged such that it curls around the hilum. The spleen can then be elevated on this retractor with no significant trauma, exposing the hilar vessels. Vascular staple loads (2.0 mm final compression) are used for the hilar vessels— usually only one 45 mm–long cartridge is required. Whenever the stapler is opened, the surgeon is ready to rapidly reclose the device in the rare circumstance of stapler failure or partial vascular control. It is even possible to bring a second stapler into the field to use proximal to the first when vascular control is incomplete or concerning.

Other tips:

1. Use a gauze 4 x 4 sponge to help blunt dissection and/or suction against. Tie a silk suture at one corner if desired for easy location and retrieval.

2. Don't rush the piecemeal removal of the spleen. Ring forceps work well to morcellate and remove large pieces. Morcellate-grab-remove-suction-repeat...

3. Always look for accessory spleens—present in 10% to 30% of cases, depending upon how carefully the surgeon looks!

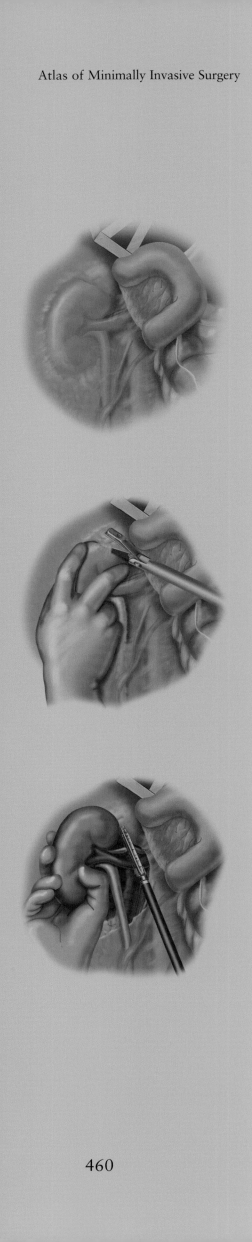

Laparoscopic Nephrectomy

Laparoscopic nephrectomy is utilized in the treatment of both benign and malignant conditions. The laparoscopic approach has also gained much favor for performing living donor nephrectomy. Anatomic differences between the right and left kidneys necessitate a slight variation in technique owing to differences in surrounding structures. Two different approaches have been described and utilized for performing a laparoscopic nephrectomy: 1) transabdominal lateral flank approach, and 2) retroperitoneal approach. Most surgeons favor the transabdominal lateral flank approach for several reasons, including a large working space, gravity retraction of surrounding structures, and easy access high in the retroperitoneum. Most indications for performing nephrectomy require the organ to be extracted intact, whether it be for pathologic investigation or for transplantation. Therefore, we recommend placing a hand port early on in the procedure to benefit from hand retraction, since an incision will have to be made to remove the specimen. This technique is described in detail.

Preoperative Preparation

1. Sequential compression stockings and subcutaneous heparin may be used for prophylaxis against deep venous thrombosis. Intravenous antibiotics, usually a first-generation cephalosporin, are administered prophylactically. After induction of general anesthesia, the bladder is emptied with a urinary catheter and the stomach is decompressed with an orogastric tube.

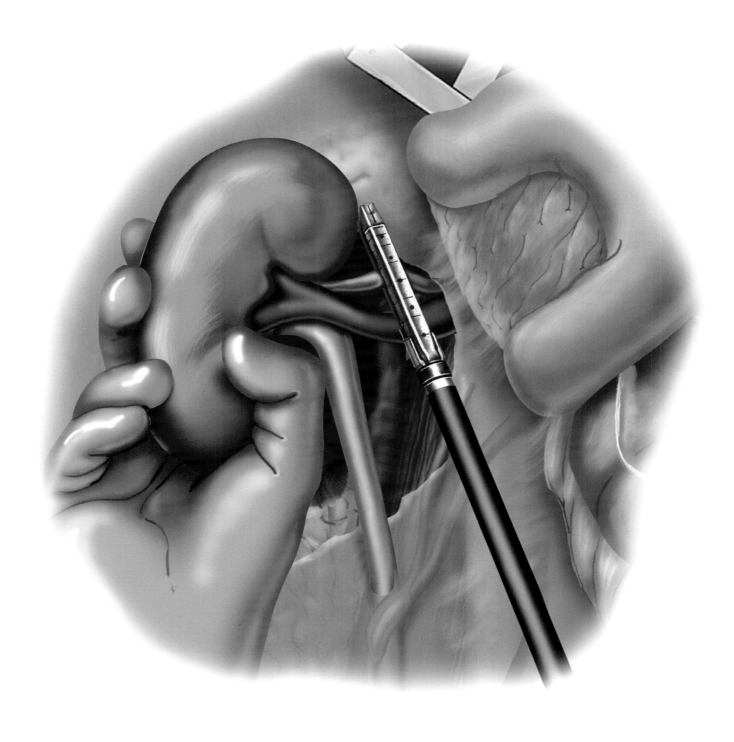

Right Nephrectomy

FIGURE A

Operating Room Setup

2. The patient is positioned in the lateral decubitus position with the right side rotated upward and the table flexed 30°at the waist. A pillow may be placed between the knees. Placing the patient in reverse Trendelenburg position further facilitates subsequent port placement and gravity retraction of adjacent organs.

3. All pressure points must be adequately padded and a bean-bag device is used to secure the patient's position when rotating the table to facilitate exposure and viewing during the procedure.

4. The surgeon and camera operator stand to the left or anterior to the patient, while the assistant stands opposite the table. The video monitors are stationed at both sides of the patient's head to facilitate adequate viewing from either side of the table. A laparotomy set should be readily available should emergent conversion be necessary secondary to uncontrolled bleeding.

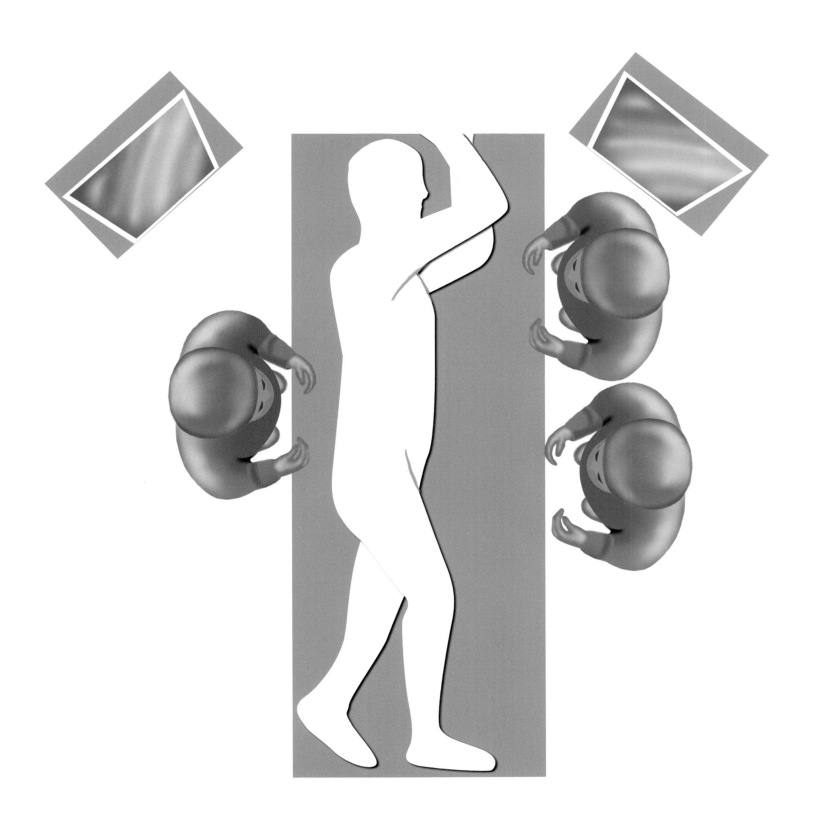

Access and Port Placement

5. Initial access is obtained just lateral to the rectus abdominus muscle at the level of the umbilicus. Pneumoperitoneum can be obtained with either an open or closed technique via a Veress needle. If a closed technique is used, a direct-view optical trocar can be utilized for placing the first port to minimize the incidence of intra-abdominal injury during this step.

6. If a 5 mm laparoscope is utilized, two 5 mm ports are placed under direct vision in the midclavicular and midaxillary lines below the costal margin. Otherwise, one of the ports should be 10 mm in size to allow for alternating the camera's position. The incision site for subsequent placement of the hand port is also shown.

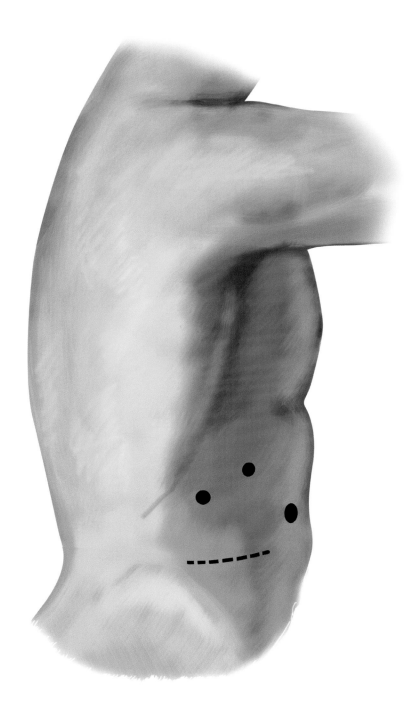

FIGURE C

Exposing the Right Kidney

7. Exploratory laparoscopy must first be performed to assess for any evidence of liver metastasis or other upper abdominal pathology.

8. Using a harmonic scalpel, the right colon is reflected medially by mobilizing the white line of Toldt, which exposes the duodenum, kidney, and ureter. The duodenum is Kocherized to allow visualization of the left renal vein emptying into the inferior vena cava (IVC). Dissection is continued along the anterior surface of the IVC until the right renal vein is identified.

9. The right lobe of the liver is mobilized anteriorly and medially by incising the triangular ligament to the level of the diaphragm. A liver retractor placed through the most medial port will adequately retract the right lobe once it has been mobilized. The assistant's hand can also be used to do this.

10. The right ureter is identified and mobilized along its length from the kidney into the pelvis. When performing a living donor nephrectomy, it is paramount to preserve the surrounding tissue containing its blood supply, including the gonadal vessel.

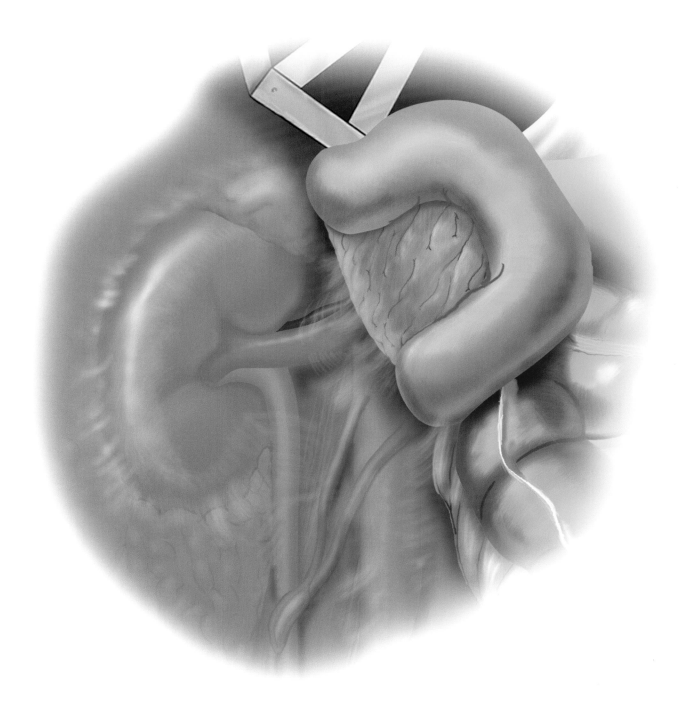

Mobilizing the Right Kidney

11. A 7 cm to 8 cm transverse incision is made in the right lower quadrant and a laparoscopic disk is placed here to allow the assistant's hand to facilitate the remaining dissection.

12. The kidney is circumferentially mobilized from its retroperitoneal attachments using ultrasonic dissection. The assistant's hand retracts the superior pole of the kidney in a caudal direction to facilitate dissecting the adrenal gland free from its renal attachments.

13. The right renal artery is identified, lying posterior to the renal vein, and mobilized to its origin from the aorta. Using a combination of medial and lateral exposure, the renal hilum is skeletonized such that the kidney is only attached by the renal artery and vein. This will require flipping the kidney medially, such that the posterior hilum can be visualized. This maneuver should be kept to a minimum when performing nephrectomy for transplantation, as it may cause renal ischemia and may jeopardize postoperative function in the recipient.

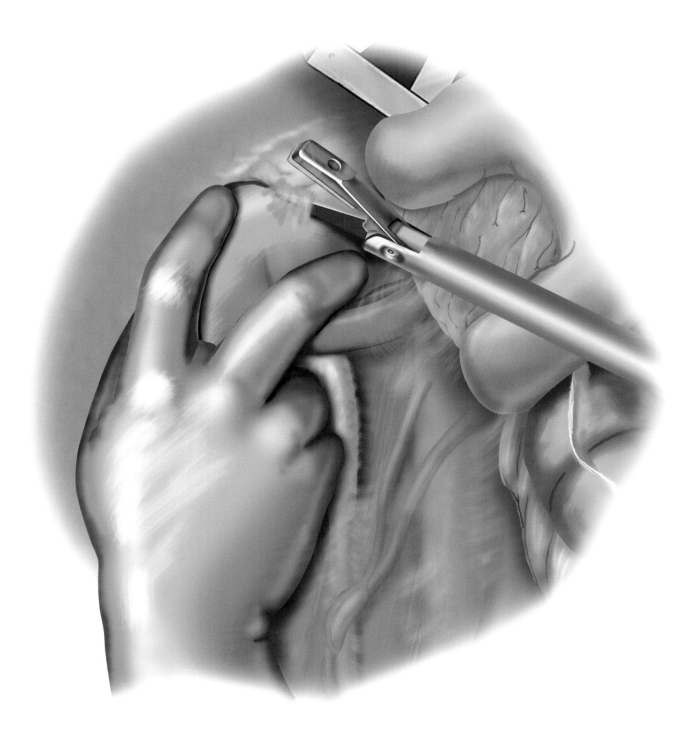

Dividing the Renal Vessels and Extracting the Kidney

14. A 30-45 mm endoscopic GIA stapler (2.5 mm staples) is used to transect the renal artery. A second firing is used to divide the renal vein. We recommend to avoid clipping the renal artery. Although this can add length to the vessel, clip dislodgement has been reported with devastating consequence.

15. The assistant delivers the kidney through the incision made for the hand port and a clamp is placed across the distal ureter and the ureter is divided proximally, thus removing the specimen from the patient. Alternatively, the ureter can be clipped in situ, prior to vessel division. If the procedure is being performed for organ donation, it is imperative to minimize the kidney's warm ischemic time.

16. A 2-0 silk tie is placed around the ureteral stump and it is allowed to retract into the abdomen. The operative field is inspected for adequate hemostasis. The ports are removed under direct vision and the fascia and skin incisions are closed in the usual manner.

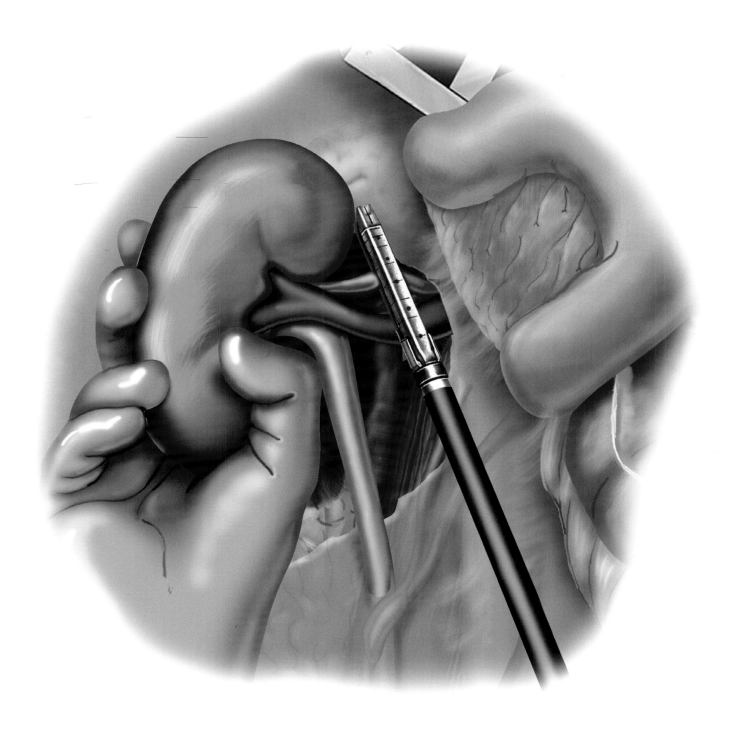

Left Nephrectomy

FIGURE F

Operating Room Setup

1. The patient is positioned in the lateral decubitus position with the left side rotated upward and the table flexed 30° at the waist. A pillow may be placed between the knees. Placing the patient in reverse Trendelenburg position further facilitates subsequent port placement and gravity retraction of adjacent organs.

2. All pressure points must be adequately padded and a bean-bag device is used to secure the patient's position when rotating the table to facilitate exposure and viewing during the procedure.

3. The surgeon and camera operator usually stand to the right or anterior to the patient, while the assistant stands opposite the table. The video monitors are stationed at both sides of the patient's head to facilitate adequate viewing from either side of the table. A laparotomy set should be readily available should emergent conversion be necessary secondary to uncontrolled bleeding.

473

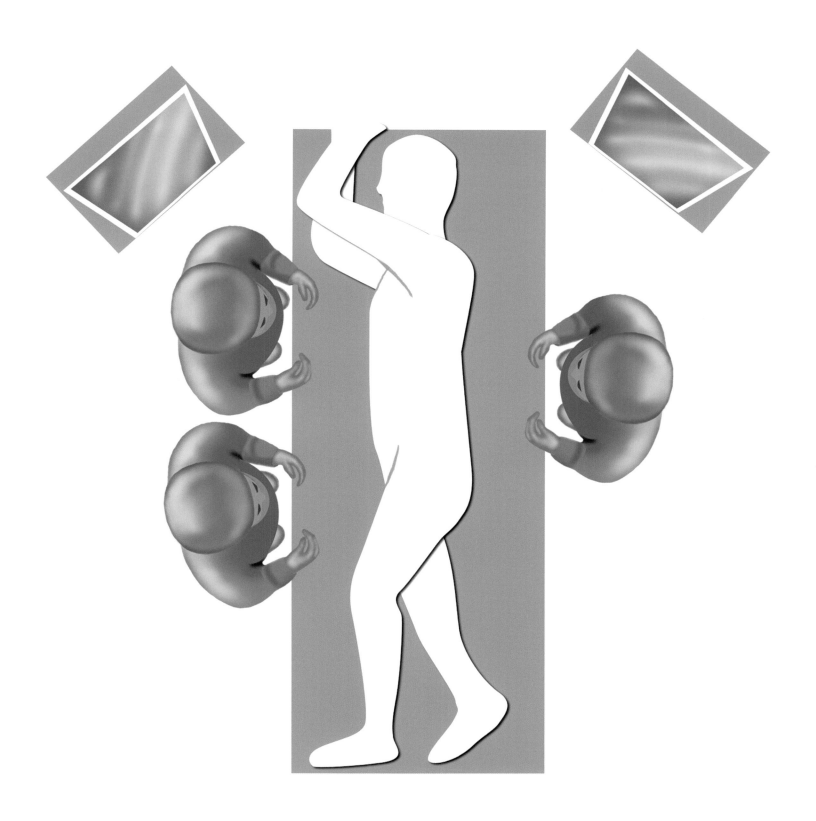

Access and Port Placement

4. Initial access is obtained just lateral to the rectus abdominus muscle at the level of the umbilicus. Pneumoperitoneum can be obtained with either an open or closed technique via a Veress needle. If a closed technique is used, a direct-view optical trocar can be utilized for placing the first port to minimize the incidence of intra-abdominal injury during this step.

5. If a 5 mm laparoscope is utilized, two 5 mm ports are placed under direct vision in the midclavicular and midaxillary lines below the costal margin. Otherwise, one of the ports should be 10 mm in size to allow for alternating the camera's position. The incision site for subsequent placement of the hand port is also shown.

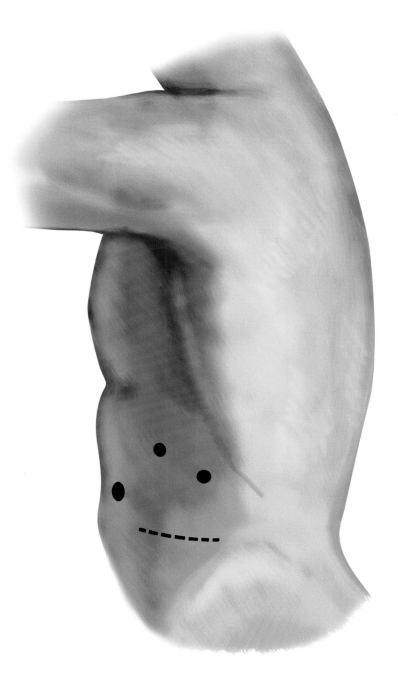

Exposing the Left Kidney

6. The splenic flexure of the colon is mobilized away from the inferior pole of the spleen by dividing the splenocolic ligament. Its lateral attachments are divided down to the level of the pelvis and gravity retraction allows the colon to fall away from the operative field.

7. The lateral attachments of the spleen and the splenorenal ligament are divided up to the level of the diaphragm. This mobilization is facilitated by gravity, allowing the spleen to fall anteriorly and medially away from the retroperitoneum. This greatly improves exposure of the upper pole of the kidney.

8. The left adrenal gland is contained in the perinephric fat at the superomedial pole of the left kidney. The tail of the pancreas often needs to be somewhat mobilized as well in order to clearly visualize the renal hilum, inferior aspect of the adrenal gland, and left adrenal vein.

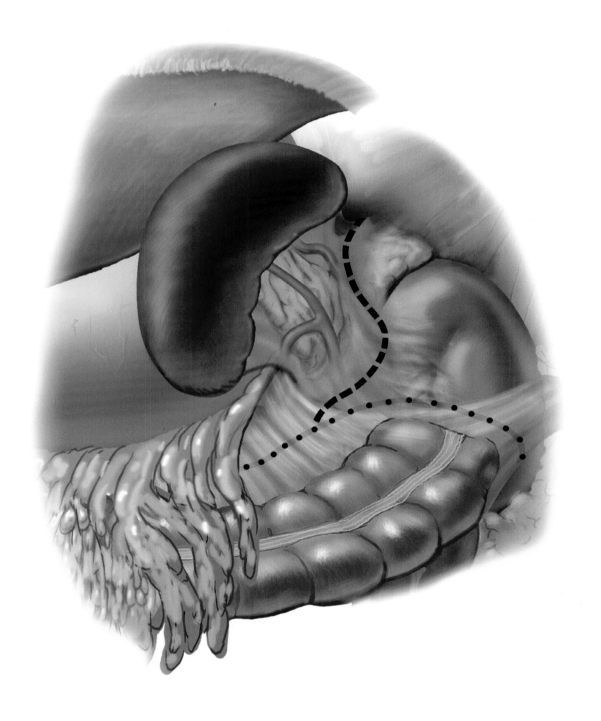

FIGURE I

Mobilizing the Left Kidney and Extraction

9. The left adrenal vein courses from the inferomedial aspect of the adrenal gland and empties into the left renal vein. The adrenal vein should be localized, circumferentially dissected free, and divided between surgical clips (two clips are placed on each side). The inferior phrenic vein usually drains into the left adrenal vein proximal to its junction with the left renal vein. The left gonadal vein emptying into the inferior aspect of the left renal vein is similarly identified, circumferentially mobilized, and divided between doubly placed surgical clips. Additional length on the cut end of the gonadal vein can be used for cranial retraction of the renal vein. This facilitates exposure behind the renal vein and will greatly help in exposure and control of any lumbar veins.

10. The left ureter is identified and mobilized along its length from the kidney into the pelvis. When performing a living donor nephrectomy, it is paramount to preserve the surrounding tissue containing its blood supply.

11. A hand port is placed in the left lower quadrant and the assistant's hand is used to facilitate circumferential mobilization of the left kidney and its hilum. Hilar vessel division, specimen retrieval, ureteral ligation, and closure are identical to that as previously described for a right nephrectomy.

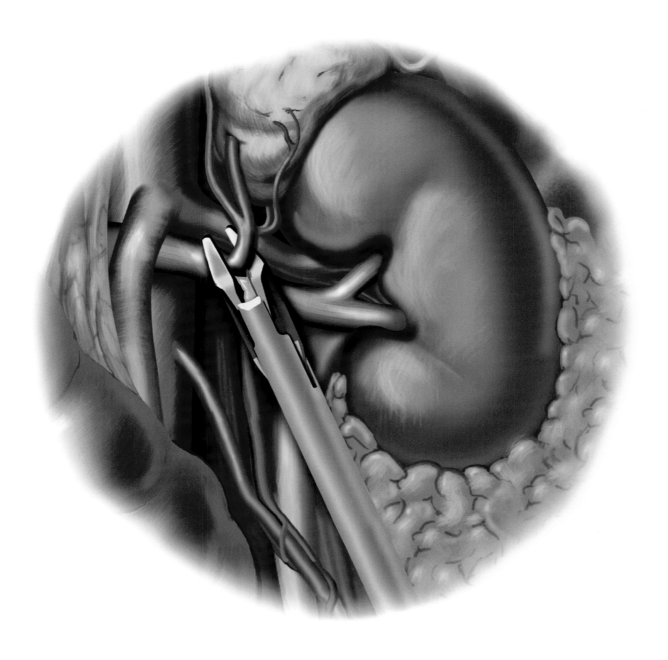

Postoperative Care

Sequential compression devices and/or subcutaneous heparin are continued postoperatively. Provided there was no colonic injury during splenic mobilization, postoperative antibiotics are usually not necessary. Oral intake is advanced as tolerated.

Suggested Reading

1. Jacobs SC, Cho E, Dunkin BJ, et al. Laparoscopic live donor nephrectomy: the University of Maryland 3-year experience. *J Urol*. 2000;164:1494-1499.

2. Kuo PC, Johnson LB, Sitzmann JV. Laparoscopic donor nephrectomy with a 23-hour stay: a new standard for transplantation surgery. *Ann Surg*. 2000;231:772-779.

3. Portis AJ, Yan Y, Landman J, et al. Long-term follow-up after laparoscopic radical nephrectomy. *J Urol*. 2002;167:1257-1262.

Commentary

Khalid Khwaja, M.D., Beth Israel Deaconess Medical Center
Harvard Medical School

Various techniques for laparoscopic donor nephrectomy have been described. The approach is either transperitoneal or extraperitoneal. The latter approach is more tedious, but has the theoretical advantage of avoiding intra-abdominal adhesions. Port placement varies, not just in location, but also size and number. The use of a hand port facilitates the dissection and adds a measure of safety. Some surgeons prefer a totally laparoscopic dissection, extracting the kidney, upon completion, through a Pfannenstiel-type incision. Robotic laparoscopy has also been successfully used for performing donor nephrectomies. Regardless of the method used, care must be taken to avoid damage to the kidney, ureter and renal vasculature. Warm ischemia, which begins after division of the renal artery, must be minimized by expeditious removal and flushing of the donor kidney.

For left nephrectomies, I position the patient at a 70° tilt rather than a complete decubitus position; this allows the colon to fall away without having the kidney fall forward and obscure the hilum. I begin with hand-port placement, via a 6 cm or 7 cm midline incision and then place two or three 12 mm, nonbladed ports in the left flank, all below the level of the umbilicus and "triangulated" toward an imaginary renal hilum. The surgeon's left hand is then placed in the hand port, and the dominant hand used for controlling the laparocopic instruments. After mobilizing the colon, I identify the ureter (it can readily be located just superficial to the bifurcation of the common iliac artery) and the gonadal vein. These structures are mobilized together if possible, thus keeping intact the periureteric tissue. The gonadal vein is then followed cephalad to its junction with the renal vein. The rest of the dissection proceeds as described by the authors.

For right nephrectomies, I prefer a subumbilical midline incision for the hand port, with trocars placed just above the umbilicus, and in the right flank region. After mobilization of the cecum and right colon, the ureter and gonadal vein are identified. The gonadal vein is traced to its caval junction; the renal vein can then be identified by continuing the dissection upwards along the right caval border. A fan-type retractor placed through the lateral-most flank port helps retract the right lobe of the liver, allowing exposure of the hilum and upper pole of the kidney. The renal artery is best dissected from "behind", with the kidney retracted toward the midline. Use of a vascular TA stapler on the renal vein will yield more length of vein for the recipient operation.

Finally, donor safety during this operation is of utmost importance. The threshold for conversion to laparotomy should be low if there is excessive bleeding, the anatomy is unclear, or the procedure is taking too long.

Jeffrey A. Cadeddu, M.D., Parkland Hospital
University of Texas Southwestern Medical Center

Laparoscopic nephrectomy, for benign disease, most malignant conditions, and kidney donation is now the standard of care. As one might expect there are numerous technical variations in the surgical technique that such an atlas cannot be expected to address. However, for the surgeon early in his/her learning curve, I believe it is critical that they are aware of the different surgical approaches.

To highlight, though a hand-assist technique is advocated in this chapter, many surgeons find the hand obtrusive and cumbersome. Similar to laparoscopic cholecystectomy, the novice should know that the kidney can be safely removed with a "pure" laparoscopic technique. Also, trocar placement varies tremendously. Those surgeons who do not use a hand-assisted technique usually place the camera port at the umbilicus with a second port midway between the xyphoid and umbilicus and the third lateral to the rectus below the umbilicus. Finally, unless a donor nephrectomy is performed, it is my opinion that the renal artery and vein need not be skeletonized routinely. Rather, once identified they can be safely divided with separate loads of the endovascular stapler. This simplifies the procedure, reducing the risk of vascular injury. Finally, in the case of malignancy, it important to use an entrapment sack to minimize the potential of tumor seeding.

The authors are to be congratulated for crafting a clear and straightforward description and illustration of laparoscopic nephrectomy.

Scott R. Johnson, M.D., Beth Israel Deaconess Medical Center
Harvard Medical School

Lap donor nephrectomy has made significant strides in the transplant community since its humble beginnings in 1995. While initially viewed by many skeptics as unnecessary, it has quickly become the standard of care in most transplant centers. Over the past decade, the number of living-donor renal transplants has increased substantially, such that in the last 2 years the number of living donors has exceeded the number of deceased donors performed in this country. While this cannot be attributed entirely to widespread use of laparoscopic donor nephrectomy, a number of centers have published single-center experience documenting increased volume with institution of a laparoscopic donor program. The benefits of laparoscopic donor nephrectomy are similar to those seen for other minimally invasive techniques as compared to the more traditional approach with one notable exception. In a single center study, donors were asked about their recovery after traditional and open nephrectomy. Surprisingly, at 1 year, open donors had not felt that they had returned to their predonation level of health, whereas laparoscopic donors reported that they had returned to baseline health status at 33 days.

A number of techniques have been described to complete the procedure, including a total laparoscopic approach and renal extraction via a Pfannenstiel incision once renal hilar vasculature has been divided, and hand-assisted techniques. Two hand-assisted techniques utilized either place the hand port in a midline supraumbilical location or via a lower abdominal incision placed lateral to the rectus sheath. The former technique permits the operating surgeon to assist himself, while the latter requires an assistant to perform the hand assist. While the self-assisted technique is faster, the downside is that upper pole dissection is more difficult, due to camera location. The benefit of the assistant surgeon performing the hand assist is that the camera can be placed more cephalad, facilitating exposure of the upper pole of the kidney. The other benefit of this technique is in training residents and fellows. With the senior surgeon guiding the procedure via a hand assist, the pace and sequence of the procedure can be controlled by the most experienced member of the surgical team.

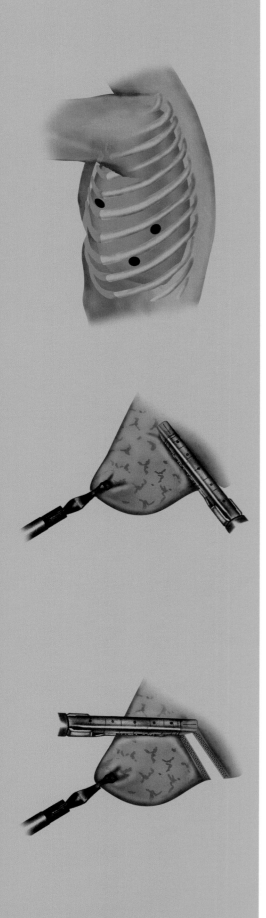

Thoracoscopic Pulmonary Wedge Resection

Video-assisted thoracic surgery (VATS) techniques can be used for pulmonary nodulectomy, lung biopsies, management of pleural and pericardial effusions, management of persistant pneumothorax, pleural decortication, sympathectomy, and esophageal myotomy.

Preoperative Preparation

1. Sequential compression stockings and subcutaneous heparin may be used for prophylaxis against deep venous thrombosis. A first-generation cephalosporin is administered prophylactically. After induction of general anesthesia, a double-lumen endotracheal tube is placed and its position is confirmed with flexible bronchoscopy. The bladder may be emptied with a urinary catheter.

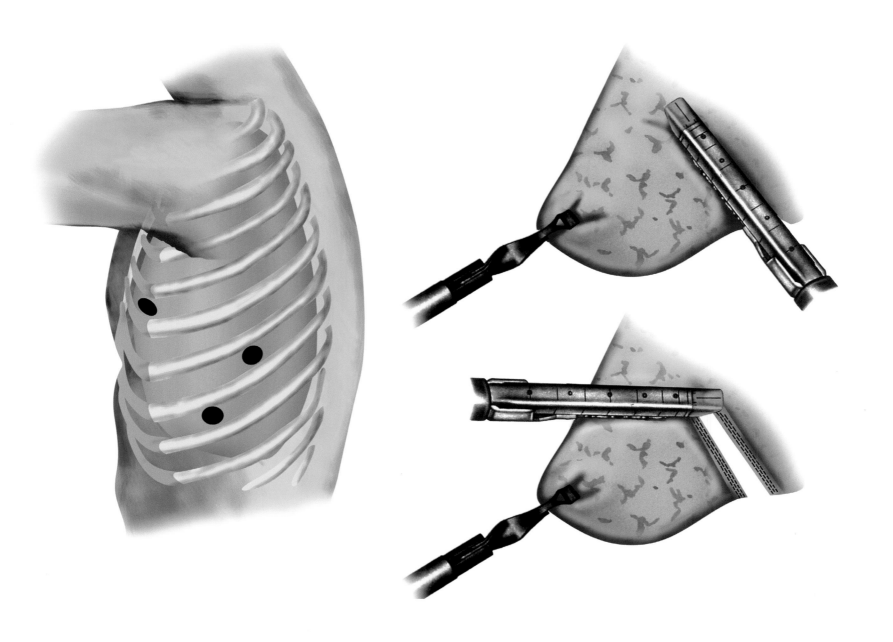

Operating Room Setup

2. The patient is placed in a lateral decubitus position on a bean-bag device with the side of interest directed upward. All pressure points are padded. The patient's positioning should facilitate a thoracotomy, if necessary.

3. The surgeon and camera holder stand facing the patient's back, while the assistant stands opposite the table.

4. The video monitors are stationed at both sides of the patient's head to facilitate adequate viewing from either side of the table. For lower-lobe targets or procedures at the base of the thorax, placement of video monitors toward the patient's feet facilitates viewing.

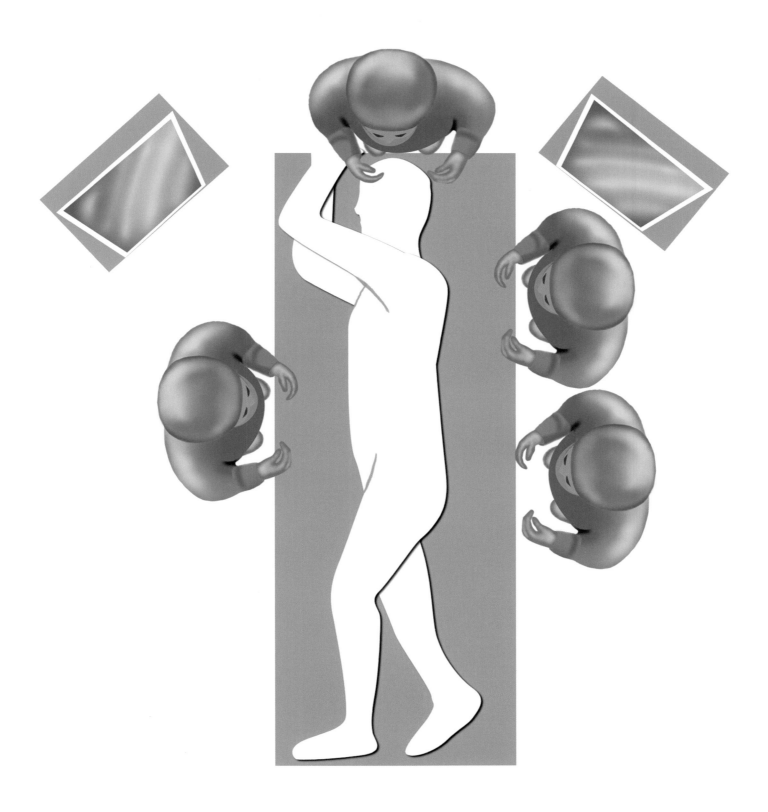

Access and Port Placement

5. The lung of interest is deflated by having the anesthesiologist remove it from the ventilatory circuit. The rigid thorax creates an adequate working space without the need for carbon dioxide insufflation.

6. Ports should be placed in order to provide the best view of the surgical field and to create the widest possible triangle centered on the area of interest. Consideration should also be made to the subsequent placement of a chest tube. The camera port is placed in the midaxillary line between the fourth and ninth intercostal spaces, depending on the area of interest. Two working ports should be inserted anteriorly and posteriorly respective to the camera in order to create a wide working triangle.

7. The technique for port insertion resembles that for placing a chest tube. Specifically, dissection should be made along the superior border of the rib to avoid injury to the neurovascular bundle and digital palpation should be used to assess for pleural adhesions prior to port placement. Once the camera is inserted, subsequent ports are placed under direct vision.

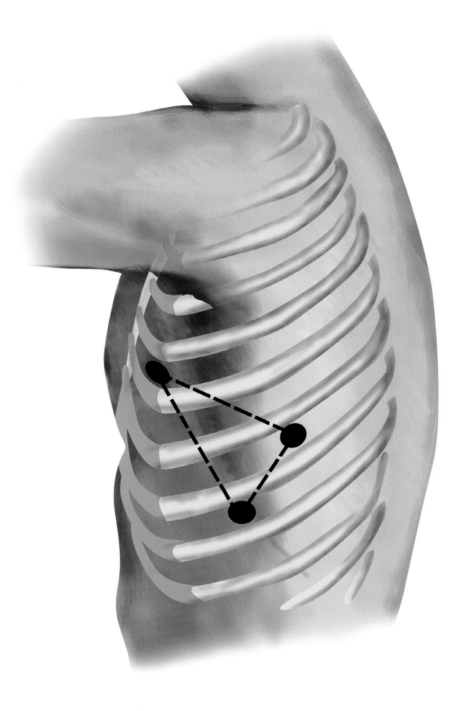

FIGURE C

Pulmonary Wedge Resection

8. A thorough visual exploration of the thoracic cavity should be conducted. The area of interest intended for resection is grasped by an atraumatic grasper. Any adhesions that interfere with proper exposure are divided.

9. Repeated fires of an endoscopic linear stapler (usually with blue 3.5 mm or green 4.8 mm staple cartridges) is used to resect the portion of lung tissue. The use of a reticulating stapler facilitates resection of targets at the extremes of the lung (apex, basilar, or medially abutting the mediastinum). Staple-line buttressing (bovine pericardium, ePTFE, etc.) may be used to help seal staple lines and reduce postoperative air leak. If necessary, hemostasis is obtained with controlled application of electrocautery.

10. The lung is returned to the ventilatory circuit under direct vision to assess for significant air leaks. If present, these should be controlled with another firing of the stapler. A single chest tube (range 20-28 Fr) is placed via the original camera port. The ports are withdrawn, and incisions closed with absorbable sutures.

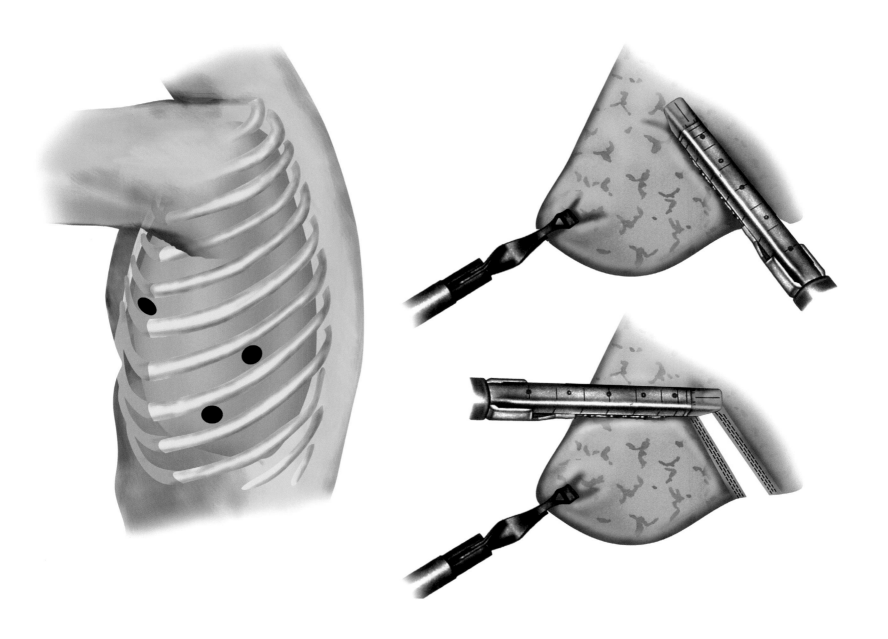

Postoperative Care

Sequential compression devices and/or subcutaneous heparin are continued postoperatively. Antibiotics may be continued for 24 hours at the surgeon's discretion. The chest tube is maintained on 20 cm to 25 cm of water suction. A chest x-ray in the PACU confirms lung expansion. Once there is no air leak and drainage is less than 200 to 300 cc/day, the chest tube may be removed. Patients are usually able to tolerate oral nutrition the evening of surgery and are advanced as tolerated.

Suggested Reading

1. DeCamp MM, Jaklitsch MT, Mentzer SJ, Harpole DH, Sugarbaker DJ. The safety and versatility of video-thoracoscopy: prospective analysis of 895 consecutive cases. *J Am Coll Surg*. 1995;181:165-167.

2. Hazelrigg SR, Nunchuck SK, LoCicero J 3rd. Video Assisted Thoracic Surgery Study Group data. *Ann Thorac Surg*. 1993;56(5): 1039-1043.

Commentary

Malcolm DeCamp Jr., M.D., Beth Israel Deaconess Medical Center
Harvard Medical School

Thoracoscopy or video-assisted thoracic surgery (VATS) has gained widest acceptance among pulmonary surgeons for excisional biopsy of peripheral pulmonary nodules, apical bullectomy or surgical lung biopsy. For each of these indications, the thoracoscopic approach has replaced thoracotomy as the contemporary standard of care. In their chapter on thoracoscopic pulmonary wedge resection, Dr. Jones et al have successfully distilled the details of this versatile operation to its essential elements.

Cancer diagnosis, staging, treatment, or palliation are common indications for VATS. As such, I consider all general thoracic surgical patients to be hypercoaguable and at high risk for perioperative thromboembolism. Dual prophylaxis with weight-based subcutaneous heparin and pneumatic compression boots is essential.

Successful thoracoscopy requires consistent split-lung ventilation. Frequent and clear communication between surgeon and the thoracic anesthesiologist is critical. VATS procedures for peripheral targets in either lung can always be accomplished with a left-sided double lumen endotracheal tube. A left-sided bronchial blocker can be used for left lung lesions but may lengthen operative time, as atelectasis is passive and dependent on pulmonary blood flow. For anatomic reasons, right-sided double lumen tubes or blockers should rarely be used. Tube position should be checked bronchoscopically both after initial placement and after turning the patient into the lateral decubitus position.

For target lesions in the mid to upper thorax, I agree with the authors that a monitor position at the patient's head works best. However, for basilar lesions, I prefer to have the camera oriented inferiorly, making it optimal to have the video monitors at the level of the patient's hips.

A wide triangular port configuration provides the greatest flexibility for access to all areas of the lung. I prefer the judicious use of a long-acting local anesthetic (bupivacaine with epinephrine) at each port site prior to incision. Excessive subcutaneous tunneling of port incisions should be avoided as it leads to increased torque on the thoracoscope or instruments, which in turn increases intercostal neuralgia. Recall that anterior interspaces are generally wider and allow for more digital or instrumental manipulation than a posterior placed port.

A single reuseable metal port for the camera is ideal for thoracoscopy. As the pneumothorax is passive, additional port sites do not need cannulas. Instruments and staplers can be passed directly through the chest wall.

Most surgeons, myself included, use either the blue 3.5 mm or green 4.8 mm staple cartridges. I would not single out bovine pericardium for buttressing as there are several products available, including ePTFE. Neither has been shown to be superior to the other. I favor routine buttressing only for patients with significant emphysema.

Roticulating staplers facilitate resection of targets at the extremes of the lung (apex, basilar, or medially abutting the mediastinum). They may add unnecessary expense for other lesion locations.

We use a single chest tube for most VATS wedge resections, usually placed via the original camera port. The patient's size and the magnitude of the resection dictate chest tube size though the range is 20 Fr to 28 Fr In keeping with MIS philosophy, we tend to use smaller drains and occasionally substitute Blake or JP drains for chest tubes.

The chest tube is maintained on 20 cm to 25 cm of water suction. A chest x-ray in the PACU confirms complete lung expansion. When there is no air leak and the drainage is less than 200 to 300 cc/24 hours, the tube can be removed. Daily chest x-rays are not necessary.

The duration of chest-tube drainage is the major driver of hospital length of stay after VATS wedge resection. Early chest drain removal allows for the immediate conversion from parenteral narcotics to oral analgesics. I will often remove drains while the patient is in the PACU if there is no air leak and the radiograph shows no pneumothorax. Eight in ten patients without major comorbidities managed accordingly can expect discharge on the first postoperative day and return to normal activities within 2 weeks.

J. Michael DiMaio, M.D.
University Of Texas Southwestern Medical Center

This is a very well-written chapter describing video-assisted thorascopic surgery for various procedures, including wedge resections, decortication, sympathectomy, and myomectomy. There are several additional points that I might bring to the attention of the reader, which may be of some use.

In a patient with severe lung disease and poor gas exchange, it may be possible and in fact necessary to use intermittent apnea instead of lung isolation. To this end, it is useful to ask the anesthesiologist to temporarily occlude the ventilation to the affected side as early as possible in the operation. This allows the anesthesiologist and the surgeon the knowledge of whether the surgery can be conducted with lung isolation or whether intermittent apnea is necessary.

The author suggests the use of three port sites for the majority of the procedures. In fact, most procedures that I perform use two port sites, which is sufficient to perform wedge resections. You may place more than one instrument within a single port site to minimize the necessity for the third one. You may use a Maryland retractor or another small instrument within the same site as the one used for the endoscopic stapler. Occasionally, I will often use a stab incision in the posterior area and simply place a Maryland retractor within that small stab incision rather than place a full port site. That small stab incision may be closed with simply a Steri-Strip or even a small chromic suture to minimize the pain associated with it.

Another additional point is that the positioning of the surgeon in the operating room setup in Figure A suggests that the surgeon be toward the patient's back. In fact, there are many procedures where the surgeon is best positioned in the patient's front.

An additional point to bring up in terms of chest tube placement is that a 28-Fr chest tube may be placed through the trocar used for camera placement. This allows the ability to direct the chest tube anteriorly and toward the apex for the proper positioning of the chest tube.

In summary, this is a very well-written chapter discussing various techniques for minimally invasive thoracoscopic surgery.

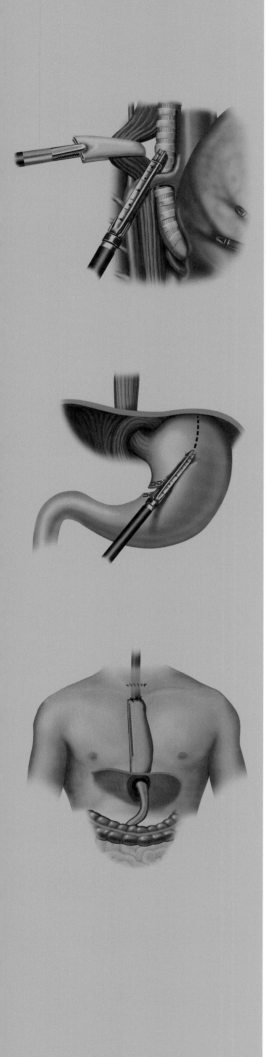

Thoracoscopic/Laparoscopic Esophagectomy

Minimally invasive esophagectomy may be performed for both benign and malignant disease, including esophageal strictures refractory to endoscopic treatment, Barrett's esophagus with pathologic evidence for the presence of high-grade dysplasia, and esophageal cancer. Palliative esophagectomy for Stage IV neoplastic disease is rarely performed due to the procedure's associated high morbidity. Traditional approaches to esophagectomy include a transthoracic, transhiatal, or a combination of an abdominal and thoracic approach (Ivor-Lewis procedure). The minimally invasive approach to esophagectomy involves a combination of all three, including laparoscopy, thoracoscopy, and a cervical neck incision.

Preoperative Preparation

1. Sequential compression stockings and subcutaneous heparin may be used for prophylaxis against deep venous thrombosis. Intravenous antibiotics are administered prophylactically. Anaerobic bacterial coverage is important to cover oral and upper esophageal bacterial flora. After induction of general anesthesia and placement of a double-lumen endotracheal tube, esophagoscopy can be performed to assess the proximal and distal extent of disease. The bladder is emptied with a urinary catheter and the stomach is decompressed with a nasogastric tube.

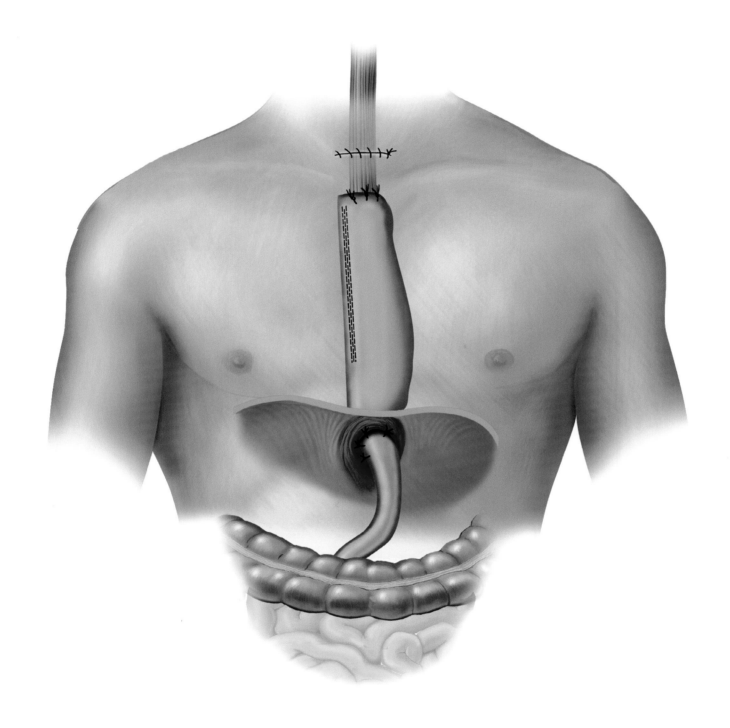

Operating Room Setup

2. The patient is placed in a left lateral decubitus position on a bean-bag device. All pressure points must be adequately padded.

3. The surgeon stands to the patient's right, while the assistant is situated to the patient's left.

4. The video monitors are stationed at both sides of the patient's head to facilitate adequate viewing from either side of the table.

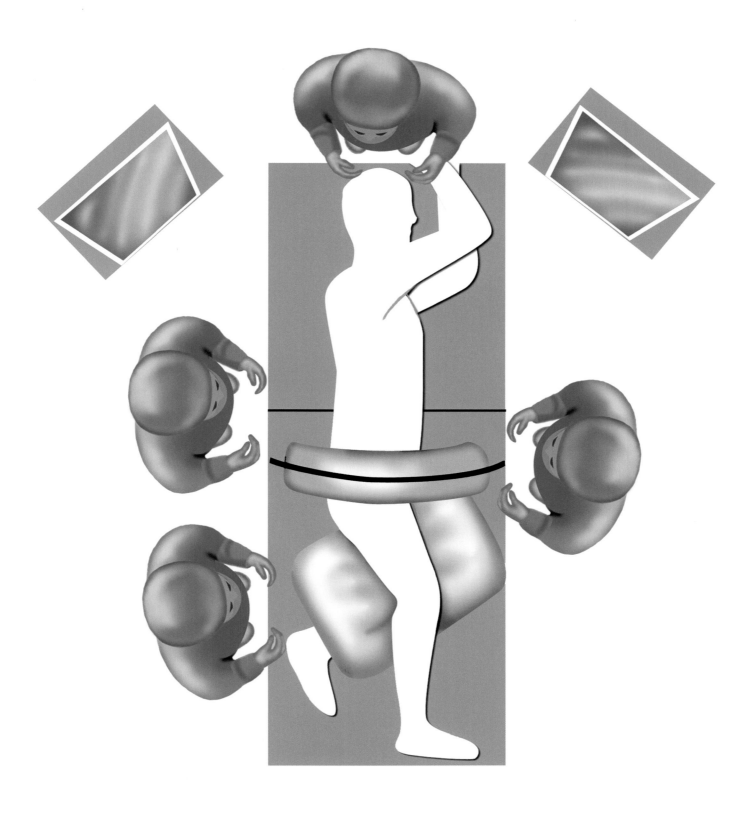

Access and Port Placement–Thoracoscopy

5. The right lung is deflated by having the anesthesiologist remove it from the ventilatory circuit. Four thoracic trocars are introduced in the right chest as depicted in Figure B.

6. A 30° angled camera is inserted in the eighth or ninth intercostal space below the tip of the scapula. A second port is placed behind the posterior axillary line just below the tip of the scapula. Two more anterior ports are placed as depicted. Carbon dioxide insufflation is not necessary for thoracoscopy.

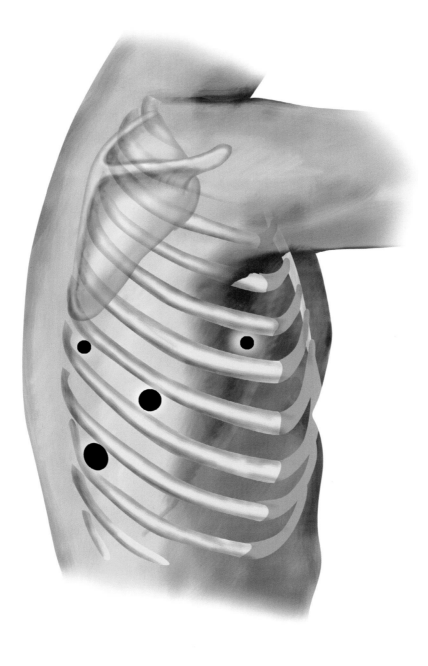

FIGURE C-a,b

Exposing the Esophagus

7. A careful exploration is conducted to assess for any evidence of metastatic disease (Figure C-a).

8. The right lung is retracted anterolaterally in order to visualize the esophagus (Figure C-b), and the inferior pulmonary ligament is divided using an ultrasonic coagulator. While the fan gives fine exposure, it is less versatile than a Duval clamp or suction device.

9. The pleura is incised to expose the intrathoracic esophagus.

FIGURE C-a

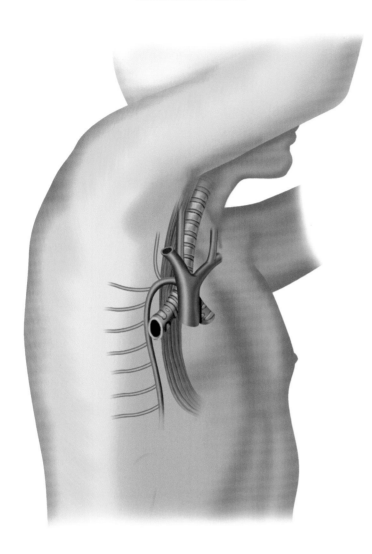

FIGURE C-b

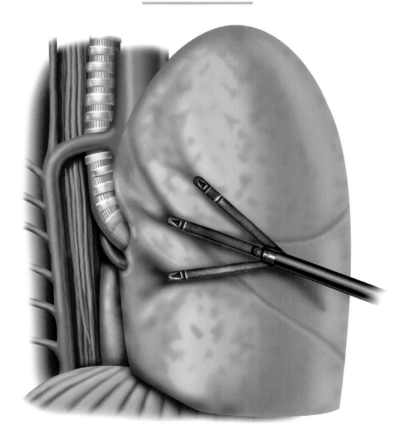

Mobilizing the Esophagus and Dividing the Azygous Vein

10. The esophagus is circumferentially mobilized using a combination of blunt and ultrasonic dissection and a Penrose drain is placed around this area to facilitate subsequent retraction (Figure D-a).

11. The azygous vein is localized, dissected free with the ultrasonic coagulator, and divided using an endoscopic linear stapler loaded with 2.5 mm staples (Figure D-b).

12. The esophagus is then circumferentially mobilized from the level of the thoracic inlet down to the esophageal hiatus. Paraesophageal lymph nodes are included in the dissection. Because the arterial supply to the esophagus is via numerous small branches, this dissection can be safely performed with a combination of ultrasonic coagulation and blunt dissection.

13. The thoracic duct should be clearly visualized so as to avoid inadvertent injury. Once the intrathoracic esophagus is completely mobilized, the Penrose drain is left in place at the level of the cervical esophagus. A 28-32 Fr chest tube is inserted through the camera port and the incisions are closed in the usual manner.

FIGURE D-a

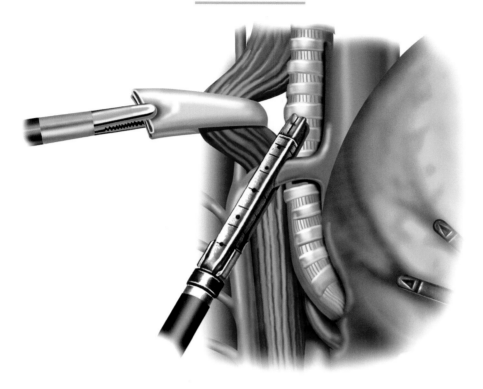

FIGURE D-b

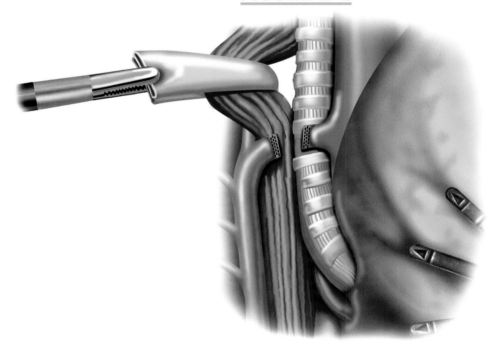

Access and Port Placement–Laparoscopy

14. The patient is switched to a supine position and prepared from the neck down to the level of the pubic symphysis. The double lumen endotracheal tube is changed to a single lumen tube.

15. The surgeon and assistant remain standing on their respective sides of the patient as during thoracoscopy. Pneumoperitoneum is obtained with either an open or closed technique (Veress needle).

16. An 11 mm trocar is placed in the left midclavicular line above the level of the umbilicus. Using a 30° angled camera, the abdomen is inspected for adhesions or injuries.

17. Under direct vision, four abdominal trocars are then inserted in a configuration as depicted in Figure E. Two 5 mm ports are placed in the anterior axillary line below the costal margin on both sides. A third 5 mm port is placed in the right midclavicular line below the costal margin. Finally, a 12 mm port is placed above the umbilicus near the midline, keeping adequate distance from the camera to avoid obstructing view. The most inferior port should be placed no more than 15 cm below the xiphoid process in order to facilitate maximal manipulation and range of motion of the instruments.

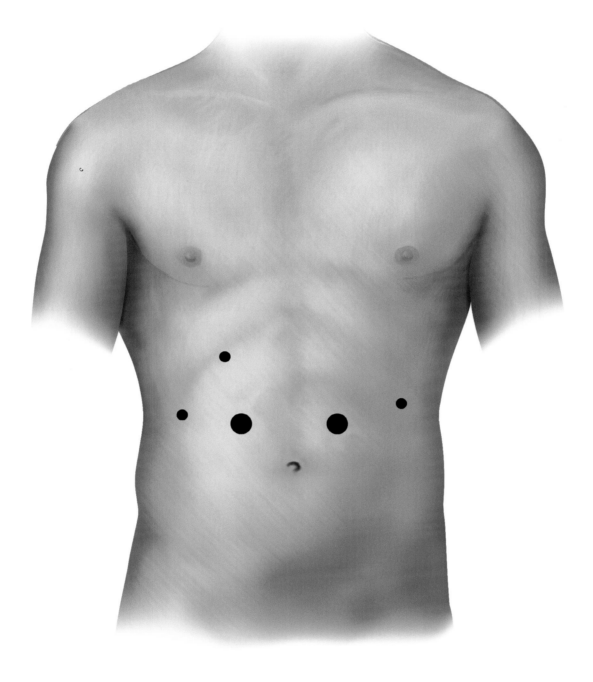

Creating the Gastric Conduit

18. A jejunostomy feeding tube is placed approximately 30 cm distal to the ligament of Treitz (see "Laparoscopic Jejunostomy" for a detailed description).

19. The patient is placed in the reverse Trendelenburg position to provide gravity retraction. A self-retaining liver retractor is used to displace the left lateral lobe of the liver anterolaterally.

20. The greater curvature of the stomach is dissected free from its omental attachments, being careful not to injure the right gastroepiploic vessels, as these will serve as the main arterial supply to the gastric conduit. The gastrosplenic ligament and short gastric vessels are divided as well with an ultrasonic coagulator. Any posterior retroperitoneal adhesions to the stomach must also be divided.

21. The first portion of the duodenum is mobilized by dividing any attachments with an ultrasonic coagulator.

22. The hepatogastric ligament along the lesser curvature is also divided and the left gastric artery is isolated and divided with an endoscopic linear stapler. At this time, a laparoscopic pyloroplasty or pyloromyotomy drainage procedure may be performed at the surgeon's discretion, although it is not routinely performed.

23. Finally, a 5 cm to 7 cm wide gastric conduit is created using multiple fires of an endoscopic linear stapler (3.5–4.5 mm staples) starting from the distal aspect of the lesser curvature and traveling along the greater curvature toward the angle of His. The nasogastric tube must be pulled back by the anesthesiologist so that it is not included in the staple line.

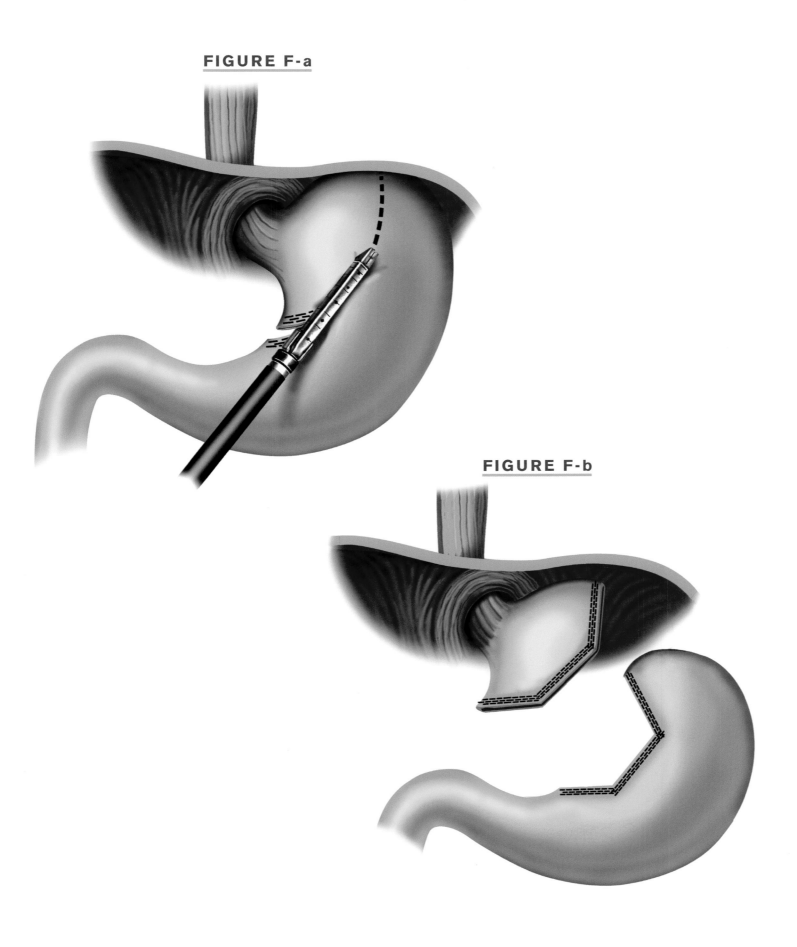

FIGURE F-a

FIGURE F-b

Preparing for Mobilizing the Conduit

24. The proximal aspect of the gastric conduit is sutured to the distal aspect of the surgical specimen using either intracorporeal or extracorporeal knot-tying techniques.

25. Next, the esophageal hiatus is circumferentially mobilized, thus entering the pleural cavity, in order to complete the abdominal dissection.

26. If needed, part of the diaphragmatic crus may be divided in order to enlarge the hiatus to facilitate delivery of the specimen and gastric conduit.

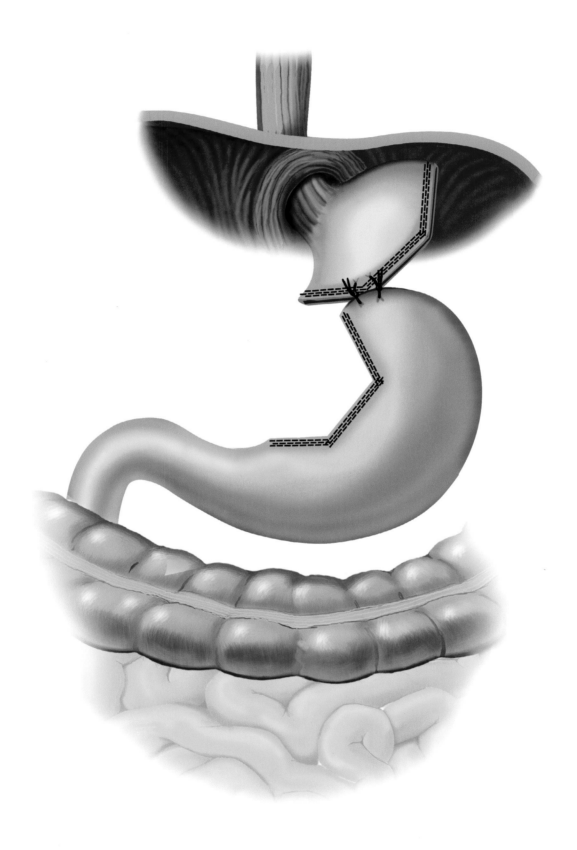

Extracting the Specimen

27. A transverse neck incision is made above the suprasternal notch. The platysma muscle is divided and the sternocleidomastoid muscle is retracted laterally.

28. The cervical esophagus is circumferentially mobilized to connect the dissection with the already mobilized thoracic esophagus. The Penrose drain previously left in the right chest is grasped through the neck incision and used to facilitate placing upward retraction on the esophagus. Care is taken not to damage the reccurent laryngeal nerve.

29. Under laparoscopic guidance, the surgical specimen is slowly pulled upward through the neck incision, while the gastric conduit is pulled into the chest ensuring that no torsion or twisting occurs.

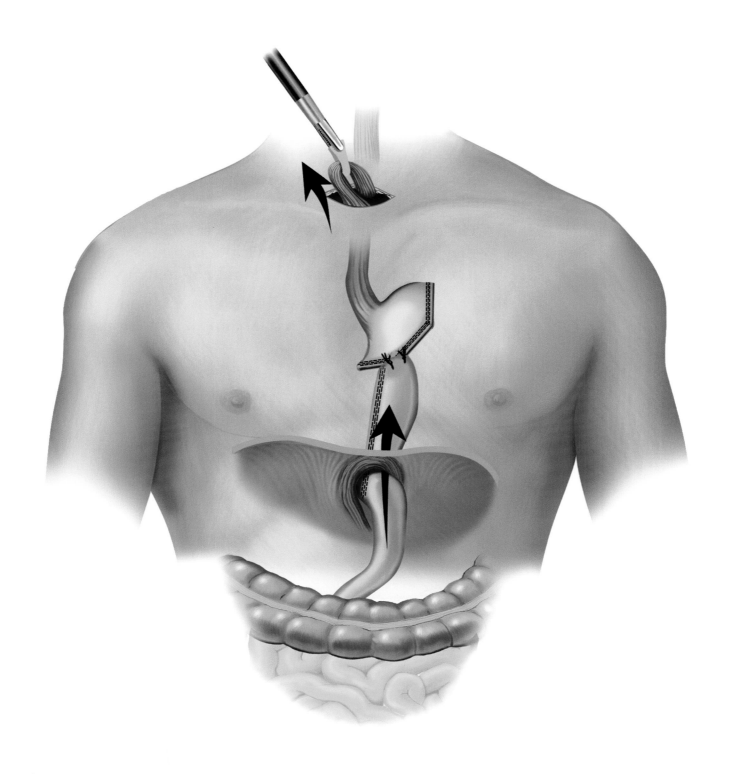

FIGURE I

Creating the Cervical Anastomosis and Closure

30. The cervical esophagus is divided and the surgical specimen is extracted by disconnecting it from the gastric conduit by cutting the previously placed sutures.

31. The nasogastric tube is passed from the cervical esophagus into the gastric conduit and a two-layer, hand-sewn esophagogastric anastomosis is created. Once complete, the neck incision is irrigated with antibiotic solution.

32. The platysma muscle is reapproximated and the skin incision is closed. The abdominal operative field is inspected for adequate hemostasis.

33. The gastric conduit is sutured to the right and left crus in order to alleviate tension on the cervical anastomosis and prevent the subsequent herniation of abdominal contents into the chest.

34. The ports are withdrawn under direct vision to ensure hemostasis at each port site. The fascial and skin incisions are closed in the usual manner.

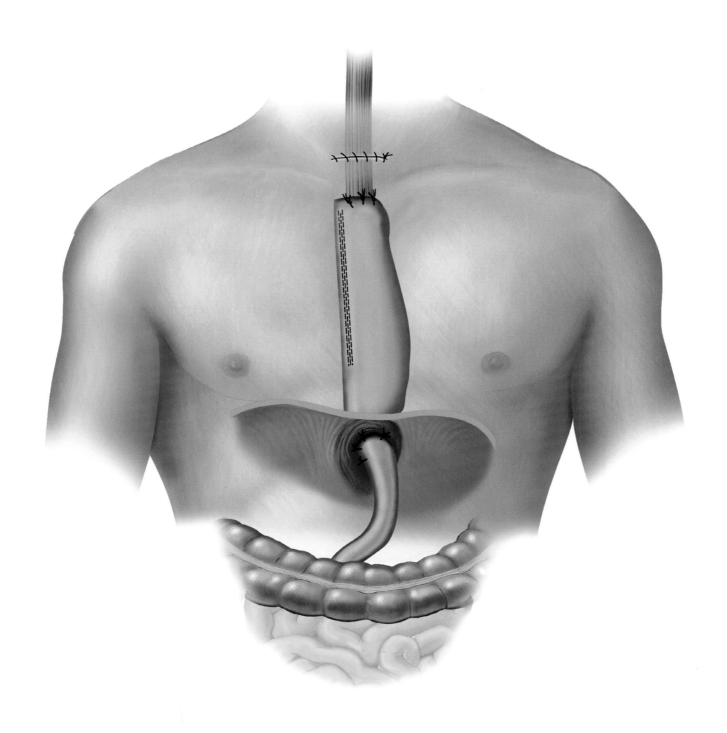

Postoperative Care

Sequential compression devices and/or subcutaneous heparin are continued postoperatively. Antibiotics are continued at the surgeon's discretion. The chest tube and nasogastric tube are maintained on wall suction. Tube feeding may be initiated through the jejunostomy tube at the surgeon's discretion. A contrast study is performed around postoperative day 5 to assess for any evidence of anastomotic leak. If no leak is demonstrated, the nasogastric tube and chest tube may be removed. Oral intake is initiated with clear liquids and advanced as tolerated.

Suggested Reading

1. Luketich JD, Alvelo-Rivera M, Buenaventura PO, et al. Minimally invasive esophagectomy: outcomes in 222 patients. *Ann Surg.* 2003;238(4):486-494.

2. Jobe BA, Reavis KM, Davis JJ, Hunter J. Laparoscopic inversion esophagectomy; simplifying a daunting operation. *Dis Esophagus* 2004;17(1):95-97.

3. Nguyen NT, Follette DM, Lemoine PH, Roberts PF, Goodnight JE. Minimally invasive Ivor Lewis esophagectomy. *Ann Thorac Surg.* 2001;72:593-596.

Commentary

Ninh Nguyen, M.D., Irvine Medical Center
University of California

Open transhiatal esophagectomy and Ivor-Lewis esophagectomy are complex operations that can be associated with significant morbidity and mortality. In an effort to limit the physiologic stress associated with an open esophagectomy, minimally invasive surgical approaches to esophagectomy were developed. Minimally invasive esophagectomy can be defined as any technique attempting to reduce the size of the surgical incision and hence the surgical insult to the host. With minimally invasive approaches to esophagectomy, the abdominal laparotomy is often substituted by laparoscopy and the right thoracotomy is often substituted by thoracoscopy. The initial minimally invasive approach to esophagectomy was a hybrid operation consisting of thoracoscopy for esophageal mobilization to reduce the morbidity associated with a right thoracotomy. Thoracoscopic esophageal mobilization, however, still required a standard midline laparotomy for construction of the gastric conduit in combination with a cervical esophagogastric anastomosis. An alternative minimally invasive hybrid technique for esophagectomy is laparoscopic gastric mobilization followed by a right thoracotomy. These two hybrid approaches utilize minimally invasive technique in only one of the two body cavities (chest or abdomen) during esophagectomy and continue to require either a thoracotomy or laparotomy.

In 1995, DePaula et al was the first group to report a small series of laparoscopic transhiatal esophagectomy performed totally via laparoscopy. Their approach consisted of laparoscopic construction of the gastric conduit followed by laparoscopic mobilization of the mediastinal esophagus through the esophageal hiatus. A neck incision was performed for construction of an esophagogastric anastomosis. Laparoscopic transhiatal esophagectomy is indicated for patients requiring total esophagectomy, especially for patients with lower- or middle- third tumor and for patients with esophageal cancer in conjunction with a long-segment of Barrett's esophagus. Limitations of this technique include the limited view of the mid and upper mediastinum leading to difficulty in performing mediastinal mobilization of the middle-third esophagus and limited ability to perform a mediastinal lymphadenectomy. Advantages of this technique are that it does not require repositioning of the patient for a thoracotomy or thoracoscopy, thereby possibly reducing the operative time. In addition, since the chest is not being entered, single lung ventilation is not required.

In 1998, Luketich reported the combined thoracoscopic and laparoscopic approach to esophagectomy. Their technique consisted of thoracoscopic esophageal mobilization followed by laparoscopic construction of the gastric conduit and a neck anastomosis. Thoracoscopic and laparoscopic esophagectomy was originally developed to overcome one of the major limitations of laparoscopic transhiatal esophagectomy, which is the laparoscopic transhiatal mobilization of the mediastinal esophagus. Unlike laparoscopic transhiatal esophagectomy, the intrathoracic segment of the esophagus is first mobilized using thoracoscopy. Thoracoscopy enables the surgeon to perform a wide mediastinal lymphadenectomy under direct visualization. Thoracoscopic and laparoscopic esophagectomy is indicated for patients requiring total esophagectomy. The esophagogastric anastomosis is performed in the neck. One advantage of a neck anastomosis is that an anastomotic leak can be drained easily through the cervical incision. This technique should not be performed in patients with prior right thoracotomy or in morbidly obese patients, as thoracoscopy would be technically difficult.

The minimally invasive Ivor-Lewis procedure was later reported by Watson; this approach involves laparoscopic construction of the gastric conduit and is followed by thoracoscopic construction of an intrathoracic esophagogastric anastomosis. Laparoscopic and thoracoscopic Ivor-Lewis resection is indicated in esophageal cancer cases whereby there is cancer involvement of the gastric cardia. In this scenario, a wide resection of the proximal gastric cardia is required to obtain a negative distal margin. The shortened length of the gastric conduit precludes construction of a neck anastomosis and an intrathoracic anastomosis is mandated to create a tension-free esophagogastric anastomosis. Laparoscopic and thoracoscopic Ivor-Lewis resection should not be performed for middle- or upper-third esophageal cancer. Any tumor located endoscopically proximal to 35 cm from the incisors should undergo total esophagectomy with a neck anastomosis to ensure adequate proximal margin of resection. Lastly, hand-assisted laparoscopic transhiatal esophagectomy has been described. The entire intra-abdominal phase of the procedure is performed laparoscopically, including mobilization of the distal esophagus and placement of the needle-catheter jejunostomy. Subsequently, an upper midline incision (8 cm) is made to perform a blunt dissection of the middle-third esophagus and the anastomosis is performed via a cervical incision.

Minimally invasive esophagectomy is technically feasible and can be performed as safely as conventional esophagectomy. There are many minimally invasive surgical options described for esophagectomy. The decisions to use a particular method are often based on the location and extension of the tumor and experience of the surgeon with a particular technique.

Lee L. Swanstrom, M.D., Legacy Health System
Oregon Health Sciences University

The importance of having a less traumatic alternative to standard esophagectomy needs to be stressed–whether for benign or malignant indications, patients and their referring physicians have alternatives to resection. Medical or endoscopic palliations, ablative techniques, and chemoradiation therapies have become preferred options to resection, in part because of the only too-real complications and prolonged recovery seen with open resection. Unfortunately, avoiding surgery means that patients with debilitating benign problems like end-stage achalasia or esophageal spasm end up suffering a decreased quality of life longer than needed. Even more importantly, surgery remains the only chance for a cure in esophageal cancer–all nonresection treatments condemn the patient to death from their disease. Clearly, a resectional therapy that minimizes the physiologic trauma of open resection will be a boon to patients and possibly restore surgeons as the primary treaters of esophageal disease.

Three different endoscopic resection techniques have been described: 1) a totally laparoscopic transhiatal approach, 2) a laparoscopic/ thoracoscopic approach with an intrathoracic anastomosis, and 3) a thoracoscopic/ laparoscopic approach as described by the authors. Overall, the currently described approach seems to have become the most widely applied as it is technically less difficult though more demanding in terms of operating room logistics and anesthesia management. In the future, as technology and techniques evolve, the other two approaches may become more popular; in particular, new flexible stapling devices may make intrathoracic anastomosis more feasible while new techniques like the "inversion" technique may make transhiatal procedures easier.

Although it was not discussed in this description, minimally invasive techniques also play a role in the preoperative evaluation of esophageal cancers. When indicated, laparoscopy for distal tumors and thoracoscopy for middle and upper cancers is a valuable adjunct for the determination of resectability. Best done as a separate, outpatient procedure peritonoscopy/laparoscopy, especially with ultrasound, is the single most accurate staging tool. If a patient has no obvious extraesophageal disease, one can perform a D-2 lymph-node dissection to look for micrometastases, divide the left gastric artery to precondition the future gastric conduit, and place the feeding jejunostomy to allow nutritional supplementation and to save time at the resection surgery.

An alternative to the use of standard thoracoscopy ports is to use standard laparoscopic ports and CO_2 insufflation. This provides excellent exposure and decreases operating room time by avoiding the complexities of double lumen anesthesia. At completion of the procedure, it is possible to use only a standard closed suction drain in the chest as opposed to a chest tube as long as there was no injury to the lung. Port placement for the laparoscopic portion of the procedure is, as described, somewhat lower than is standard for laparoscopic fundoplication. This is required to allow dissection of the lower stomach and duodenum, but can make the upper portions of the procedure more difficult to reach with standard instruments. Having extra-long laparoscopic tools and a laparoscope, as commonly used in bariatric surgery, is very helpful for this part of the operation. The majority of the dissection is done with an ultrasonic shears as described. It is generally necessary to divide the left gastric vessels with either a suture ligature or a vascular staple load. The left gastric artery should be taken at its origin from the celiac plexus so that the primary lymph nodes are removed with the specimen. For curative cancer cases, consideration can be made to place the cancerous part of the specimen in a retrieval bag before pulling it out the neck. Either a large purse-stringed specimen bag or a disposable camera sleeve can be used for this. Finally, the cervical anastomosis is well performed using a hand-sewn technique, but surgeons should also be familiar with the various staple techniques, which are sometimes preferable, especially in deep, short necks.

Jonathan F. Critchlow, M.D., Beth Israel Deaconess Medical Center Harvard Medical School

This is an excellent technique for either benign or malignant disease, affording complete exposure and the ability to do an adequate nodal clearance in malignant disease. It is a formidable operation requiring advanced laparoscopic skills and considerable experience with open techniques of esophagectomy, postoperative care, and the management of complications. A convenient way to begin is with a team of a thoracic surgeon and gastrointestinal laparoscopic surgeon.

Preoperative administration of cream by mouth or jejunostomy tube (in patients after neoadjuvant therapy) will facilitate identification of the thoracic duct or injuries to its branches. Mobilization of the esophagus should begin in the midesophagus then moving cephalad, clearing the subcarinal pocket. The azygos vein is divided, then a wide pleural envelope should be preserved above the vein to encircle the graft and exclude any potential leakage in the neck from the pleural space. Dissection above the vein should continue directly on the esophageal musculature to minimize the potential for damage of the recurrent laryngeal nerves. Dissection of the lower esophagus can be facilitated by the placement of a traction suture on the diaphragm pulled through the lowest thoracic port. A Penrose drain may be left on the lower esophagus next to the diaphragm, which facilitates identification of the esophagus and any undissected tissue when mobilizing from the abdominal approach.

During the laparoscopic portion, a sequential and complete dissection of the posterior gastric attachments is key to identification of the origin of the right gastroepiploic artery and avoids injury. Full mobilization of the duodenum can be assessed by the ability to move the pylorus with a grasper up to hiatus. The hiatus must be dissected last, after the neck dissection has been opened. The entry of carbon dioxide into the right chest may cause hypotension and hypercarbia. A communication with the left chest must also be entertained in patients with refractory hypotension. The cervical anastomosis may also be created with the stapler. The relatively thin, elongated graft will come well up into the neck with redundancy. A purse-string applier may be applied to the esophagus and the esophagus cut. The head of a 25 mm end-to-end stapler is placed into the esophagus and then tied down. The stomach is then opened at the apex and the stapler introduced. The pin then penetrates the back wall. The stapler is approximated and fired. The extra stomach is trimmed with a linear stapler. A drain is often left in the neck as the incidence of leak is considerably higher in cervical than thoracic anastomosis. The patient should be observed for complications such as leak, recurrent laryngeal nerve injury, delayed gastric emptying, and pulmonary complications.

James D. Luketich, M.D., Heart, Lung and Esophageal Surgery Institute University of Pittsburgh Medical Center

Minimally invasive esophagectomy, similar to open esophagectomy, is a complex operation that requires detailed attention to virtually every step to avoid complications. Our group at Pittsburgh has explored several approaches to minimally invasive esophagectomy and at the present time use primarily the technique described, that is a thoracoscopic, laparoscopic approach with a cervical anastomosis. This is assuming a tumor at the gastroesophageal junction, with little or no cardia or gastric extension. Significant cardia extension will many times require more of a gastric resection margin and may prevent the construction of a gastric conduit that will reach the neck. Thus for these cases, we prefer the laparoscopic mobilization followed by an upper thoracic anastomosis, generally performed thoracoscopically. Mid- or upper-thoracic esophageal squamous cell cancers are not frequently seen in our referral pattern and the ideal approach to these lesions would require a discussion beyond the scope of this commentary.

Our initial experience with the totally laparoscopic approach was limited primarily by the hiatal opening and poor visibility and technical maneuverability. However, other surgeons have been successful with this approach, but having tried both, I continue to recommend the laparoscopic/thoracoscopic combination.

The approach described is accurate to a great degree but deserves several points of emphasis and comment. The authors wisely advise esophagoscopy, but I would emphasize this should include esophagogastroscopy. If gastric extension is suspected, we would consider another operative approach or at least laparoscopic staging to more formally address the extent of gastric involvement.

During the thoracoscopic mobilization, care must be taken as the dissection continues above the azygous vein. At this level and above, we carry the dissection directly on the esophagus to avoid potential injury to the recurrent laryngeal nerves. In general, this is facilitated by dividing the vagus nerves above the azygous vein and avoiding any further traction on these structures. In addition, during mobilization of the esophagus from the thoracic duct area, we generously apply metal clips to minimize any subsequent thoracic duct leaks. If an injury to the main thoracic duct or a significant tributary is suspected, we ligate the thoracic duct near the diaphragmatic hiatus.

The laparoscopic mobilization of the pyloroantral area must be meticulous. During this part of the procedure, we periodically grasp the antrum, near the pylorus and carefully lift it toward the diaphragmatic hiatus. When sufficiently mobilized, the pylorus should easily be elevated to the right crus in a tension-free manner. If this cannot be accomplished, or there is tension during this maneuver, further Kocherization is needed. During the creation of the gastric tube, we have found it beneficial to have the first assistant grasp the tip of the fundus and gently stretch it toward the spleen, a second grasper is placed on the antral area and a slight downward retraction is applied. This places the stomach on slight stretch, and facilitates a straight staple-line application, which should be parallel to the gastroepiploic arcade.

After the neck anastomosis is completed, attention must be directed to reducing any excess gastric conduit pulled into the thoracic cavity, which invariably occurs during the pull-up and anastomosis. This can be achieved by grasping the antral area firmly, but carefully and gently tugging downward toward the abdomen, often several centimeters will reduce before the anastomosis is observed to move slightly caudad—when this occurs, one can generally assume the redundant gastric tube in now within the abdomen. Failure to perform this step may lead to a slight sigmoid curve of the redundant gastric antrum within the chest and leads to poor gastric emptying and a potential cause for subsequent revision. We then proceed to the tacking described to the right and left crus.

The closure of the platysma, and skin at the cervical level need not be meticulous, and aggressive closure here may lead to drainage of a subsequent anastomotic leak into the thoracic inlet along the plane of the thoracoscopic dissection. To avoid this southward drainage of an occasional leak from the neck into the chest, several points may minimize this tendency: during the upper part of the thoracoscopic drainage, we attempt to leave the mediastinal pleura intact to seal this area, the neck is only loosely closed to encourage the easy exit though this area, and the anastomosis is performed high, within 2 cm to 3 cm of the cricopharyngeus. Performing the anastomosis lower allows the anastomosis to lie very near the thoracic inlet or lower, leading to a tendency to thoracic soilage in the event of a neck leak.

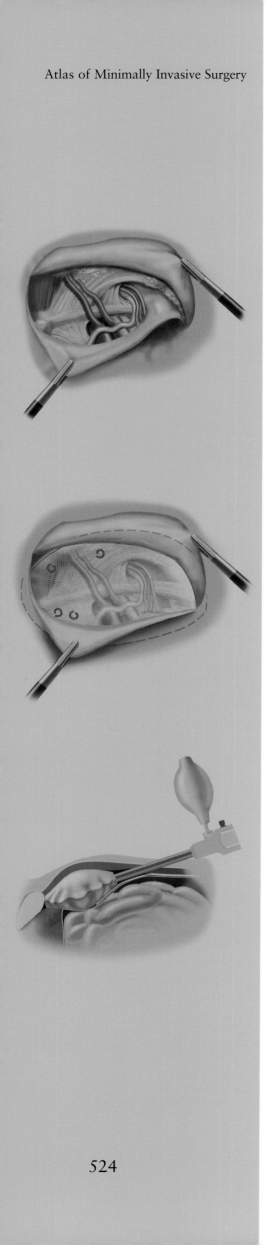

Laparoscopic Inguinal Hernias

Two different laparoscopic techniques have evolved to repair inguinal hernias, which include the transabdominal preperitoneal (TAPP) and totally extraperitoneal (TEP) approaches. The laparoscopic approach is especially useful for recurrent and/or bilateral hernias and for those patients who seek an early return to rigorous physical activity. The laparoscopic approach also allows visualization and repair of direct, indirect, femoral, and obturator hernias.

FIGURE A

Review of the Anatomy

The anatomy must be understood in order to successfully perform a laparoscopic hernia repair.

Preoperative Preparation

1. Sequential compression devices and subcutaneous heparin may be used for prophylaxis against deep venous thrombosis. We administer a first-generation cephalosporin prophylactically. After induction of general anesthesia, the bladder is emptied with a urinary catheter selectively.

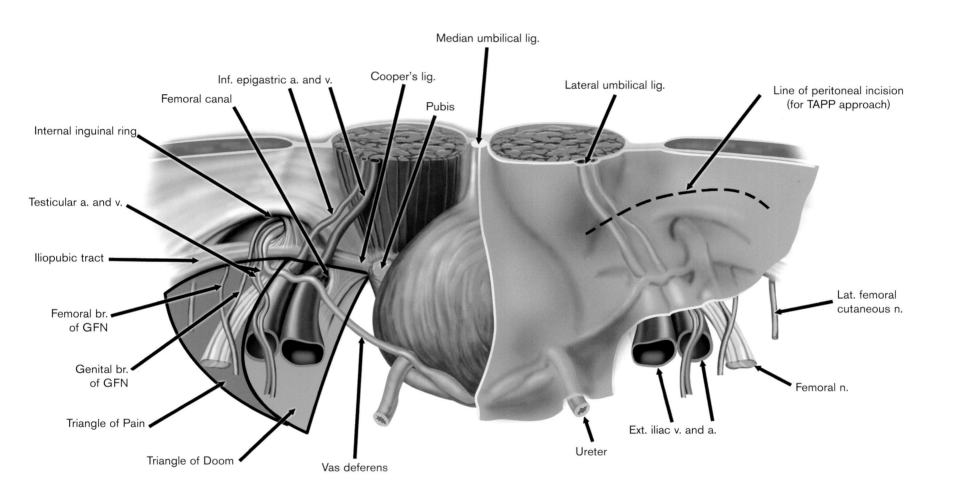

Internal inguinal ring

Testicular a. and v.

Iliopubic tract

Femoral br.
of GFN

Genital br.
of GFN

Triangle of Pain

Triangle of Doom

Femoral canal

Inf. epigastric a. and v.

Cooper's lig.

Pubis

Median umbilical lig.

Lateral umbilical lig.

Line of peritoneal incision
(for TAPP approach)

Lat. femoral
cutaneous n.

Femoral n.

Ext. iliac v. and a.

Ureter

Vas deferens

Transabdominal Preperitoneal Repair (TAPP)

Operating Room Layout

2. The patient is positioned in the supine Trendelenburg position. The arms are tucked, secured, and padded.

3. The surgeon stands on the side opposite the hernia. The assistant and scrub nurse stand opposite the surgeon.

4. The video monitors are placed at the foot of the table.

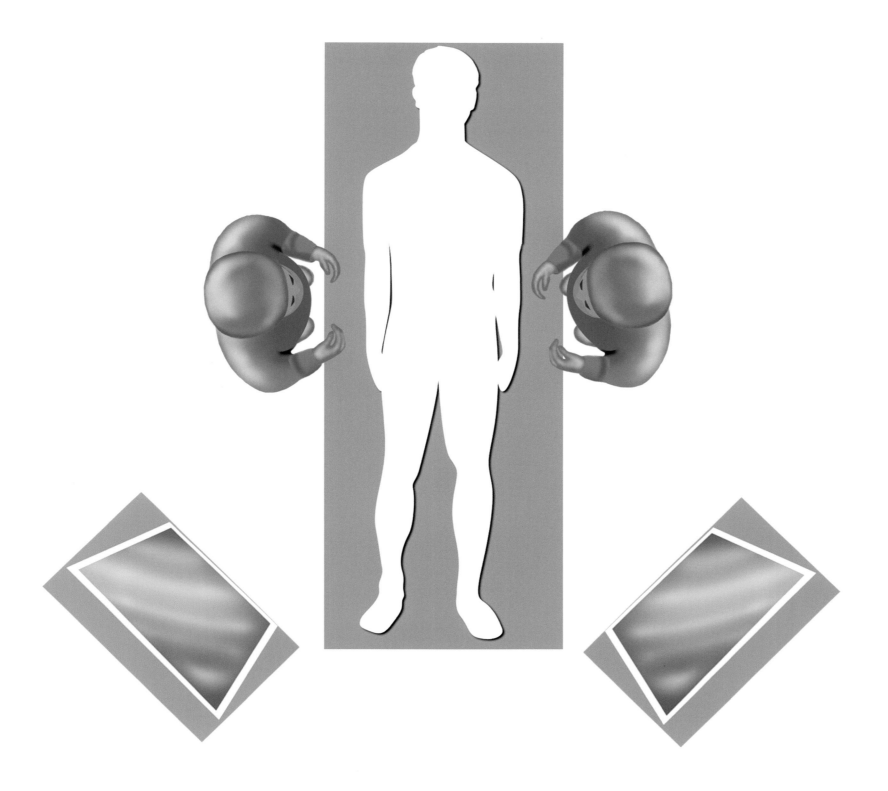

FIGURE C

Access and Port Placement

5. An infraumbilical incision is used to establish pneumoperitoneum, setting a maximum pressure limit of 12 mm Hg. This is established either with an open or closed technique. A 10/11 mm port is placed here and the laparoscope is inserted. Either a straight or 30° angled scope can be used, although the angled scope, if available, is preferred. A careful exploration is performed to ensure that no injury occurred during port insertion and that no other abnormalities are present.

6. Two 5 mm ports are placed under direct vision in the midclavicular line as shown.

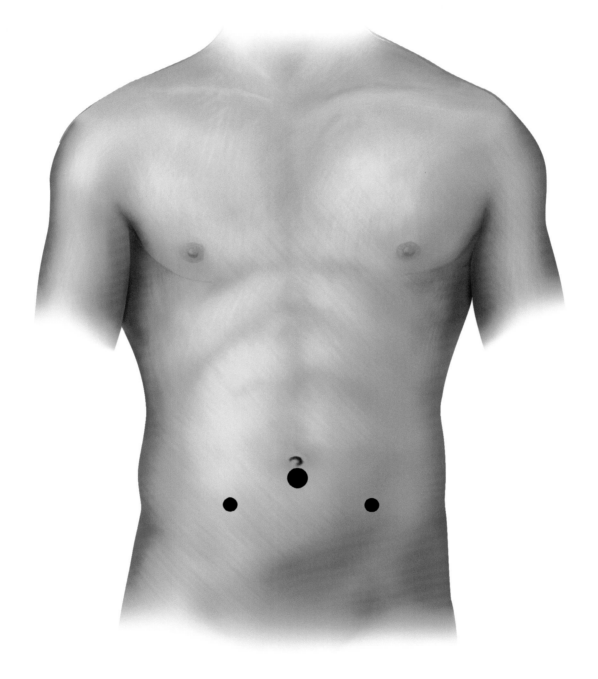

Reducing the Hernia

7. After the hernia is identified, the peritoneum overlying its superior edge is incised transversely. This should extend from the medial umbilical ligament to the anterior superior iliac spine to provide adequate exposure of the preperitoneal space.

8. The inferior epigastric vessels should be identified early and protected. Peritoneal flaps are developed. Other landmarks including the pubic symphysis, Cooper's ligament, and the iliopubic tract, are also identified.

9. The hernia sac is reduced using blunt dissection. The vas deferens and gonadal vessels should be skeletonized and clearly visualized to avoid missing a small hernia or cord lipoma. The peritoneum should be dissected away from these structures to facilitate proper mesh placement.

10. Alternatively, if a large indirect hernia is present, the hernia sac can be divided to minimize the extent of distal dissection. Care must be taken during this dissection to avoid injury to the external iliac vessels located in the "triangle of doom" (bounded by the vas deferens medially and the gonadal vessels laterally.

11. If identified, femoral and obturator hernias should also be reduced.

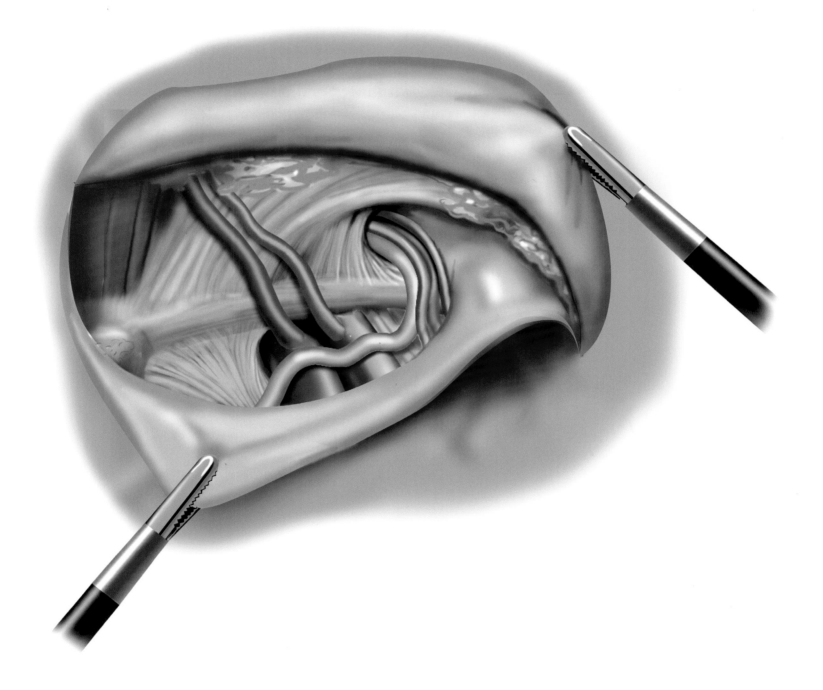

Placing and Fastening the Mesh

12. We recommend using a large (10 x 12 cm) polypropylene or polyester mesh for the repair. The mesh is introduced through the 10 mm port and is unfolded to cover each of the hernia defects with at least a 2 cm to 3 cm overlap.

13. If the spermatic cord has been adequately separated from the peritoneum, the mesh can be placed directly over the cord without having to cut a slit to encircle the cord, which is usually associated with increased postoperative pain and a higher rate of recurrence.

14. Spiral fasteners are used to fixate the mesh to the anterior abdominal wall and medially to Cooper's ligament. Additional fixation points can be applied to the rectus muscle and/or transversus abdominis arch. No fasteners should be applied posterior to the iliopubic tract to avoid nerve entrapment in the "triangle of pain" (bounded by the gonadal vessels and iliopubic tract). Alternatively, some advocate mesh placement without any fixation provided that a large enough mesh is used for the repair.

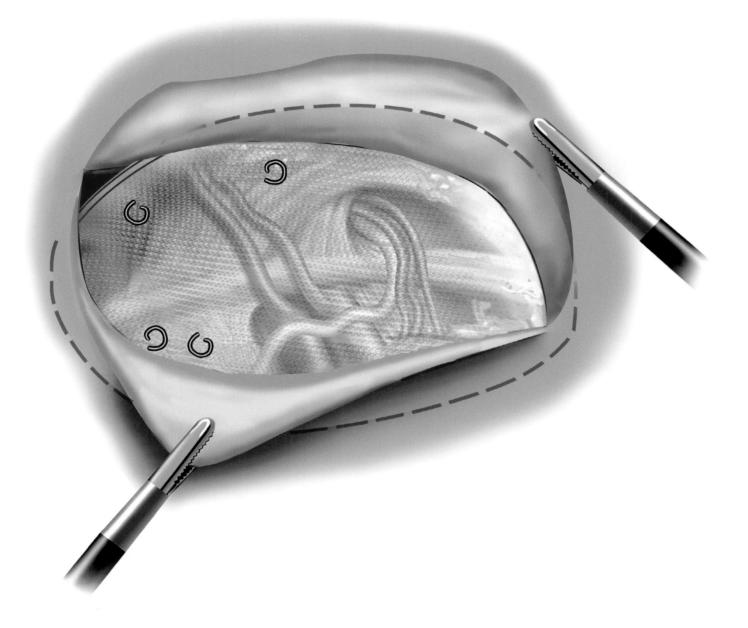

Closing the Peritoneum

15. Once the mesh is in place, the peritoneum is closed with a running suture. Care must be taken to avoid leaving gaps that could allow for formation of adhesions between the mesh and loops of bowel.

16. The ports are removed under direct vision, and the fascia and skin are closed in the usual manner.

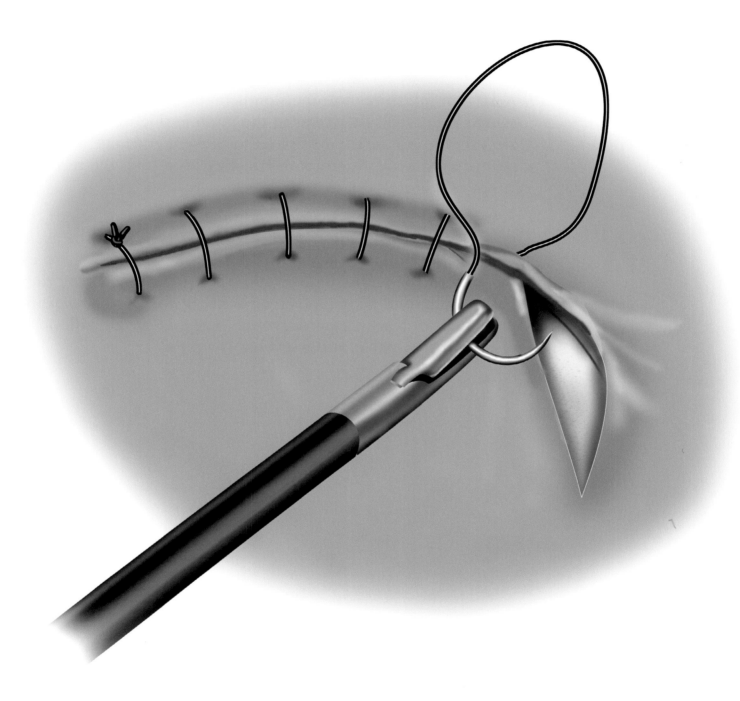

Totally Extraperitoneal Repair (TEP)

The preoperative preparation and operating room layout are identical to that of a TAPP repair.

FIGURE G, H, I

Access to the Preperitoneal Space and Port Placement

1. A 10 mm infraumbilical incision is made and the anterior rectus sheath is incised just lateral to the midline (Figure G). The linea alba should not be divided so as to prevent entrance into the peritoneal cavity. S-retractors are used to retract the rectus muscle laterally (Figure H).

2. A balloon dissector is placed along the anterior surface of the posterior rectus sheath and advanced inferiorly past the arcuate line (line of Douglas), where the posterior sheath ceases to exist, to the level of the pubic bone (Figure I). Generally, placing the patient in a mild degree of Trendelenberg will facilitate proper placement of the balloon dissector. The end of the balloon dissector is palpable at the level of the pubis.

FIGURE G

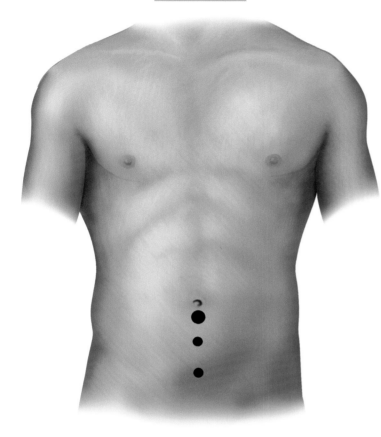

FIGURE H

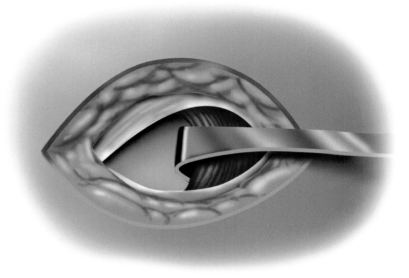

FIGURE I

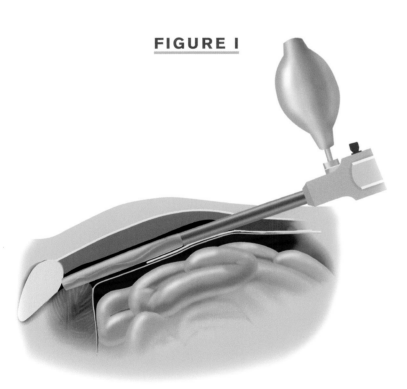

Access to the Preperitoneal Space and Port Placement, Part II

3. The balloon dissector is inflated to create a working space (Figure J). Adequate inflation usually requires 30 to 40 "pumps" of the balloon, while inspecting progress with a 0° laparoscope.

4. The balloon is then deflated and removed, and the preperitoneal space is inflated to 10 mm Hg to 12 mm Hg. A 45° 10 mm laparoscope is used and the area is inspected (Figure K). Two 5 mm ports are placed under direct visualization in the midline as previously shown (Figure G). The most inferior port is located three fingerbreadths above the pubis.

FIGURE J

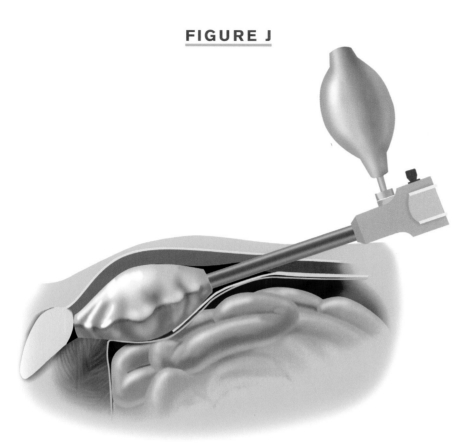

FIGURE K

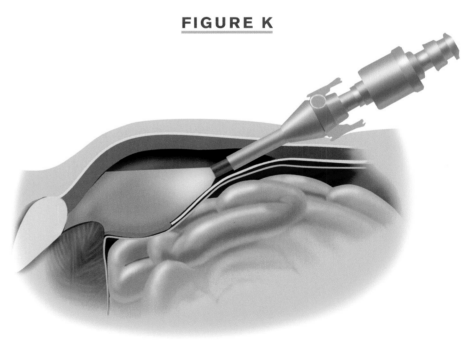

FIGURE L

Hernia Repair and Mesh Placement

5. Hernia reduction and repair for the TEP repair is nearly identical to that of the TAPP approach. The same landmarks are identified to provide the crucial orientation necessary to successfully perform a TEP repair. The pubis is initially identified in the midline, after which Cooper's ligament is clearly exposed. Dissection should not continue too lateral of Cooper's ligament for fear of injuring the external iliac vein.

6. Next, the space lateral to the anterior superior iliac spine is separated bluntly. The structures that remain between Cooper's ligament and this lateral space are the hernia sac and its contents, the vas deferens, and the gonadal vessels.

7. An indirect hernia sac should be reduced and separated from the cord structures as described for the TAPP repair (Figure L). The peritoneal edge of the hernia sac must be dissected below the bifurcation of the vas deferens and gonadal vessels to ensure an adequate dissection. Alternatively, if a large indirect hernia is present, the hernia sac can be divided to minimize the extent of distal dissection.

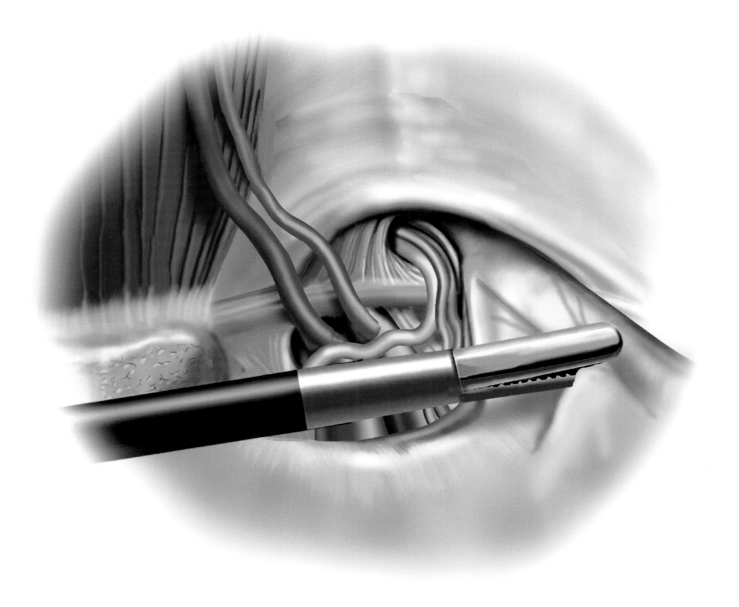

Hernia Repair and Mesh Placement, Part II

8. A direct hernia often will be reduced with the balloon dissector, but if not, must be completely reduced (Figure M). Femoral and obturator hernias should be reduced at this time as well.

9. If an inadvertent tear is created in the peritoneum during dissection, a competing intra-abdominal pneumoperitoneum may inhibit visualization of the preperitoneal space. A Veress needle placed in the upper abdomen usually allows for sufficient decompression. The peritoneal defect may be closed with sutures, endoloops, or clips to avoid the potential of postoperative adhesions of loops of bowel to the mesh. Alternatively, the procedure can be converted to a TAPP repair.

10. A 12 x 15 cm mesh is inserted through the 10 mm port and situated to cover all the hernia defects with ample overlap. The same fixation points are used, thus avoiding the same potential complications of nerve entrapment; some surgeons advocate avoiding fixation altogether.

11. The inferior and lateral aspects of the mesh are held in place while the pneumopreperitoneum is evacuated under direct visualization to ensure that the peritoneum does not slip underneath the mesh and cause an immediate recurrence.

12. The ports are removed and CO_2 released. The fascia and skin incisions are closed in the usual manner.

FIGURE M-a

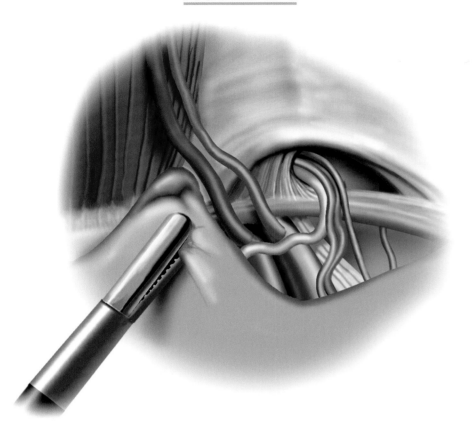

FIGURE M-b

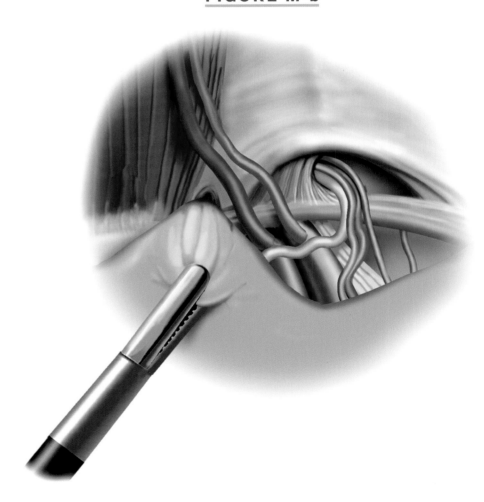

Postoperative Care

The patient can usually be discharged home the day of surgery, after adequate recovery from the general anesthetic and once they are able to void spontaneously. If, for whatever reason, the patient requires admission to the hospital, pneumatic compression devices and/or subcutaneous heparin are continued postoperatively. Additional administration of antibiotics is usually not necessary. Oral intake can be advanced as tolerated.

Suggested Readings

1. EU Hernia Trialists Collaboration. Laparoscopic compared with open methods of groin hernia repair: systematic review of randomized controlled trials. *Br J Surg.* 2000;87:860-867.

2. Scott DJ, Jones DB. Hernia. In: McClelland RN, ed. *Selected Readings in General Surgery.* 1999;26, No.4 (1-2).

3. Wright D, Paterson C, Scott N, et al. Five-year follow-up of patients undergoing laparoscopic or open groin hernia repair: a randomized controlled trial. *Ann Surg.* 2002;235:333-337.

4. Grunwaldt LJ, Schwaitzberg SD, Rattner DW, Jones DB. Is laparoscopic inguinal hernia repair an operation of the past? *J Am Coll Surg.* 2005;200(4):616-620.

5. Jones SB. Choice of anesthesia for surgical endoscopy patients. In: Soper NJ, Swanstrom CC, Eubanks WS, eds. *Mastery of Endoscopic and Laparoscopic Surgery.* 2nd ed. Philadelphia: Lippincott, Williams & Wilkins; 2005:15-22.

6. Hamilton EC, Scott DJ, Kapoor A, Jones DB. Improving operative performance using a laparoscopic hernia simulator. *Am J Surg.* 2001;182:725-728.

7. Memon MA, Cooper NJ, Memon B, Memon MI, Abrams KR. Meta-analysis of randomized clinical trials comparing open and laparoscopic inguinal hernia repair. *Br J Surg.* 2003;90:1479-1492.

8. McCormack K, Scott NW, Go PMNYH, Ross S, Grant AM. Laparoscopic techniques versus open techniques for inguinal hernia repair. *Cochrane Database of Syst Rev.* 2003;CD001785.

9. Scott DJ, Jones DB. Hernias and abdominal wall defects. In: Norton JA, Bollinger RR, Chang AE, et al, eds. *Surgery: Scientific Basis and Current Practice.* New York: Springer-Verlag, 2000:787-823.

Commentary

David W. Rattner, M.D., Massachusetts General Hospital
Harvard Medical School

Few operations have engendered as much controversy as the laparoscopic repair of inguinal hernias. The procedure was originally developed as the transabdominal preperitoneal approach (TAPP) nicely described by the authors in this chapter. Subsequently, the totally extraperitoneal preperitoneal approach (TEP) was developed and this is currently the most widely used method. In accomplished laparoscopic surgeons' hands, patients return to work faster and have less pain than if they had had a traditional open repair. However, the difference is small and therefore for laparoscopic repairs to achieve superior results, they must be performed in a precise, careful, and correct manner. The learning curve for laparoscopic herniorrhaphy is longer than what it might seem and this probably accounts for the mixed results that have been reported in large series with relatively inexperienced laparoscopic surgeons.

It is not always necessary to insert a urinary catheter at the start of the operation and, in fact, catheterizing male patients can increase the incidence of urinary retention. It is our practice to have patients void just prior to surgery and avoid the use of urinary catheters. The authors very nicely depict the steps in performing both TAPP and TEP repairs, but I would make one modification to the instructions and that is to avoid placing any staples or tacks lateral to the epigastric vessels. The lateral component of the mesh used in these repairs will lie flat and be held in place easily by the peritoneum as the pneumopreperitoneum or pneumoperitoneum is released. If one places tacks only medial to the epigastric vessels, it is virtually impossible to injure the ilioinguinal or genitofemoral nerve. Another important technical point to avoid nerve injury is the avoidance of monopolar cautery and the use of bipolar cautery only medial to the epigastric vessels. In the vast majority of dissections, cautery is completely unnecessary. In order to reduce the costs created by disposable instruments, many experienced laparoscopic hernia surgeons do not perform balloon dissection of the preperitoneal space. Rather, they use the laparoscope itself to develop the plane between the peritoneum and the posterior surface of the rectus muscle. The scope is swept side to side and then a standard Hasson trocar is used to seal the subumbilical incision and create the pneumopreperitoneum. By following the steps outlined by the authors, avoiding placement of tacks lateral to the epigastric vessels, and avoiding the use of cautery lateral to the epigastric vessels, complications should be rare and excellent results should be achieved.

Daniel J. Scott, M.D., Charity Hospital
Tulane University School of Medicine

Although a controversial topic, numerous prospective randomized trials have demonstrated decreased pain and a faster recovery following a laparoscopic approach compared to conventional open hernia repairs. Since laparoscopic repairs are tension-free and reinforce the entire myopectineal orifice with a large mesh prosthesis, a very sturdy repair can be achieved, as indicated by Level I data showing recurrence rates of 2% at 5-year follow-up. Thus, for unilateral nonrecurrent hernias, laparoscopic repairs may be offered to patients fit for general anesthesia. Additionally, laparoscopic repairs are especially advantageous for bilateral hernias, as the need for two open groin incisions is obviated, and for recurrent hernias, as anterior scar tissue is avoided. Surgeon experience is important for appropriate patient selection, as very large hernias, incarcerated hernias, and prior lower abdominal incisions may be considered relative contraindications.

The TAPP procedure uses traditional intra-abdominal laparoscopic access and affords the benefits of easier visualization, rapid inspection of both groins, reduction of incarcerated hernia contents, and performance of additional procedures simultaneously. However, many surgeons feel that the TEP procedure is preferable, due to the decreased risk of visceral injury and adhesion formation. The TEP approach is somewhat more difficult due to the limited working space; the learning curve has been estimated to be 30 cases or higher, but may be offset by simulator-based training. A clear understanding of the anatomy and operative technique is crucial in order to perform a safe and effective repair via either laparoscopic method.

As outlined, the key components of the TAPP repair involve establishing access, creating a peritoneal flap, reducing all hernias, skeletonizing the cord structures, placing mesh, and closing the peritoneum. Anatomic landmarks help maintain orientation and guide the dissection. Kittner and/or blunt-tip dissectors with fine serrations are used to reduce the hernia. Electrocautery should be very sparingly used to avoid inadvertent injuries to the numerous nerves and vital structures that are inevitably in close proximity. If the dissection is performed in the correct tissue planes, very little bleeding occurs. Special attention should be paid to full skeletonization of the cord to avoid missing small indirect components and to maximize space for mesh placement. To provide a secure repair, the mesh should generously overlap all defects, and usually spans from midline to the anterior superior iliac spine. During mesh fixation (optional if a sufficiently large prosthesis is used), fasteners must not be placed in the triangle of doom or in the triangle of pain (posterior to the iliopubic tract), to avoid vascular injury (external iliac artery and vein) or nerve entrapment (lateral femoral cutaneous and femoral branch of the genitofemoral nerves). The peritoneal flap must be completely closed using sutures (as described) or, alternatively, tacks or staples so that viscera are not exposed to the mesh.

For the TEP repair, access to the preperitoneal space is most easily achieved using a balloon dissector, as shown. The key components are essentially the same as for the TAPP approach, but the working space is smaller and familiarity with this perspective is important. During dissection, care should be taken to dissect the flimsy attachments tethering the sac to the groin while avoiding tearing of the sac itself. Tears result in a competing pneumoperitoneum, which often compromises visibility; although sometimes difficult, these tears should be identified and closed to avoid potential adhesion formation to the mesh. To avoid postoperative pain, intraperitoneal gas should be released using a Veress needle or by incising (followed by closure) the posterior rectus sheath at the umbilicus at the end of the case. Since fasteners cannot be placed posterior to the iliopubic tract, the posterior edge of mesh must be held in place at the conclusion of the procedure to ensure that the visceral sac lies on top of the mesh and does not slide underneath, elevating the mesh, and rendering the repair ineffective.

Following these principles and using sound surgical judgment, laparoscopic repairs may be safely performed with a low incidence of complications and durable results.

Antonio Garcia-Ruiz, M.D., Hospital Central Militar

My experience with laparoscopic inguinal hernia repair has been restricted to the TAPP approach. Being in an academic position, it has been much easier to teach my fellows this apparently "complex" technique and for them to get over the learning curve. Also, I can review the contralateral inguinal region and have a quick view of the abdominal cavity.

Regarding port placement, I keep the 12-mm umbilical port, but I change the position of my lateral ports depending on the side of the inguinal hernia. To get a better visualization, I use a 5-mm angular scope inserted through the lateral port on the side of the hernia. Therefore, I have to place this port 1 inch above the umbilical plane and the contralateral port 1 inch below the umbilical plane. Then, I can comfortably work with both hands using the umbilical and the contralateral ports. If the case is bilateral, I place both lateral ports above the umbilical plane.

At the beginning of the operation, I start the transverse peritoneal incision right at the anterosuperior iliac spine and elevate the lower peritoneal flap caudally, keeping almost all the preperitoneal fat on the abdominal wall side. The preperitoneal dissection medial to the hernia (Retzius' space) down to the pubic bone is usually simple, but here it is important to recognize that there is a plane between the preperitoneal fat (which will remain on the side of the abdominal wall) and the prevesical fat (which will stay with the urinary bladder after the dissection).

Reducing the hernia sac is typically easier in direct hernias. Dissection of the sac from the elements of the inguinal cord may be very difficult in large indirect hernias. I do my best to totally reduce the sac on all cases because I don't like to leave any chance for a postoperative scrotal fluid collection. Also, oftentimes I find a large lipoma accompanying the inguinal cord, which has to be carefully resected to avoid any palpable inguinal lump after surgery. Finally, in direct hernia cases I like to invert the transversalis fascia of the inguinal defect and tack it to the Cooper's ligament before placing the mesh in order to eliminate the potential space for a seroma. When elevating the inferior peritoneal flap, care has to be taken to prevent injury to the ductus deferens and to avoid the iliac vessels. In female patients, I have found it easier to divide the round ligament than to separate it from the peritoneum at this point.

I don't agree that the mesh can be placed without any fixation in the preperitoneal space. I believe it can migrate and leave potential for recurrence. Closing the peritoneal flaps with sutures may be time consuming; instead I use the same spiral fasteners to close the peritoneal flaps and to fix the inverted peritoneal sac to the lateral abdominal wall.

On the postoperative care, I advise my patients to use an ice bag over the inguinal region for 24 to 48 hours as this may reduce postoperative bleeding and inflammation.

Stephanie B. Jones, M.D., Beth Israel Deaconess Medical Center Harvard Medical School

Opponents of laparoscopic inguinal hernia repair often support their argument by citing the benefits of open hernia repairs performed under local anesthesia with sedation. Conventional wisdom among both surgeons and anesthesiologists seems to support the notion that local anesthesia with sedation is always safer than general anesthesia, especially in the geriatric population. This is not validated by the scientific literature. On the contrary, inadequate local anesthesia can result in far more surgical stress and attempts to compensate for this with sedative agents may lead to respiratory and cardiovascular compromise.

The majority of laparoscopic inguinal hernia procedures are done under general anesthesia for a variety of reasons. These include ability to control ventilation and compensate for the increased carbon dioxide load, optimization of the surgical view with full muscle relaxation, and patient comfort. Spinal anesthesia is an underutilized option for preperitoneal repairs, which do not require as high a dermatomal level as the transabdominal operation. The decision to select an open or laparoscopic hernia repair should be based upon the relative benefits of the surgical procedure, rather than solely upon the possible anesthetic options.

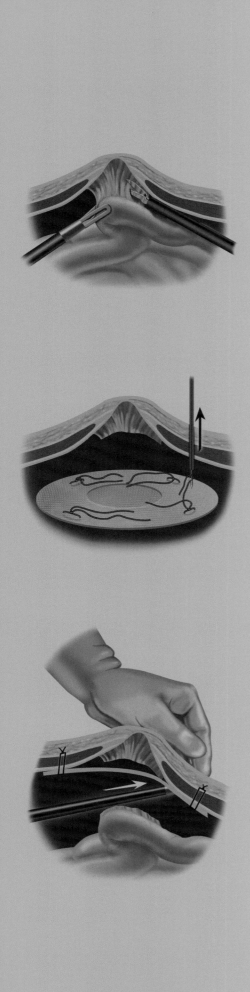

Laparoscopic Ventral Hernia Repair

Ventral hernia repair is the second most common type of abdominal hernia operation performed each year in the United States. When approaching the hernia with the traditional open technique, the fascial defect is ideally reinforced/repaired with a prosthetic mesh placed in a subfascial position. The recurrence rates with this technique are lower than compared to a simple overlay mesh. However, this appropriate positioning of the mesh usually involves a large incision and a fair amount of dissection, often complicated by the patient's body habitus. The laparoscopic approach to ventral hernia repairs offers a minimally invasive technique to repair these hernias that facilitates ideal mesh placement in the subfascial position and reduces recurrence rates.

Preoperative Preparation

1. Sequential compression stockings and subcutaneous heparin may be used for prophylaxis against deep venous thrombosis. Intravenous antibiotics, usually a first-generation cephalosporin, are administered prophylactically. Some may choose to also empirically cover enteric gram-negative organisms in the event of an inadvertent enterotomy. A preoperative bowel preparation, although advocated by some surgeons, is usually not necessary.

2. After induction of general anesthesia, the bladder is emptied with a urinary catheter and the stomach is decompressed with an orogastric tube. Following preparation of the skin, the abdomen may be covered with an Ioban skin barrier to limit contact of the mesh with the patient's skin during the procedure.

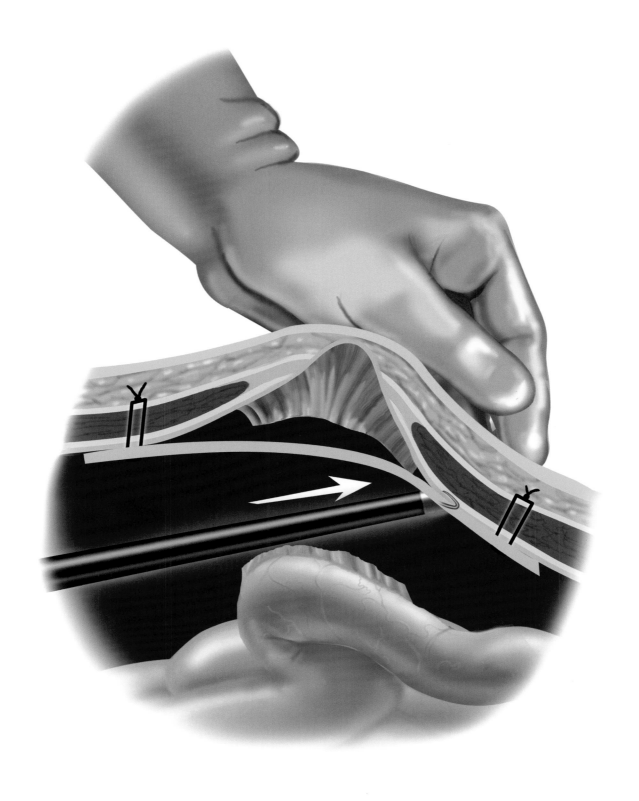

Operating Room Setup

3. The patient is positioned supine.

4. The surgeon usually stands on the patient's right side while the assistant is to the left, although the surgeon may choose to alternate sides later in the procedure to facilitate adequate mesh fixation.

5. The video monitors are stationed at both sides of either the patient's head or feet, depending on surgeon preference and position of the hernia, in order to facilitate adequate viewing from either side of the table.

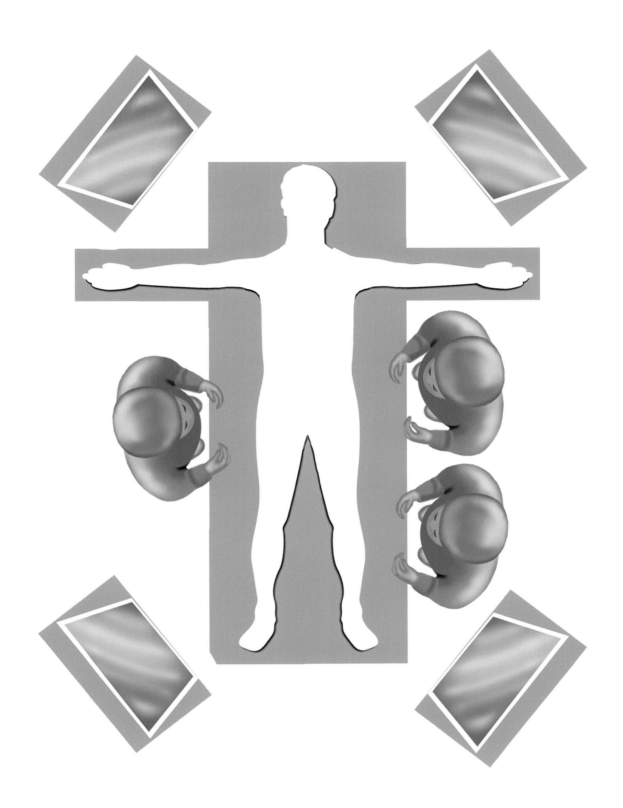

Access and Port Placement

6. Appropriate port placement varies with each individual operation, depending on the size and position of the hernia, as well as the patient's body habitus. However, general principles apply that facilitate adequate exposure and placement of the intra-abdominal mesh. Pneumoperitoneum of 15 mm Hg is obtained with either an open or closed technique (e.g., Veress needle) via an incision placed at least 10 cm lateral to the closest margin of the fascial defect.

7. An angled laparoscope is inserted to assess the extent of adhesions and size of the fascial defect. A 5 mm 30° angled scope is ideal as it can be placed through any of the trocars during the procedure to maximize visibility. A radially expanding 12 mm port and two 5 mm ports are then placed under direct vision. Some surgeons advocate the use of only 5 mm ports. These ports must be lateral enough to the fascial defect to allow for adequate manipulation of the laparoscopic instruments. For midline hernias, the anterior axillary line usually suffices.

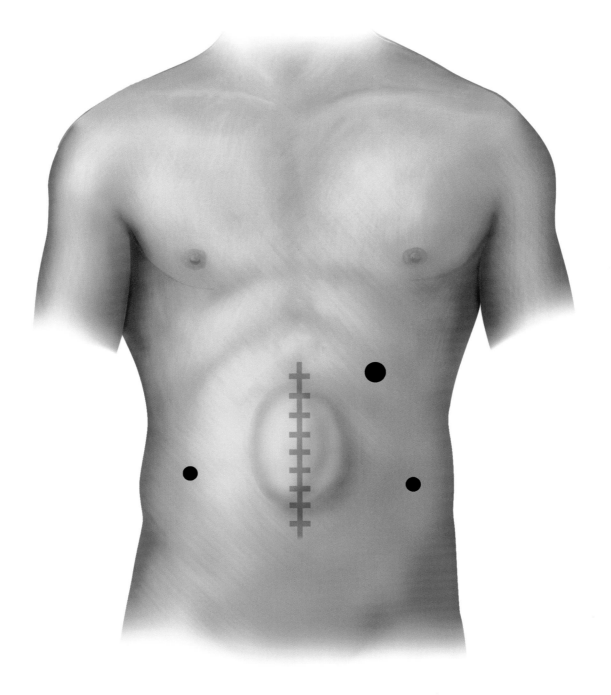

FIGURE C

Reducing the Hernia

8. Using a traction/countertraction technique, adhesiolysis is performed using primarily sharp dissection. Electrocautery is usually not necessary due to the relatively avascular nature of these adhesions, and should be kept to a minimum to avoid occult or delayed bowel injury. All adhesions between intestine and/or omentum and the abdominal wall should be lysed within a 5 cm circumferential margin to the fascial defect.

9. It is important to completely expose all fascial defects, as it is not uncommon to have multiple defects resembling a "Swiss cheese" pattern. The circumferential margin is crucial for adequate mesh placement. The peritoneal sac can be left in place unless tenacious adhesions between the bowel and sac necessitate excision of the sac from the fascial edge.

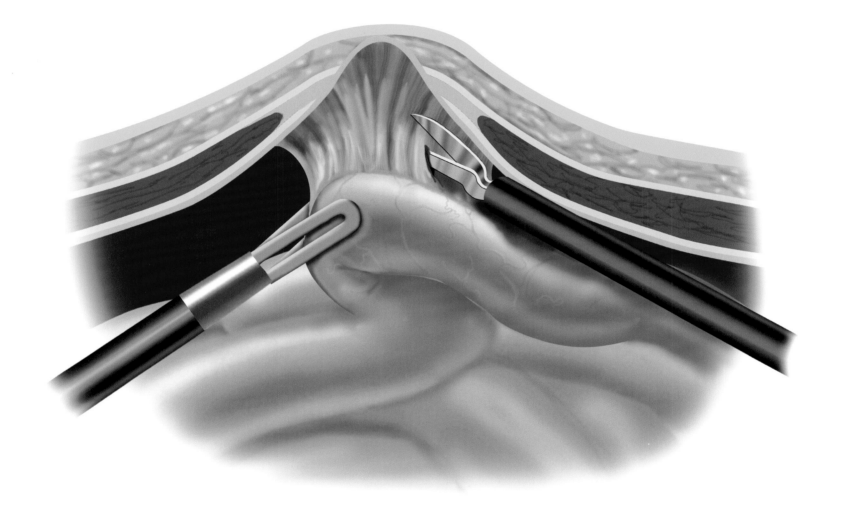

Preparing the Mesh

10. The extent of the fascial defect is clearly identified by passing a spinal needle through the abdominal wall and marking the borders upon the patient's abdomen with a pen. A dual-sided mesh (smooth side facing the abdominal viscera and rough side oriented toward the abdominal wall) is cut to allow a 3 cm circumferential overlap from the edges of the fascial defect.

11. A 2-0 polypropylene or Gortex suture is then placed in each of the four quadrants in a horizontal mattress fashion, with the tails of the suture oriented toward the rough side of the mesh. The location of these sutures relative to the proposed area for mesh placement is clearly marked on the patient's abdomen.

12. The mesh is rolled with the suture tails oriented inward and is inserted into the abdomen via the 12 mm port. For larger mesh, the port is removed and mesh passed through the skin incision directly. The mesh is then unfolded and oriented appropriately to cover the entire fascial defect while aligning the previously placed sutures with their corresponding marked positions on the abdomen.

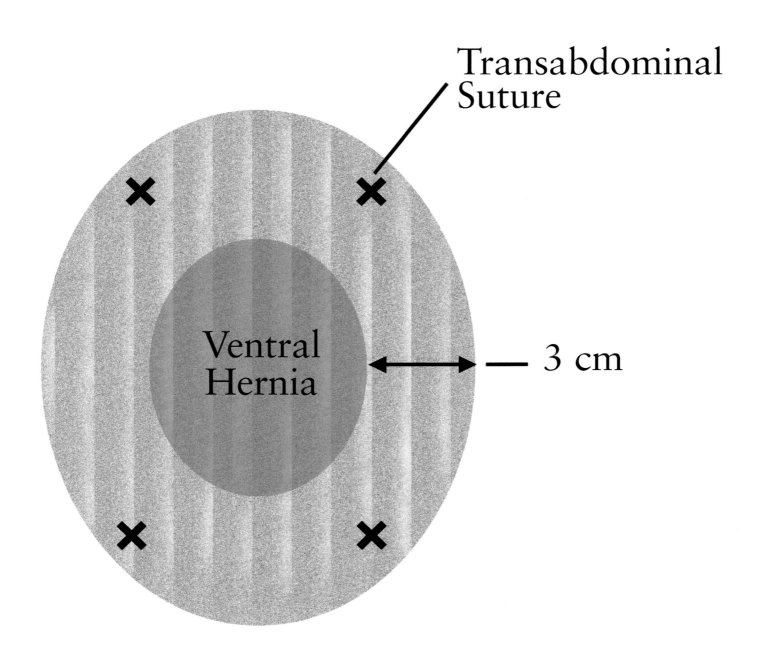

Fixating the Mesh

13. Skin incisions of 1 mm are made in each of the four quadrants over the previously marked areas (Figure inset top). A suture grasper, or fascial closure device, is inserted (Figure inset bottom) and both tails of the sutures are grasped and retrieved with separate passes through separate points on the fascia, utilizing the same skin incision (Figure E).

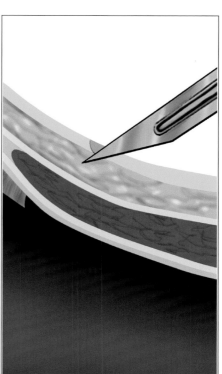

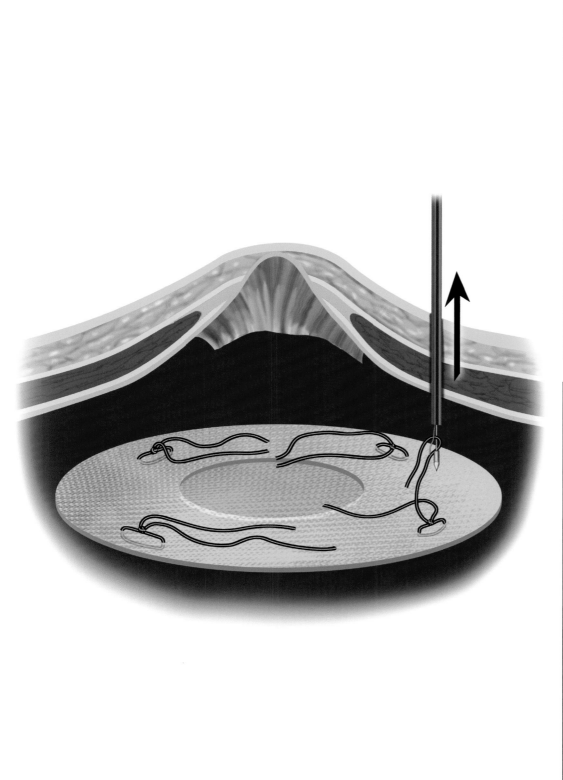

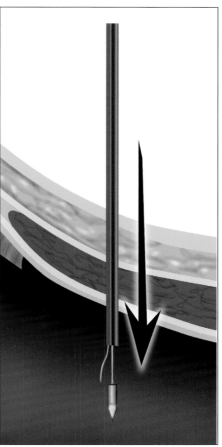

Fixating the Mesh, Part II

14. The sutures are tied extracorporeally, with the knots lying in the subcutaneous tissue, thus providing transabdominal fixation of the mesh at each of these points. For large hernias, additional transfascial sutures can be placed so that there is one suture every 5 cm around the mesh.

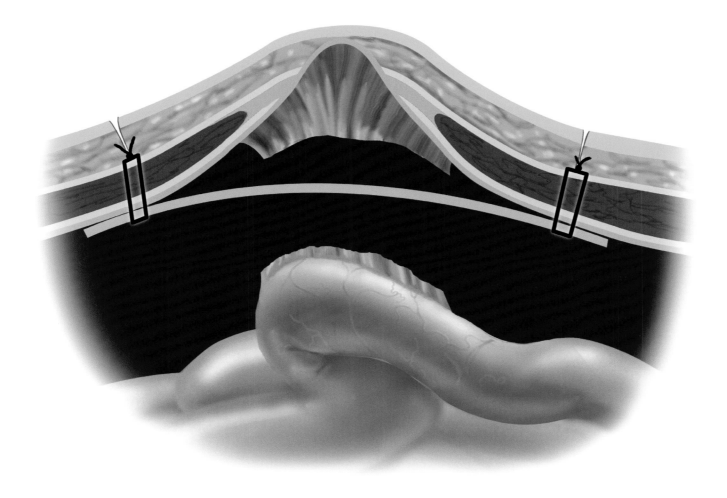

Fixating the Mesh, Part III

15. The mesh is additionally secured by placing 5 mm surgical tacks circumferentially at intervals of 1 cm to 2 cm. This close interval of tack placement is crucial to prevent the formation of folds in the mesh once pneumoperitoneum is released, which could lead to hernia recurrence. Alternatively, some surgeons choose to secure the mesh with only surgical tacks, without the use of secondary reinforcement of the sutures in each of the four quadrants. We recommend using a combination of tacks and sutures for mesh fixation.

16. The trocars are removed under direct vision and pneumoperitoneum is released. Fascial defects greater than 5 mm should be closed in the usual fashion. The skin is closed with 4-0 absorbable subcuticular sutures.

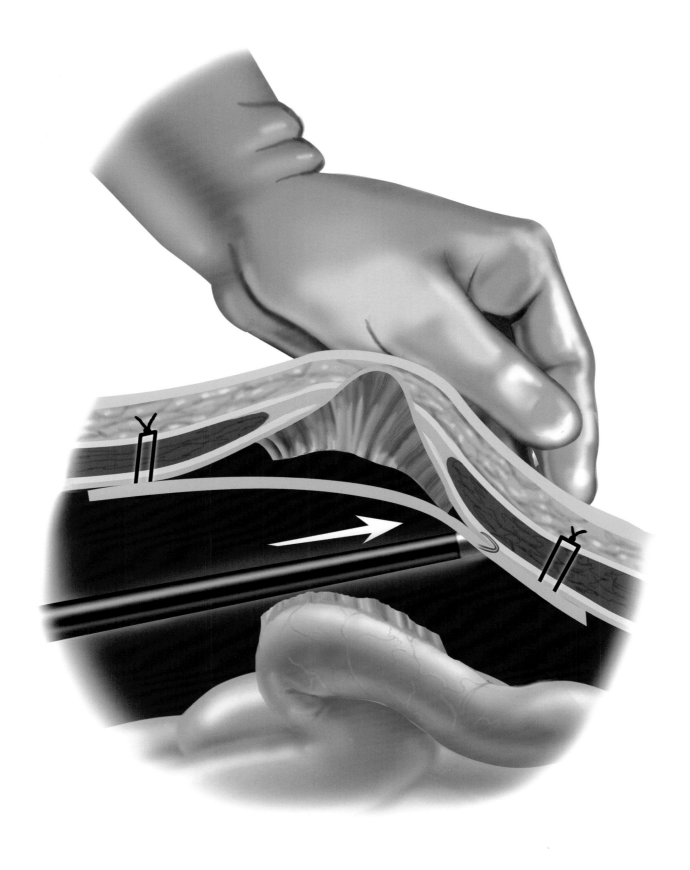

Postoperative Care

An abdominal binder is placed and should be continued postoperatively to assist with patient comfort and to minimize seroma formation. Sequential compression devices and/or subcutaneous heparin are continued postoperatively. Provided there was no enteric injury, postoperative antibiotics are usually not necessary. Patients are usually admitted for observation and pain control. Oral intake is advanced as tolerated. Occasionally, patients will develop an ileus which may delay discharge from the hospital.

Suggested Reading

1. Park A, Birch DW, Lovrics P. Laparoscopic and open incisional hernia repair: a comparison study. *Surgery*. 1998;124:816-822.

2. Toy FK, Bailey RW, Carey S, et al. Prospective multicenter study of laparoscopic ventral hernioplasty: preliminary results. *Surg Endosc* 1998;12:955-959.

3. Scott DJ, Jones DB. Hernias and abdominal wall defects. In: Norton JA, ed. Surgery: Scientific Basis and Current Practice. 2nd ed. New York: Springer-Verlag; 2006. In press.

Commentary

Kenric M. Murayama, M.D., John A. Burns School of Medicine University of Hawaii

Ventral hernias, particularly incisional hernias, are a common problem. The laparoscopic approach has provided an improved technique for repair of these sometimes difficult hernias with lower recurrence rates. The authors have identified the standard method for performing laparoscopic ventral hernia repair.

Regarding placement of trocars, there are two other important factors I consider at the time of placement. If the hernia is an incisional hernia, I place the initial trocar contralateral to the majority of the previous intra-abdominal dissection (e.g., on the left side if the patient had a previous right hemicolectomy). This increases the likelihood of placing the initial trocar into a space with fewer adhesions. It is also important to place the trocars an adequate distance away from the costal margin, the iliac crest, and the upper thigh to facilitate anterior mobility of the intra-abdominal tips of the instruments.

Although a polypropylene or Gortex suture is frequently used, I prefer a braided polyester suture because it has less "memory" and "glare," making it easier to deal with inside the abdomen.

Finally, when placing the tacks to secure the mesh, it is helpful to place pressure against the tip of the tacking device with the opposite hand on the outside of the abdomen. This results in more secure placement of tacks without the tip of the tacking device slipping off the mesh.

Adrian E. Park, M.D. University of Maryland Medical Center

Laparoscopic ventral hernia repair (LVHR) is a procedure that is very much on the rise in terms of numbers of cases performed across the country. There are several reasons for its ascendance. Ventral or incisional hernia is a common problem facing all abdominal surgeons and one that lends itself very well to a laparoscopic approach for repair. Furthermore, LVHR is a technique that can realistically be assimilated into most surgeons' clinical practice because of the frequency with which such patients present and because the procedure can be mastered by surgeons possessing fundamental laparoscopic skills who are taught the technique and then appropriately proctored.

Several elements of the technique of LVHR, which are discussed by the authors, bear further emphasis. Although some may quibble over the choice of biomaterial to be used in the repair, few would argue that a tension-free technique employing a mesh, containing an adhesion barrier, placed in a subfascial or "underlay" position must increasingly be considered the standard of care in ventral herniorrhaphy. There must be adequate overlap of all defect margins by the mesh (minimum of 3.0-5.0 cm), which must be secured by sutures, as well as tacks or staples to ensure long-term durability of the repair.

The authors rightly recommend limited use of energy sources during adhesiolysis to reduce the risk of recognized or, worse, occult bowel injury. Preoperatively, patients need to be made aware of the possibility of inadvertent enterotomy and that should it happen, they may have their hernia repair delayed or staged to avoid even a remote possibility of mesh infection.

LVHR is a procedure that warrants such widespread adoption by surgeons. It offers our patients a surgical solution to a common yet difficult problem that is truly minimally invasive and results in a minimally morbid, durable hernia repair.

Vivian Sanchez, M.D., Beth Israel Deaconess Medical Center Harvard Medical School

Laparoscopic ventral hernia repair has emerged as a safe, effective means of repairing ventral hernias. Although prospective, randomized trials are lacking, LVHR has acceptable and equitable recurrence rates, lower wound infection rates, and shortened hospital stays.

When attempting a laparoscopic hernia repair, the preferred method of entering the abdomen is through a Veress needle in the left upper quadrant followed by controlled entry via a clear port. One must then assess the location of the hernia defect prior to placement of the rest of the trocars to ensure adequate distance from the edge of the defect to allow at least a 3 cm underlay of mesh. If using a 5 mm 30° camera, I use at least two 5 mm ports and one 12 mm port on one side to allow the surgeon to work with two hands, as well as a third 5 mm port on the opposite side to allow for proper tack fixation. If using a 10 mm 30° camera, I would use two 12 mm ports and one 5 mm port on one side to allow the camera angle to change, as well as a second 5 mm port on the opposite side for tack fixation.

Once the abdomen is entered, adhesions are lysed bluntly, and electrocautery is rarely used unless certain there is no bowel. When measuring the defect, it is important to insert the spinal needle/angiocatheter perpendicularly so as to not overestimate the size of the defect. The abdomen can be deflated and the defects remeasured extracorporeally. At least a 3 cm overlap of mesh on each side is key. After the appropriate-size mesh is utilized, sutures are placed around the periphery. Although there are some surgeons who use no transfascial sutures, and those that only anchor in four corners, the trend is toward utilization of sutures at least every 5 cm to 7 cm to improve the strength. After the sutures are placed, the mesh and abdominal wall are labeled, as well as each of the suture locations, to facilitate mesh placement. One should intermittently assess the tautness or flaccidness of the mesh as each of the transfascial sutures are placed. Typically, tie the sutures only after satisfied with proper mesh and suture placement. Tacks should be placed at 1 to 2 cm intervals around the periphery. Marcaine is injected into each of the transfascial sutures for postoperative analgesia.

For hernias extending down to the pubic symphysis, it is often necessary to bring down a peritoneal flap and tack the mesh to Cooper's ligament for appropriate fixation.

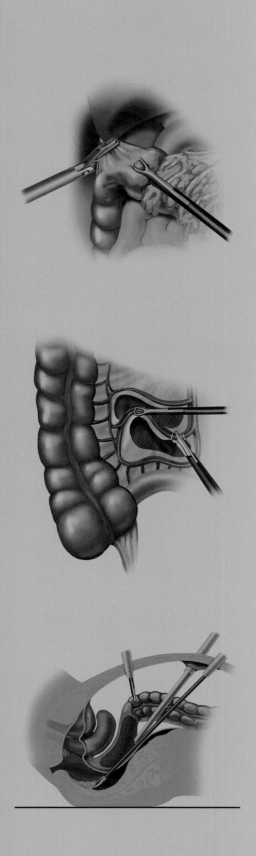

Laparoscopic Colorectal Resections

A recent multi-institutional randomized controlled trial has demonstrated comparable outcomes between the laparoscopic and open approach for colorectal malignancy. Patients have a similar incidence of postoperative complications, local recurrence, and survival. A recent consensus statement by the American Society for Colorectal Surgery (ASCRS) and the Society for American Gastrointestinal and Endoscopic Surgeons (SAGES) endorses the laparoscopic approach for malignancy after a surgeon has appropriate training and experience.

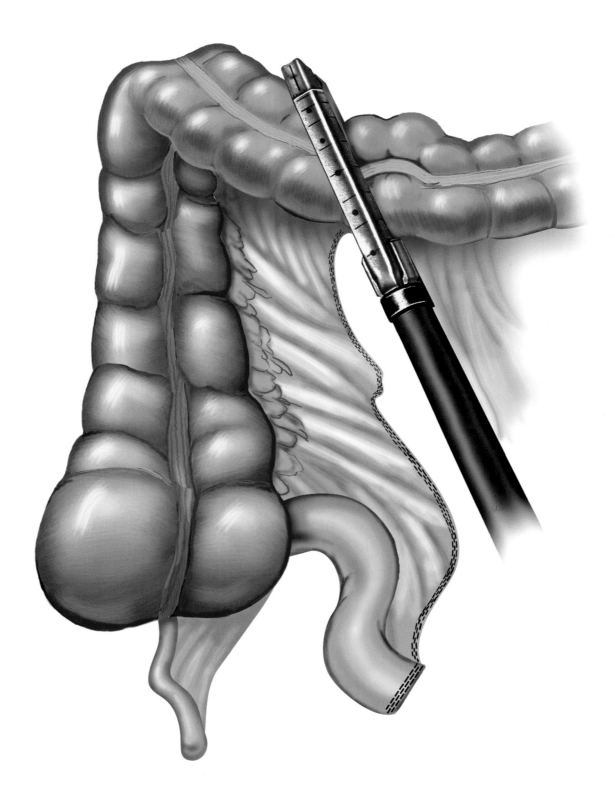

Right Colectomy

Preoperative Preparation

1. The position of tumors and/or polyps should be clearly identified with either an endoscopic tattoo or a preoperative barium enema. Sequential compression devices and subcutaneously administered heparin are used for prophylaxis against deep venous thrombosis. Perioperative antibiotics are administered. Our preference is to have the patient undergo a mechanical bowel preparation. After induction of general anesthesia, the stomach is decompressed with an orogastric or nasogastric tube and a urinary catheter is placed. If severe inflammation is expected or encountered, ureteral stents may be placed to help identify the ureters intraoperatively and prevent complications.

FIGURE A

Operating Room Setup

2. The patient is placed in a modified lithotomy position with the legs in stirrups, being careful to appropriately pad all prominences as to avoid pressure injuries. The arms are tucked to the sides. Care is taken to avoid excess flexion of the hips or knees as this limits the mobility of the laparoscopic instruments.

3. The surgeon and camera holder stand to the patient's left, while the assistant stands between the patient's legs. The surgeon uses a two-handed technique. The video monitors are arranged as shown.

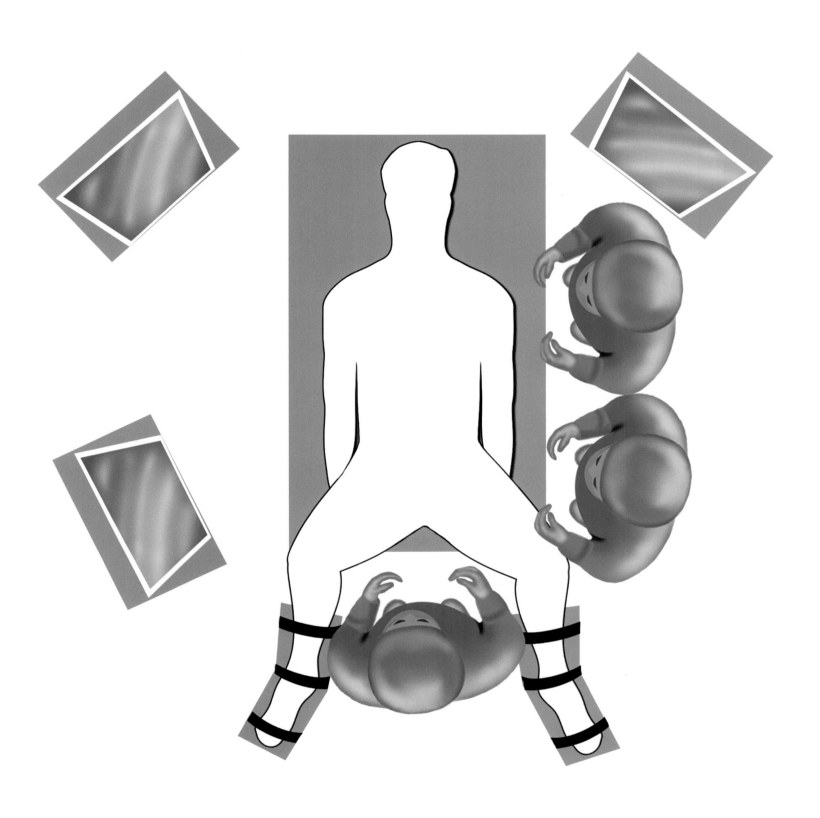

Port Placement

4. An infraumbilical incision is used to establish pneumoperitoneum, setting a pressure limit of 15 mm Hg. This may be established either with an open or closed technique. A 10/11 mm port is placed here and the laparoscope is inserted. A 30° angled scope is preferred as it facilitates obtaining crucial images during the operation. A careful exploration is performed to ensure that no injury occurred during port insertion and that no other abnormalities or metastatic disease are present.

5. Three additional 10/12 mm trocars are then placed in the suprapubic area and the left and right lower quadrants, creating an anchor shape that provides access to all sides of the abdomen (Figure B-a). An optional 5 mm port placed in the right upper quadrant midclavicular line may be necessary to assist with hepatic flexure mobilization. Alternatively, a subxiphoid port may be substituted for the suprapubic port (Figure B-b). A hand-assist port can be used as well, which will facilitate retraction, dissection, specimen extraction, and creation of an extracorporeal anastomosis.

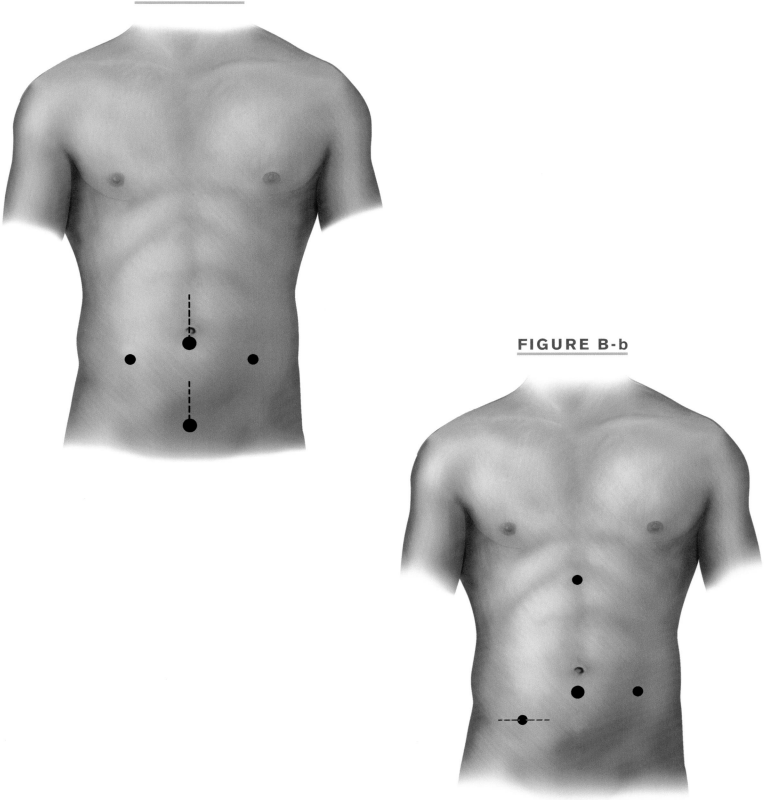

FIGURE B-a

FIGURE B-b

Lateral to Medial Approach

FIGURE C

Initiating Mobilization of the Right Colon

6. Mobilization begins at the cecum. After the patient is placed in Trendelenburg position and tilted 30° to the left, the cecum and terminal ileum are retracted in a cephalad and medial direction. The peritoneum is incised over the avascular retroperitoneal space as shown. Mobilization of the peritoneum overlying the ileal mesentery is carried out to the level of the duodenum.

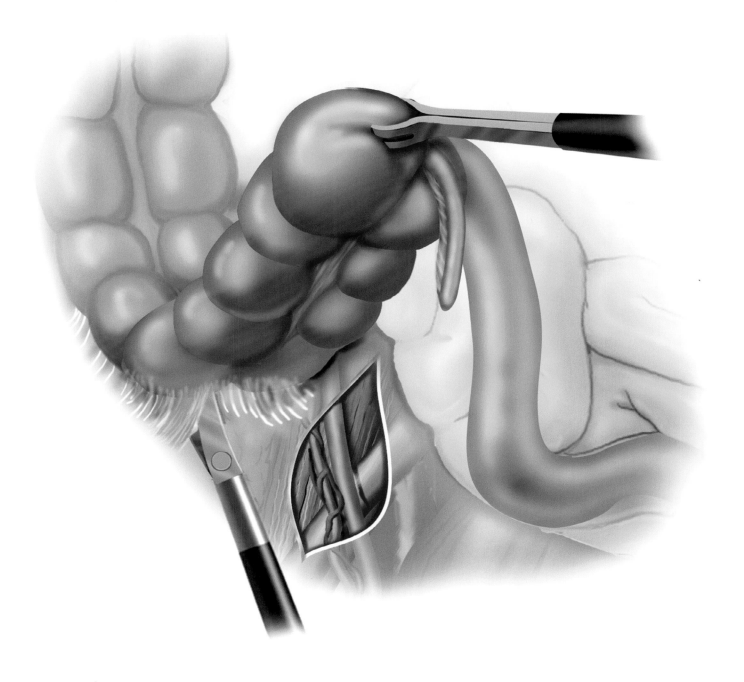

Mobilizing the Right Colon

7. With continued retraction of the ascending colon in the cephalad and medial direction, the lateral peritoneal attachments (white line of Toldt) are divided with curved monopolar cautery scissors or an ultrasonic scalpel using a traction/countertraction technique. As the dissection approaches the hepatic flexure and the ascending colon is mobilized medially, special care should be taken to avoid violating Gerota's fascia or injuring the ureter or lateral wall of the duodenum.

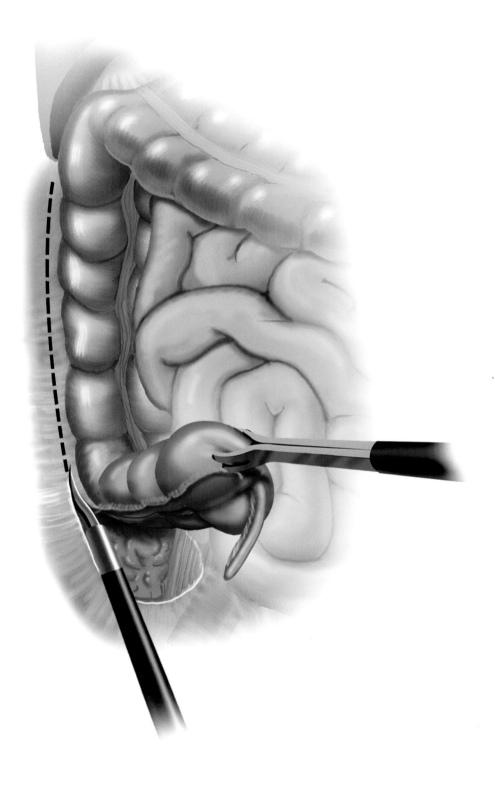

Mobilizing the Hepatic Flexure

8. The patient should be switched to the reverse Trendelenburg position. The laparoscope can be moved to the right lower quadrant position to allow for better visualization of the right gutter and paraduodenal area.

9. The hepatic flexure is retracted inferiorly and medially and the peritoneal attachments are divided. Vascular attachments may require surgical clips or the use of ultrasonic shears to obtain appropriate hemostasis. Excessive traction should be avoided as to prevent iatrogenic injury to the liver.

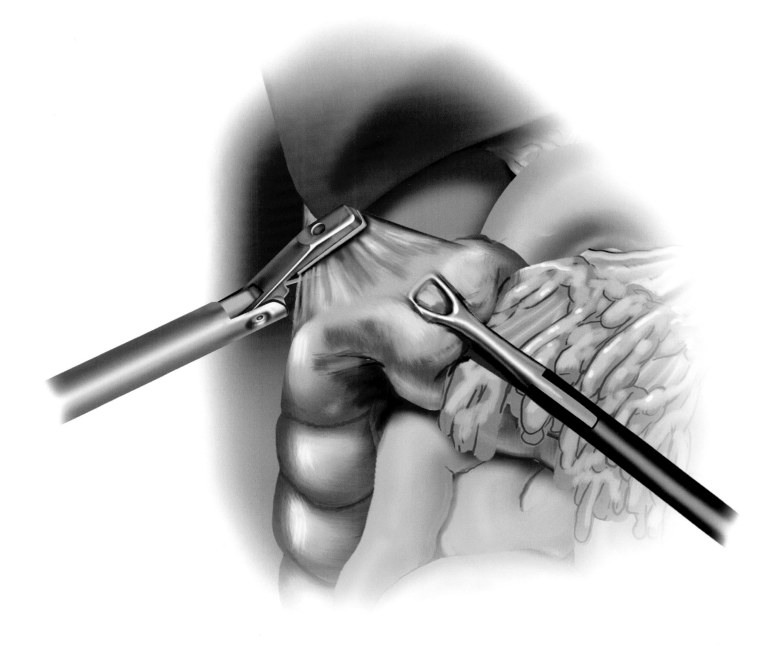

Mobilizing the Proximal Transverse Colon

10. The omentum is detached from the proximal transverse colon with an ultrasonic shears or electrocautery dissection.

11. Mobilization of the gastrocolic ligament may also be necessary to completely free the hepatic flexure from the undersurface of the liver. The duodenum is carefully separated from the colonic mesentery using blunt or sharp dissection.

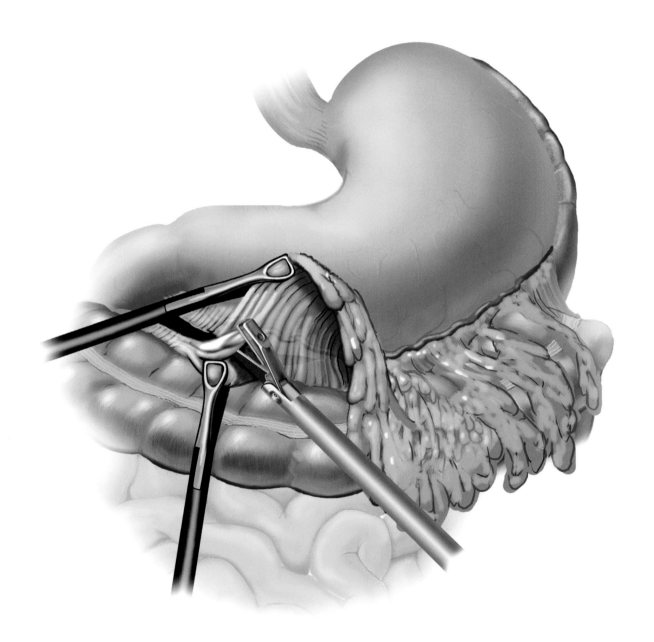

Dividing the Mesentery

12. Using electrocautery scissors, the peritoneum overlying the mesentery is scored in the window beneath the ileocolic vascular trunk of the superior mesenteric artery (Figure G-a). The vessels are skeletonized, two to three surgical clips are placed on the mesenteric side, at least one clip is placed on the specimen side, and the vessel is divided with scissors (Figure G-b). This dissection should be carried out near the root of the mesentery if the operation is being performed for malignancy.

13. This maneuver is repeated until the mesentery is divided up to and including the right branch of the middle colic artery.

14. A pretied surgical ligature (endoloop) may be placed on each mesenteric stump for additional security. Alternatively, a linear laparoscopic stapler with a vascular load (2.5 mm staples) or a LigaSure device can be used to divide the mesentery. Although this technique is usually faster than the one previously described, it is substantially more expensive. Either an extracorporeal or intracorporeal resection and anastomosis can be performed.

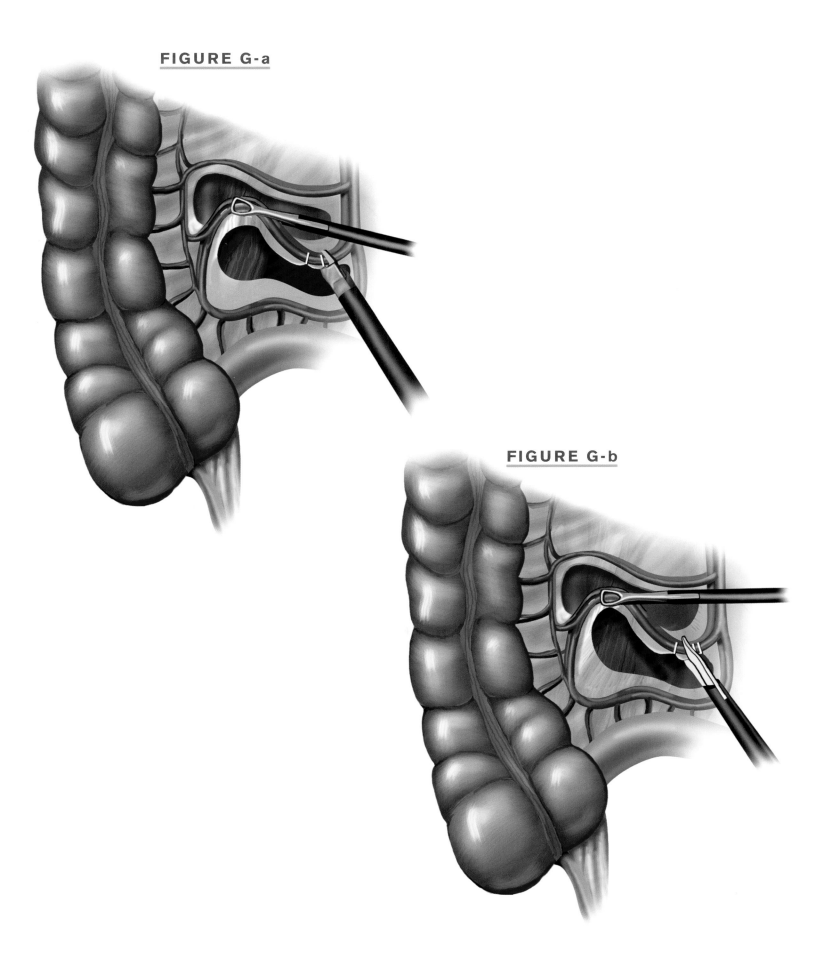

FIGURE G-a

FIGURE G-b

Medial to Lateral Approach

FIGURE H

Dividing the Mesentery and Mobilizing the Right Colon

15. Alternatively, a medial to lateral dissection can be performed where the right colon is left attached to the lateral abdominal wall while the mesenteric vessels are controlled, ligated, and divided using one of the techniques previously described. The duodeneum is clearly identified in its retroperitoneal position as it serves as a landmark for the location of the ileocolic and right colic vessels. Using this approach, great care is taken to dissect within the correct plane while mobilizing the right and proximal transverse colon, so as not to violate Gerota's fascia or injure any underlying structures (duodenum, common bile duct, kidney, ureter).

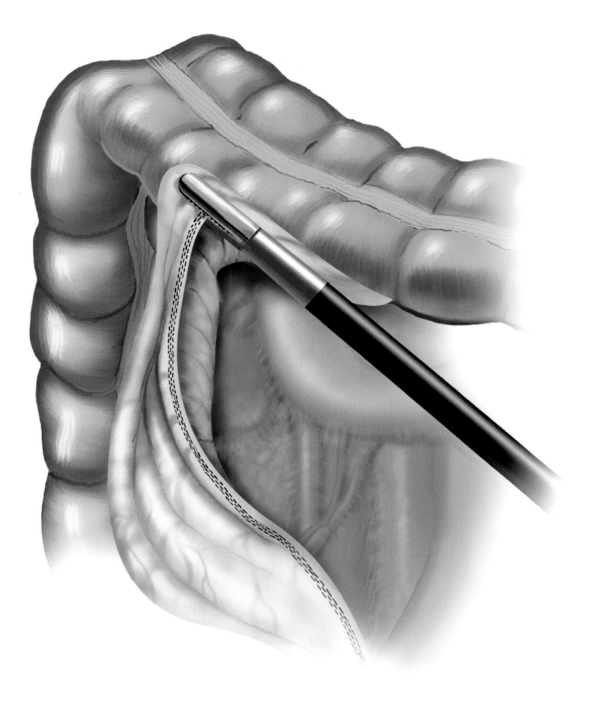

Extracorporeal Resection and Anastomosis

16. For an extracorporeal resection and anastomosis, a fascial opening of 6 cm to 10 cm is created by extending the umbilical or right lower quadrant incision. The terminal ileum and colon are eviscerated through this opening, being careful to avoid inadvertent rotation, while protecting the abdominal wall with a plastic drape, laparotomy pads, towels, or other protective material.

17. The proximal and distal margins of the specimen are then divided using a linear stapler (3.5 – 3.8 mm staples). A side-to-side, functional end-to-end, anastomosis is fashioned using either a conventional hand-sewn (Figure I-a) or stapled technique.

18. The mesenteric defect can also be closed at this time (Figure I-b). The bowel is returned to the peritoneal cavity and the fascia is closed in the usual manner. Wounds are irrigated and injected with 0.5% bupivacaine, and the skin is closed with either a skin stapler or 4-0 absorbable subcuticular sutures.

FIGURE I-a

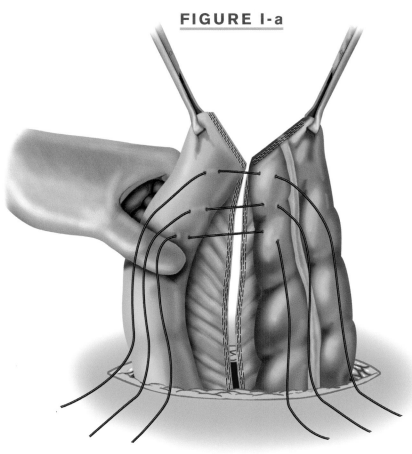

FIGURE I-b

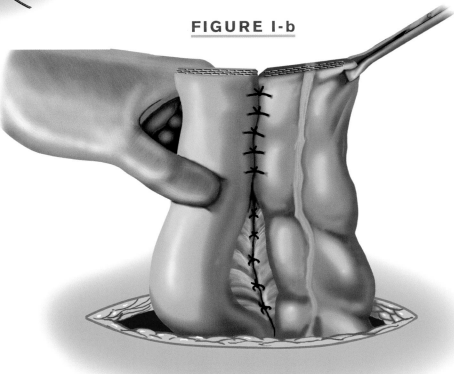

Intracorporeal Resection

19. For an intracorporeal resection and anastomosis, a 30 mm or 60 mm endoscopic linear stapler (3.5–3.8 mm staples) is used to divide the proximal and distal margins of the specimen.

20. The specimen is removed through a small fascial opening of 3 cm to 6 cm and is inspected outside the abdomen to ensure complete resection of the lesion. This fascial opening usually requires closure at this time in order to appropriately re-establish pneumoperitoneum. The mesentery is carefully inspected for hemostasis. Alternatively, the specimen can be placed in a retrieval bag and placed over the liver while the anastomosis is constructed.

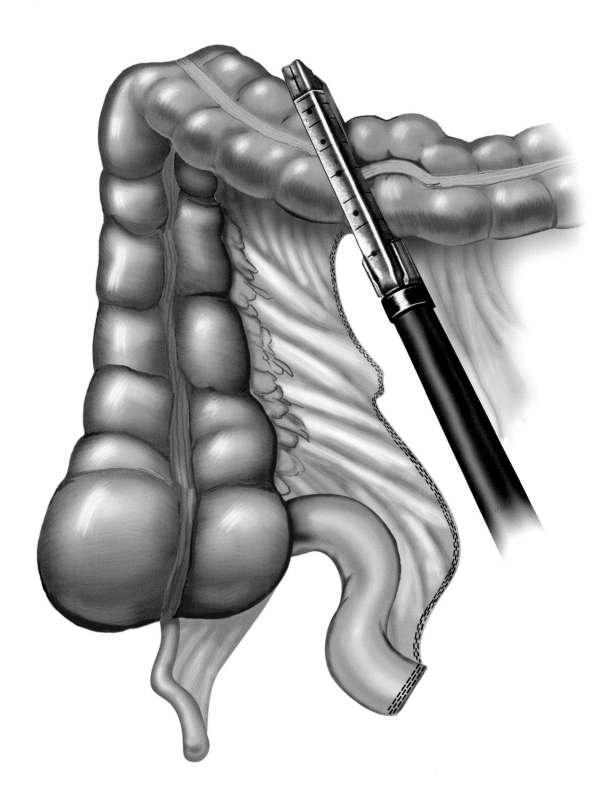

Intracorporeal Anastomosis

21. An additional 5 mm port is placed in the left upper quadrant. Each limb of the bowel is controlled with a grasper and aligned appropriately. Ordinarily, the right abdominal trocar is used to insert an endoscopic 60 mm linear stapler (loaded with 3.5-3.8 mm staples).

22. A small enterotomy is made in each limb using electrocautery scissors. Each limb of the stapling device is inserted into the enterotomies and fired (Figure K-a), being careful to exclude all mesentery from the staple line. The anastomosis is inspected for integrity and bleeding.

23. The enterotomies are closed with a second firing of the linear stapler (Figure K-b). Alternatively, the anastomosis and/or enterotomy closure can be performed with intracorporeal suturing. The mesenteric defect is usually left open. After final inspection, the abdomen is closed as described above.

FIGURE K-a

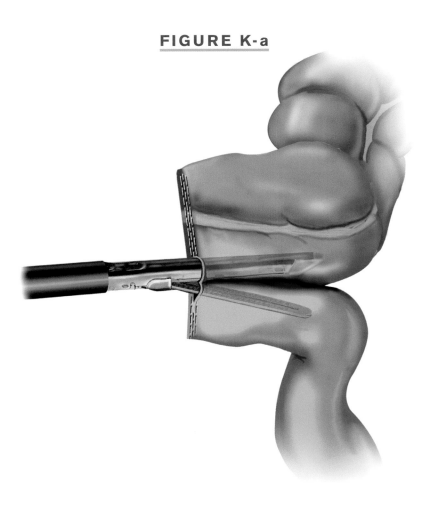

FIGURE K-b

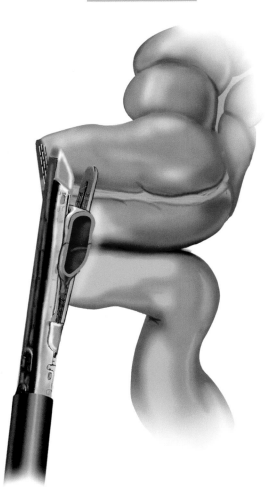

Left Colectomy

Preoperative Preparation

1. The same preparation as described for a right colectomy is performed.

FIGURE L

Operating Room Setup and Port Placement

2. A similar setup is used as described for a right colectomy, except the surgeon and camera holder stand to the patient's right and the assistant to the left.

3. The same technique and port positions as described for a right colectomy can be used.

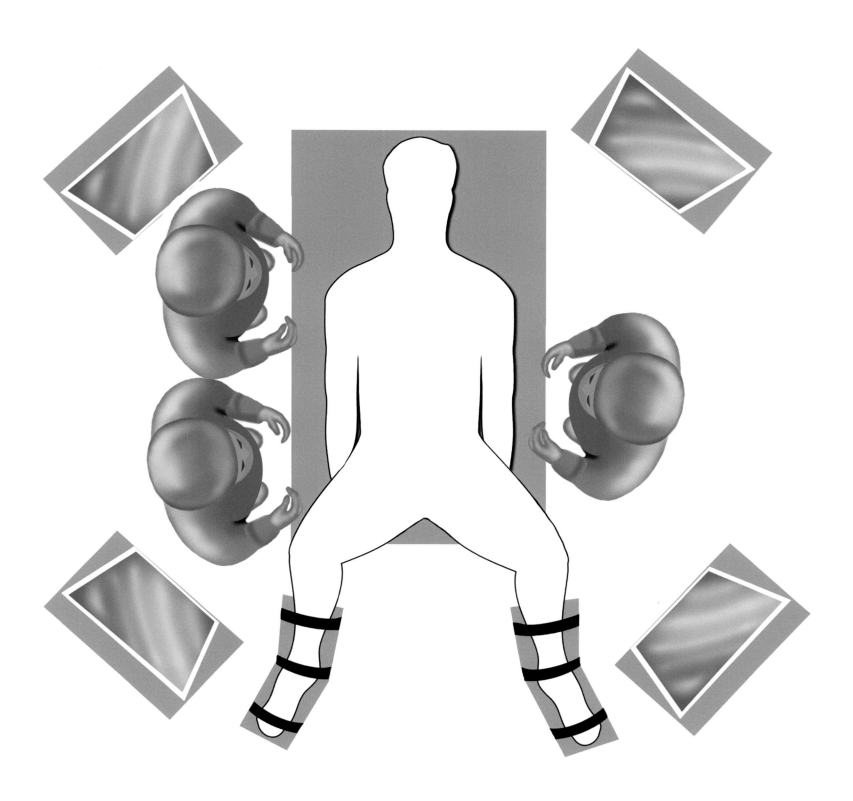

Mobilizing the Sigmoid and Left Colon

4. The sigmoid and descending colon are dissected and mobilized using a similar technique as described for a right colectomy. Care is taken to avoid ureteral injury.

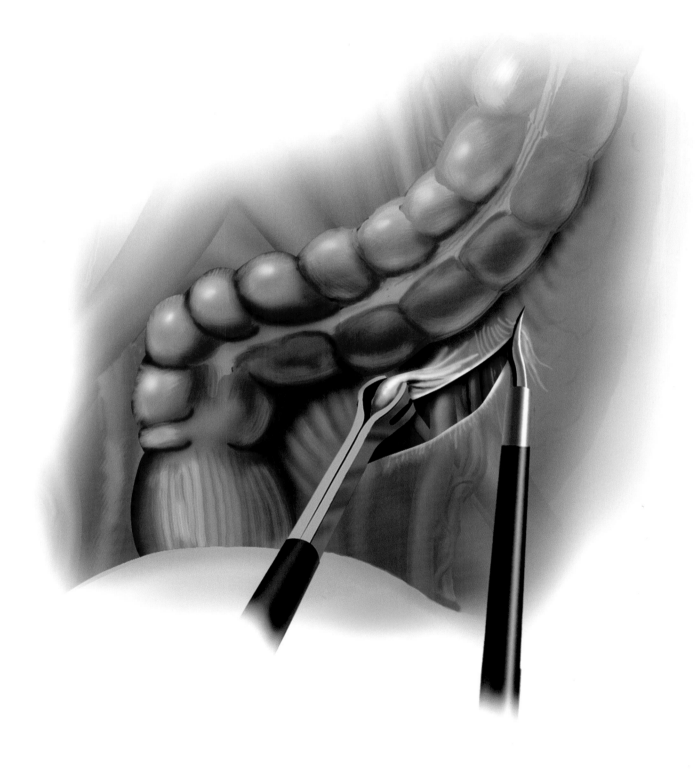

Mobilizing the Splenic Flexure and Transverse Colon

5. Similar to mobilizing the hepatic flexure, the splenic flexure is gently retracted in a caudal and medial direction as the attachments are divided. Any vascular attachments should be carefully dissected and controlled with surgical clips, sutures, or staples. Excess traction must be avoided to avoid splenic injury.

6. The transverse colon is dissected free from its attachments to the omentum as described previously.

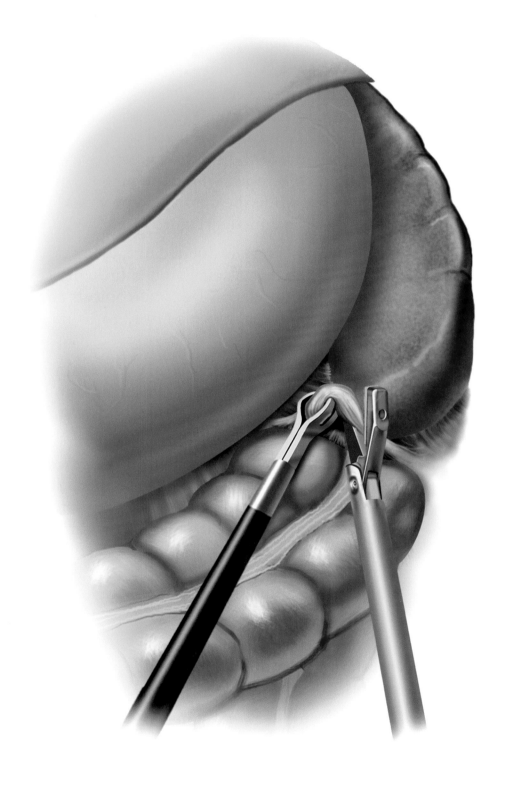

Dividing the Mesentery, Resection, and Anastomosis

7. The mesocolon is divided using a similar technique as described for a right colectomy. The position of the left ureter should routinely be identified during this stage of the operation. A window is made in the peritoneum about the inferior mesenteric vessels, allowing for ligation with clips or a stapling device (Figure O-a). Alternatively, a medial to lateral approach can be utilized for left colectomy as well. The retroperitoneal dissection is similar to that as described for a right colectomy, where the mesenteric vessels are divided first while the colon is kept intact with its lateral peritoneal attachments (Figure O-b).

8. Once the mesentery is divided and colon adequately mobilized, the transverse colon is brought down to the pelvis to ensure that a tension-free anastomosis can be constructed. The hepatic flexure may also need to be mobilized to accomplish this.

9. The bowel can be resected intracorporeally or extracorporeally after evisceration through a 6 cm to 8 cm lower midline incision. The distal bowel transection is usually performed at the level of the sacral promontory.

10. The anastomosis can be constructed intracorporeally or extracorporeally as previously described, although a distal transection line below the level of the sacral promontory makes an extracorporeal anastomosis difficult to perform. In this circumstance, one may choose to construct the anastomosis using an EEA stapler, as described for a low anterior resection. The mesenteric defect is closed with simple sutures.

11. The anastomosis should be tested with an underwater insufflation test and any leaks are repaired with simple sutures.

12. The fascia and skin incisions are closed in the usual fashion.

FIGURE O-a

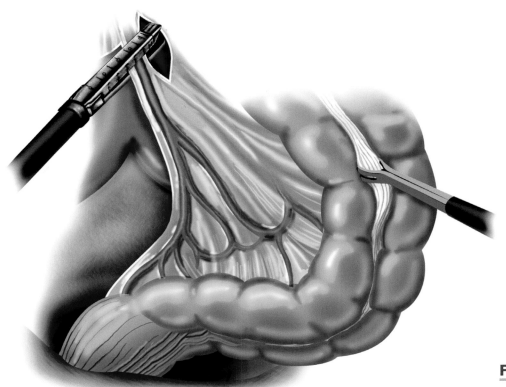

FIGURE O-b

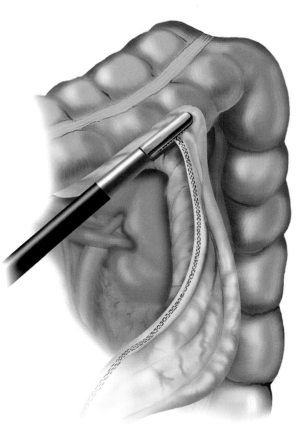

Low Anterior Resection

Preoperative Preparation

1. The same preparation as described for a left colectomy is performed.

Operating Room Setup and Port Placement

2. The same setup is used as described for a left colectomy.

3. The same technique and port positions as described for a left colectomy are used.

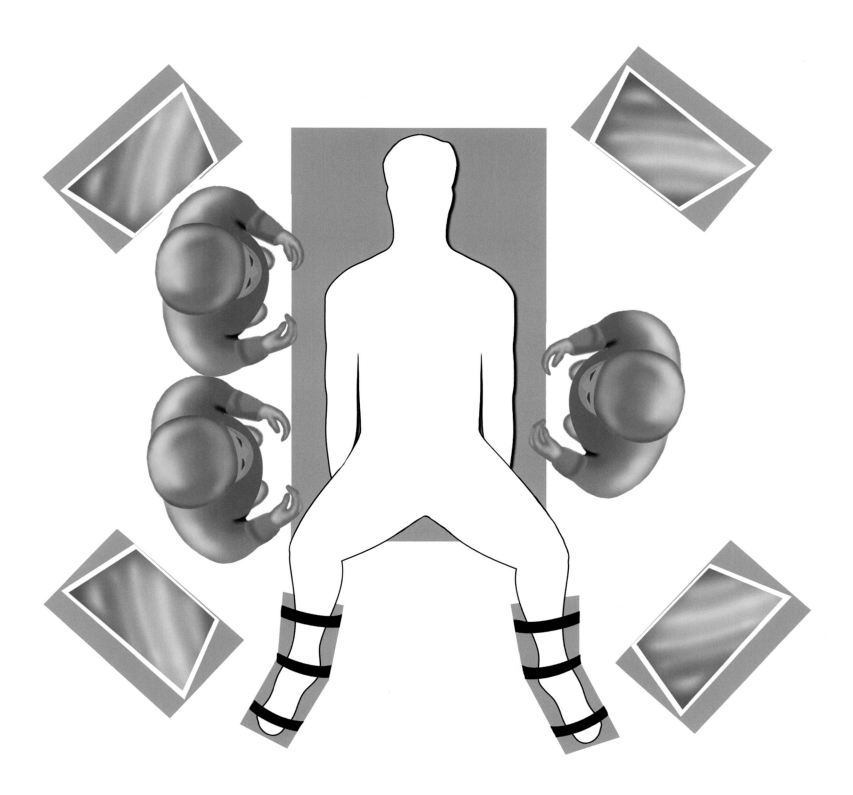

Mobilizing the Sigmoid and Left Colon

4. The sigmoid and descending colon are dissected and mobilized using a similar technique as described for a left colectomy. Careful attention must be directed toward avoiding ureteral injury.

5. The splenic flexure, transverse colon, and hepatic flexure, if necessary, are mobilized as previously described.

6. Rectal dissection begins in the posterior avascular plane between the rectum and presacral fascia.

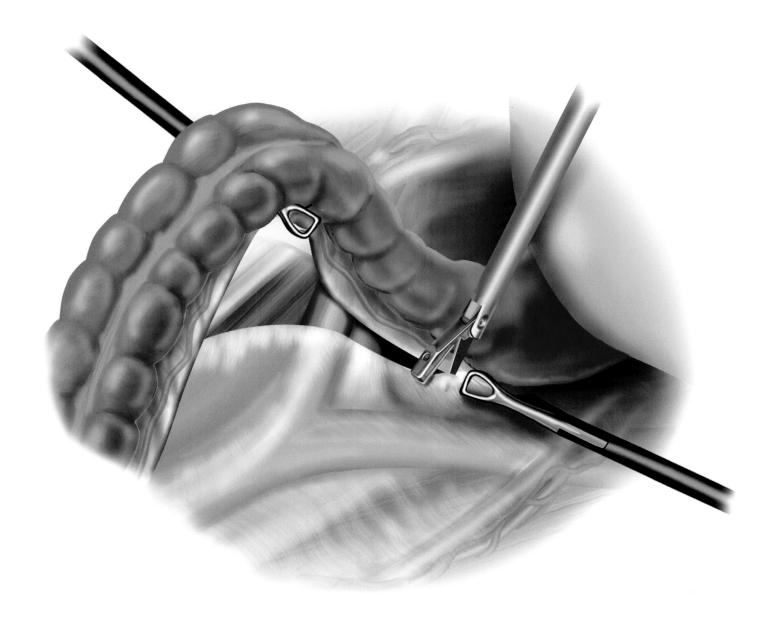

Rectal Dissection

7. The sigmoid and rectum are retracted anteriorly toward the abdominal wall and the rectal dissection continues in the avascular posterior plane down to the pelvic floor. The presacral fascia should not be violated as to preserve the pelvic nerves and presacral veins.

8. Anteriorly, the peritoneum is incised down to the peritoneal reflection to expose the lateral ligaments. Using a traction/countertraction technique, electrocautery or ultrasonic coagulation is used to transect the lateral ligaments. Surgical clips may be used to attain hemostasis. Anterior dissection should not violate the urethra in males or the posterior vaginal wall in females. A tenaculum-type retractor can be used to lift the uterus anteriorly to facilitate exposure of the anterior rectal plane.

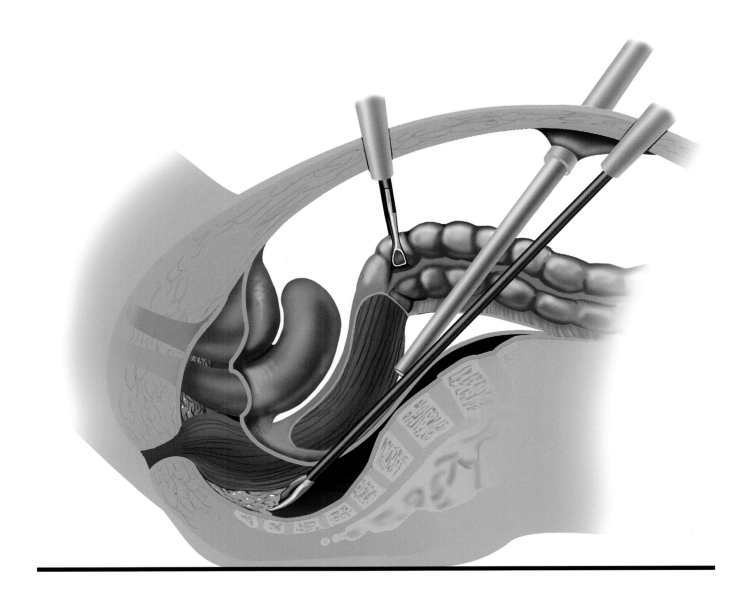

Resection and Anastomosis

9. The rectum is transected 4 cm to 5 cm above the dentate line using a reticulating transverse stapling instrument (3.5–3.8 mm staples).

10. The proximal margin of the specimen is divided and the specimen is removed through a 6 cm to 8 cm lower midline abdominal incision.

11. After sizing the anastomosis, the corresponding anvil is secured in the proximal transected end with a purse-string suture (Figure R). A conventional circular stapler is inserted transanally and the stapler spike is carefully pushed through the stapled end of the rectal stump.

12. The anvil and stapler are mated and the stapler is fired (Figure S). After the "doughnuts" of tissue are inspected, the anastomosis should be tested with an underwater air insufflation test under direct vision. Any detected leaks are repaired with simple sutures. The mesenteric defect may be approximated with silk sutures.

13. The fascial and skin incisions are closed in the usual fashion.

FIGURE R

FIGURE S

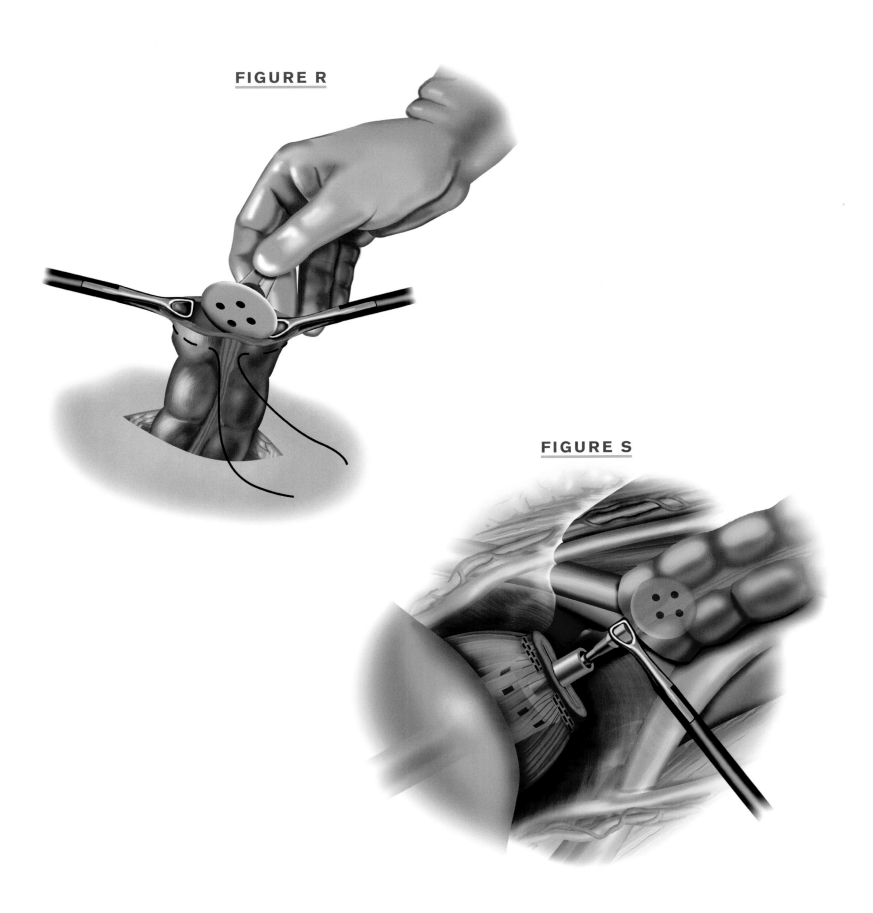

Abdominoperineal Resection

Preoperative Preparation

1. The same preparation as described for a left colectomy is performed.

Operating Room Setup and Port Placement

2. The same setup is used as described for a left colectomy.

3. The same technique and port positions as described for a left colectomy are used. The only variation is that the left lateral port should be placed at the intended position of the end-colostomy, which is usually in the left rectus muscle.

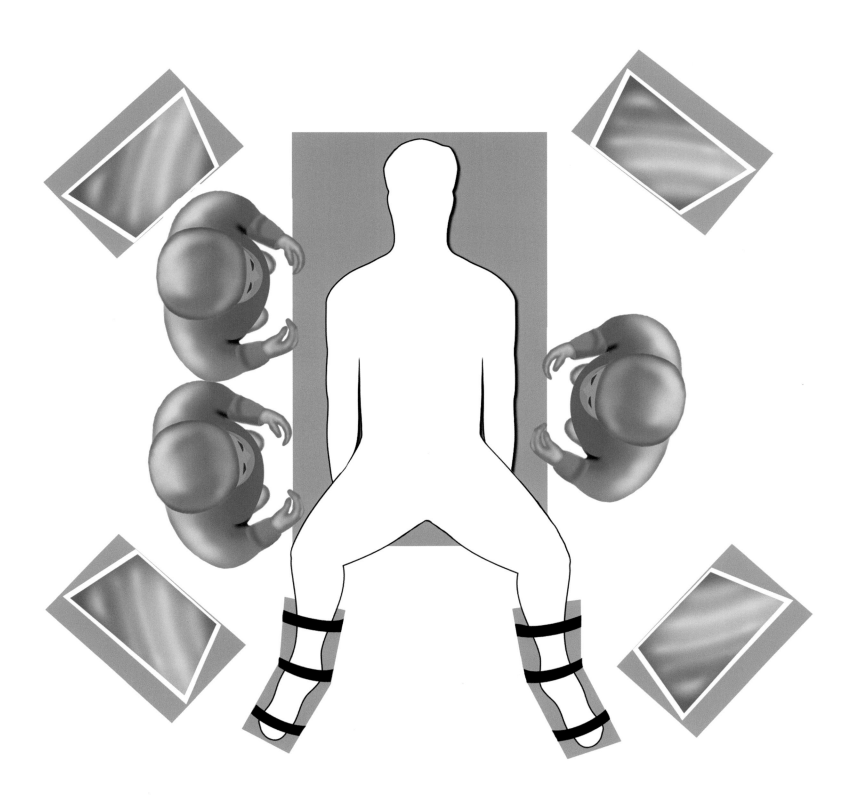

Mobilizing the Sigmoid and Left Colon and Colonic Transection

4. The sigmoid and descending colon are dissected and mobilized using a similar technique as described for a left colectomy. Careful attention must be directed toward avoiding ureteral injury.

5. The mesentery is divided as previously described. A medial to lateral approach can again be utilized.

6. Rectal dissection begins in the posterior avascular plane between the rectum and presacral fascia and continues as described for a low anterior resection.

7. The proposed area for proximal division of the colon is brought to the left lateral port site (colostomy site) to ensure a tension-free colostomy. The splenic flexure and transverse colon, if necessary, are mobilized as previously described to relieve any visible tension.

8. The bowel is then transected with a linear stapler (3.5–3.8 mm staples). Careful inspection of the abdominal and pelvic cavity is made to ensure hemostasis and assess for any inadvertent injury.

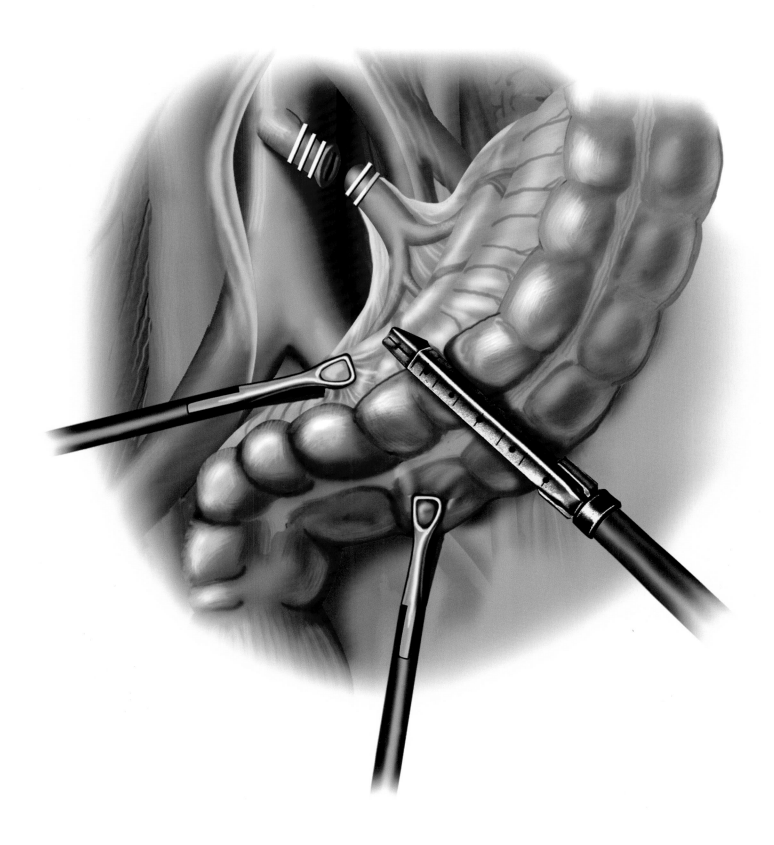

Creating the Colostomy and Perineal Dissection

9. The proximal end of the divided colon is brought out through the enlarged left lateral port site and the distal limb is retained in the abdomen.

10. The perineal dissection and stoma maturation can be performed simultaneously if a second surgeon is present. The specimen is retrieved through the perineal wound.

11. Drains are left in place either lateral to the perineal wound or through one of the port sites.

12. The perineal wound is closed in layers in the standard fashion. The fascial and skin incisions are closed in the usual manner.

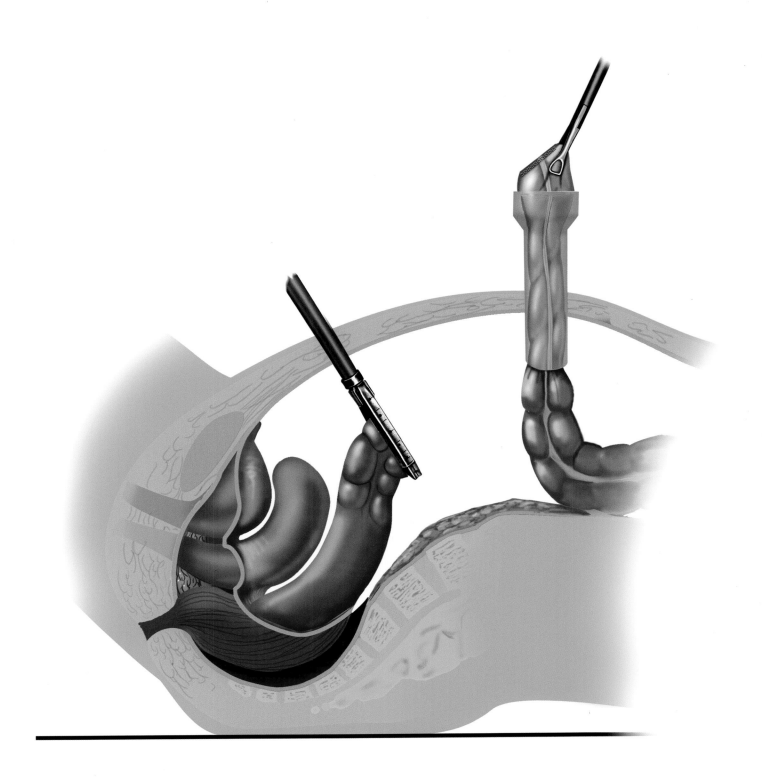

Postoperative Care

Pneumatic compression devices and subcutaneous heparin are continued postoperatively. Continued use of antibiotics is at the discretion of the surgeon. Patients are usually able to tolerate liquids within 24 to 72 hours after the operation.

Suggested Readings

1. Falk PM, Beart RW Jr, Wexner SD, et al. Laparoscopic colectomy: a critical appraisal. *Dis Colon Rectum*. 1993;36:28-34.

2. Fleshman JW, Fry RD, Birnbaum EH, Kodner IJ. Laparoscopicassisted and minilaparotomy approaches to colorectal diseases are similar in early outcome. *Dis Colon Rectum*. 1996;39:15-22.

3. Jones DB, Fleshman JW. Laparoscopic approaches to rectal cancer. In: Soper NJ, ed. *Problems in General Surgery*. Philadelphia: Lippincott-Raven Publishers; 1996;135-145.

4. Zucker KA, Pitcher DE, Martin DT, Ford RS. Laparoscopic-assisted colon resection. *Surg Endosc*. 1994;8:12-18.

Commentary

Jeffrey Marks, M.D., University Hospitals of Cleveland
Case Western Reserve University

Laparoscopic colorectal surgery is an advanced procedure requiring experienced two-handed laparoscopic skills, as well as an understanding of intra-abdominal anatomy. Although there are unique anatomical differences between the different types of surgical resections, all these procedures incorporate the use of tissue traction and retraction, alternative patient positioning, and the ability to be flexible in terms of port placement based on individual body habitus and prior abdominal surgeries. Patients must be explained the full risks, benefits, alternatives, and complications of this procedure, as well as the possibility for conversion, which should never be considered a complication, but rather a decision based on judgment for patient safety. The indications for laparoscopic colorectal surgery should be comparable to those for open surgery. Both benign and malignant diseases can be approached with laparoscopic techniques. Complex diverticular disease with associated abscess, however, has a very high rate of conversion and may be better approached with open technique. The same may be said for large bulky tumors. It is also important not to forget oncologic principles when performing laparoscopic colon surgery for cancer, including appropriate tissue margins, mesenteric resection, lymph node sampling, and wound protection to prevent trocar-site recurrences.

This chapter describes the use of a diamond shape for port setup and the use of lithotomy position. One advantage of lithotomy position is access to the anus for intraoperative colonoscopy if there is any need to reconfirm the site of needed resection. One must remember that tactile sensation is lost in laparoscopy, and the surgeon is therefore dependent on preoperative localization of the tumor. Preoperative marking with India ink or other tattooing substances are helpful to ensure appropriate resection margins.

As described in this chapter, additional techniques that can be utilized include the hand port. This can be very helpful in complex diverticular cases where tissue planes are better managed by finger fracture rather than sharp dissection. One consequence of placing a hand port is the possible obstruction in view that may occur if the port is not placed appropriately. Hand ports also provide wound protection for removal of malignant lesions. Numerous devices are available for mesenteric division, including harmonic scissors, clips, ligasure, and endoscopic staplers. The staplers will require a 12 mm port whereas the other instruments can be placed in a 5 mm port site.

Finally, the adoption of these techniques requires appropriate instrumentation and technical skills. It would be recommended to start with a less complex procedure such as a right hemicolectomy before considering advancing to more challenging surgery such as transverse colon resection or abdominal perineal resection. Requesting assistance of a more experienced peer can be beneficial, as well as having a low threshold for conversion if there is any question of anatomical variability, viscus injury, or extensive bleeding.

Steven D. Wexner, M.D., Cleveland Clinic Foundation Health Sciences Center University of South Florida

The colorectal section is a very useful introduction. While I agree with most of their principles, a few differences exist and will form the basis of my comments. For all of the sections, the authors are to be commended upon their use of ureteric catheters in inflammatory conditions. One generic comment that I would add is that I prefer an integrated operating room environment, which removes the laparoscopic carts from the floor of the operating room for better visualization.

For right colectomy, I fundamentally agree with the narrative. However, I do not feel that there is any role for a handassist port for right colectomy since, in general, these procedures can be completed through a single 5 cm incision without the need for the introduction of a hand. However, use of the hand port may be a useful "bridge" for teaching or learning laparoscopic-assisted colectomy. The second point is that I use two 12 mm left-sided ports, one in the left upper quadrant and one in the left lower quadrant, for dissection and a supraumbilical port for the camera. There are several alternative energy sources such as ultrasonic shears, the Enseal (SurgRx, Palo Alto, Calif), and the LigaSure (Tyco, Norwalk, Conn), which may be useful particularly for the dissection of the hepatic flexure. I routinely use a combination of the ultrasonic shears and the Enseal. I do not feel that intracorporeal division of the mesentery, and certainly not intracorporeal resection, has any advantage for right colectomy. In fact, I feel that these maneuvers add considerable time and expense. Generally, once intracorporeal mobilization of the entire right colon, terminal ileum, and right half of the transverse colon have been completed, even the most inflamed mesentery can be delivered through an approximately 5 cm supraumbilical incision appropriately protected during specimen extraction. The resection of the specimen, construction of the anastomosis, and, if desired, mesenteric defect closure, can all be extracorporeally performed. It is difficult for me to justify the additional time and expense of an intracorporeal procedure.

For left colectomy, once again, I agree with most of the steps as described by the authors. The fundamental difference is that whereas for right-sided lesions an intracorporeal resection seems hard to justify, for the left side, an extracorporeal resection, in my view, essentially equals a conversion. All left-sided resections should be accomplished with complete intracorporeal division of all vessels and of the distal portion of the resection (for example, the rectosigmoid junction). The proximal bowel can then be delivered through a small incision to allow placement of the circular stapler anvil and after reinsuflation, a transanal anastomosis can be performed. The fundamental difference is that while the superior mesenteric artery is mobile and thus allows the ileocolic arcade and right colic vessels to easily reach above the desufflated anterior abdominal wall, the aorta is not similarly mobile and in order to access the root of the superior mesenteric artery and similarly the root of the superior mesenteric vein near the duodenum, a 6 cm to 8 cm incision may not be sufficient, particularly in an obese patient with an inflamed mesentery (for example, diverticulitis).

For low anterior resection and abdominoperineal resection, the artist's rendition does not justify the potentially difficult technique that can be encountered in the narrow male pelvis. While Dr. Jones et al are expert at this dissection, the novice is to be cautioned that good retraction is imperative. In these instances, several additional ports are necessary. For all left-sided resections, I prefer a 12 mm right upper quadrant port, a 12 mm right paraumbilical port, and a 12 mm infraumbilical camera port. For pelvic retraction, contralateral left-sided ports may be added. I generally prefer extracorporealization of the proximal end of the bowel for anvil insertion through a suprapubic Pfannenstiel-type incision ranging from 3 cm to 5 cm in length.

Morris E. Franklin Jr., M.D., Texas Endosurgery Institute

I would reinforce the use of sequential compression devices and some mechanism and/or set of devices to prevent an intraoperative drop in the patient's body core temperature, both of which are extremely helpful. I believe that colonoscopy should be available for each and every case to help localize the lesion and/or test the anastomosis. Furthermore, we also recommend having the ultrasound device in the operating room to check the liver for possible metastatic disease. As far as the ports are concerned, we also use 5 mm ports in the umbilicus with the new, better cameras being available, and use a 5 mm port at the subxiphoid area, as this tends to facilitate dissection. An additional port in the left upper quadrant many times will allow mobilization around a particularly large transverse colon.

Our first maneuver is to identify the location of the lesion. If it has not been primarily tattooed or its location confirmed by barium enema, we may do an on-the-table colonoscopy in this situation. We usually mobilize the colon prior to this as well as isolate the vessels. We currently are utilizing a primarily medial to lateral approach, identifying and isolating the blood vessels first. This is initiated by identifying the duodenum and its retroperitoneal structure, as we feel this is the key structure to identify in right colon resections. The reason for this is that if the duodenum is identified and isolated in its retroperitoneal position, the first structure inferiorly is always the ileocolic artery and the first structure cephalad, unless there is a gross anomaly, is the right colic artery. This facilitates identification of these structures considerably.

We take great care in, and near, the hepatic flexure to ensure that the correct plane is dissected to avoid duodenal and common bile duct injury. Additionally, if there has been previous surgery in this area, the omental attachments may be particularly problematic, and one must have the ability to go lateral to medial, as well as medial to lateral, in this instance.

If the malignancy is near the distal descending colon or the hepatic flexure, we also take a generous portion of the omentum, taking this down from the gastric side as opposed to leaving a tremendous amount of omentum.

When dealing with cancer, the vessels should be taken very near the origin from the superior mesenteric artery. Therefore, the superior mesenteric artery and the immediate takeoff of the branches must be identified in that area. This is best approached with a medial to lateral dissection. We also tend to use the LigaSure device, in place of the clips and/or harmonic scalpel, as we find this greatly speeds up the process and provides a more adequate seal of the vessel.

When constructing an extracorporeal anastomosis, care must be taken to avoid rotating the small bowel and/or large bowel, which results in disorientation of the anastomosis. This can frequently be done by placing a suture intracorporeally on the two segments that are to be anastomosed prior to bringing it to the outside. This will ensure proper orientation.

As far as an intracorporeal resection and anastomosis is concerned, we place the specimen in a retrieval bag, which is then placed over the liver. This allows us to construct the anastomosis and then make a convenient muscle-splitting incision in the right lower quadrant to extract the specimen, which seems to offer some protection from postoperative pain. We also, as far as the intracorporeal anastomosis is concerned, like to use smaller trocars, and have found that the US Surgical 60 mm Endo-GIA works very well.

For mobilizing the sigmoid and left colon, we now go almost entirely from medial to lateral, leaving the specimen and the colon attached to its embryological peritoneal attachments and isolate the vessels preserving the parasympathetic nerves, which, I feel, must be identified in each case.

As far as mobilizing the splenic flexure, we will approach this from two directions. One is as described, going up the left gutter. On the other hand, we can also extend the retroperitoneal dissection going from medial to lateral to the left gutter and above Gerota's fascia to the splenic flexure. We take down the omentum first after the retroperitoneal dissection, which helps facilitate tremendously this splenic flexure mobilization.

If the patient is undergoing a colon resection for diverticulitis, care must be taken to be sure that the distal bowel transection is below the sacral promontory to allow complete removal of all diverticula. If one goes below the sacral promontory, constructing an extracorporeal anastomosis is many times extremely difficult. In this case, an intracorporeal or, at least, partially intracorporeal anastomosis utilizing an EEA stapling device, is the most convenient procedure. The specimen may be removed transanally if the distal colon is left open after confirmation of a clean colon and lavage of the colon with Betadine.

I feel strongly that anal access must be present by placing the buttocks over the edge of the table to ensure adequate placement of the EEA device. We also feel that taping the shoulders helps prevent the patient from shifting on the table while in steep Trendelenburg and/or airplane maneuvers.

For mobilizing the sigmoid colon, we again start medially just below the inferior mesenteric artery and extend our initial dissection into the pelvis, which allows for rapid dissection essentially down to the levators and adequate preservation of the parasympathetic nerves. This opens the plane quite adequately to perform lateral dissection on each side, saving the anterior dissection for last.

For the rectal dissection per se, an additional nice trick, if a female patient has a residual uterus, is to suspend the uterus with transantral sutures utilizing Keith needles inserted on each side of the midline and passing the suture around the ligaments and body of the uterus. This works very well to suspend the uterus completely out of the way.

As far as resection and anastomosis is concerned, it is imperative that the exact location of a rectal tumor be established, either by digital examination or preferably by proctoscopy and/or intraoperative colonoscopy, as this will allow more accurate distal-margin determination than palpation or guessing. We have found that one rarely needs more than a 4 cm to 5 cm incision for a laparoscopically assisted procedure and that a muscle-splitting incision in the left lower quadrant seems to be adequate. We feel that the anus should be dilated to two fingerbreadths to prevent the stapler from entering the anal muscles and result in prolonged anal dysfunction.

An additional comment that I have with regard to abdominoperineal resections is to complete the entire rectal dissection down to the levators, laterally and anteriorly prior to division of the colon. Division of the colon and construction of the colostomy can be done very easily after the rectum is completely mobilized, and having the colon attached may add retraction advantages of the rectum. The dissection plane is incredibly important to be stressed here, starting posteriorly, working laterally, and staying well below the seminal vesicles as the dissection proceeds.

James W. Fleshman, M.D., Barnes-Jewish Hospital
Washington University School of Medicine

Laparoscopic Colectomy

Techniques for laparoscopic surgery for colorectal cancer require anatomic dissection with resection of the specimen based on vascular supply and lymphatic drainage. Laparoscopic surgery is especially aligned to making this possible when anatomic planes and well-defined anatomic landmarks are used to accomplish the operation. The atlas has provided the basics for this with a starting point for the procedure and definite steps throughout the description of the procedure.

The description of the right colectomy is excellent. The setup and trocars as described are essentially the same as in my practice. There are four approaches to performing a right colectomy laparoscopically. The posterior caudad to cephalad approach and as described in the atlas, medial to lateral approach, lateral to medial approach, and cephalad to caudad approach. Anatomic landmarks are the keys to understanding each of these approaches and fortunately are the same for each approach. The landmarks are obtained at different points in the approach. The posterior approach as described in the atlas requires incision over the iliac artery all the way up to the duodenum along the mesentery fusion plane of the small bowel to the retroperitoneum. Retroperitoneal dissection over the ureter, gonadals, duodenum, and kidney to the hepatic flexure ligament is the second step in the procedure. Vascular pedicle identification with the cecum suspended to the right lower quadrant allows the ileocolic to be stretched across the field of the view in the laparoscope to expose two windows on either side of the ileocolic vessels as Dr. Jones has demonstrated. One must remember that there is the possibility of a right colic artery more proximal on the superior mesenteric artery and should always look for a second artery at the upper extent of the more cephalad window above the ileocolic vessel. It is important sometimes to take the right branch of the middle colic vessel at the pancreas head during the dissection to allow the transverse colon to reach the anterior abdominal wall for the extracorporeal anastomosis. Releasing the hepatic flexure is a sometimes treacherous procedure since heat from any electrocautery can be transmitted down to the head of the pancreas and the sweep of the duodenum. Use of non monopolar energy sources such as radiofrequency or bipolar or ultrasound should eliminate some of the issues of heat distribution and possible duodenal damage.

The approach described in the atlas is the lateral to medial approach to a left colectomy. There is also a medial to lateral and cephalad to caudad approach for the left colectomy. It is important for surgeons dealing with all aspects of colorectal disease to be able to perform each of these approaches through a laparoscopic technique and, to be able to accommodate individual patient's needs during complex operations. The key anatomic features involved in a left colectomy are the inferior mesenteric artery at the aortic bifurcation, the avascular plane at the sacropromontory, which is the starting point for the medial to lateral approach, the ureter over the left iliac at the bifurcation of the external and internal iliac, inferior mesenteric vein (IMV) at the ligament of Treitz where there is a window between the inferior mesenteric artery and aorta and the IMV runs diagonally over the window. The splenic flexure has several attachments of the colon to Gerota's fascia posteriorly and laterally, and there are attachments of the splenic flexure to mesentery to the tail of the pancreas. Occasionally there is a vessel in the mesentery of the splenic flexure, which runs from the splenic artery to the left ascending branch known as the arc of Riolan. This is an arterial supply that provides collateral blood flow and will need to be managed in those individuals because it restricts mobility of the splenic flexure to the pelvis. The window into the lesser sac from the left lateral aspect is identified with the splenic flexure pulled medially. The pancreas is located posteriorly and the omentum is overlying as the roof of the lesser sac. The window can be entered lateral and cephalad to the splenic flexure of the colon and the posterior aspect of the stomach view. This begins the dissection of the mesentery toward the midline. The final unroofing of the lesser sac is performed by freeing the omentum from the anterior surface of the transverse colon. For a left colectomy, the extraction site is most convenient at the suprapubic incision, which can be either a Pfannenstiel or a vertical midline for placement of either a hand-port access site or a wound protector.

The Low Anterior Resection and Abdominal Perineal Resection

The dissection for cancer in the rectum must follow the avascular plane to provide complete mesentery dissection to 5 cm below the distal edge of the tumor or a complete total mesorectal excision for mid- and low-rectal cancer. The position that is most advantageous for the dissection is steep Trendelenburg without airplaning the patient to either side to keep the planes clear and provide improved spatial-relationship awareness to the surgeon. This is a circular motion dissection with a cylinder of fat and rectum within a half circle of bone and muscle in the pelvis. It is important to use a pinpoint dissecting tool, such as a hook cautery with suction, to remove smoke plumes. This form of sharp dissection in the avascular areolar tissue plane is most effective. Waldeyer's fascia must be divided at the lower portion of the sacrum to enter the lower pelvis below the coccyx and this allows the pelvic floor muscles to be seen to indicate the most distal aspect of the pelvic dissection. Other areas of danger to be avoided during the dissection include the splenic nerves at the pelvic rim running along the side of the pelvis, which control bladder and genital function, the ureters along the side wall running down toward the base of the bladder, seminal vesicles and prostate, or vagina and uterine vessels anteriorly. In a male with a posteriorly placed rectal cancer, it is important to keep the dissection behind the Denonvilliers' fascia to avoid damage to nerves and vas deferens. It has been helpful to use a 10 mm Babcock or a hand through a suprapubic hand, access port to retract the rectum back and forth and provide tension during the dissection. Laparoscopic approaches to rectal cancer are not standard of care as yet and a randomized controlled trial is being considered by the American College of Surgeons Oncology Group.

I want to congratulate Dr. Jones on an excellent atlas and thank him for the opportunity to comment on the use of laparoscopic techniques and his description of them in the atlas.

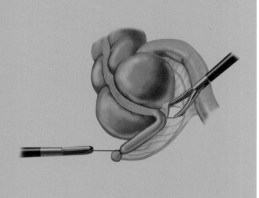

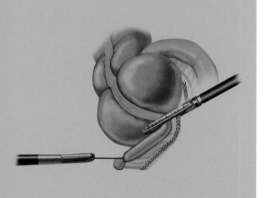

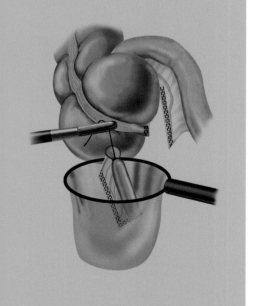

Laparoscopic Appendectomy

Laparoscopic appendectomy allows for a more thorough abdominal exploration than traditional open appendectomy though a McBurney's incision. Controversy abounds as to whether the benefits of laparoscopic surgery are worth the added costs since most patients generally tolerate the traditional approach very well. Proponents cite reduced postoperative pain, shorter hospital stays, better cosmesis, and an earlier return to work. Moreover, the laparoscopic approach may be most advantageous in patients with a questionable diagnosis, female patients with suspected gynecologic pathology, and obese patients.

Preoperative Preparation

1. Sequential compression devices and subcutaneously administered heparin may be used for prophylaxis against deep venous thrombosis. Antibiotic coverage should include gram-positive (particularly *Enterococcus*), gram-negative, as well as anaerobic organisms. The bladder should be emptied as to avoid having to place a urinary catheter during the operation.

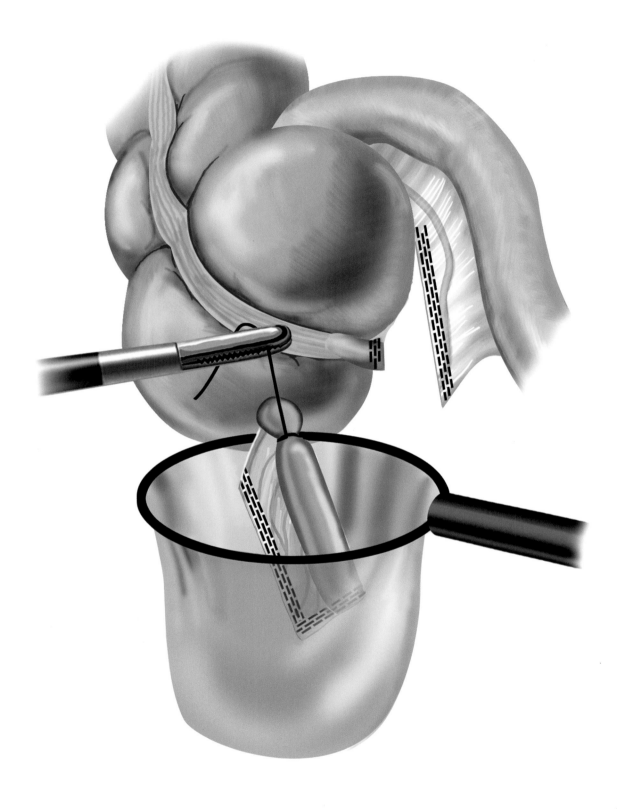

Operating Room Setup

2. The patient is positioned supine with arms tucked. If gynecologic pathology is suspected, the patient may be placed in lithotomy position to allow for use of a cervical manipulation device.

3. The surgeon and assistant stand to the patient's left; the assistant operates the camera.

4. The video monitor is arranged as shown.

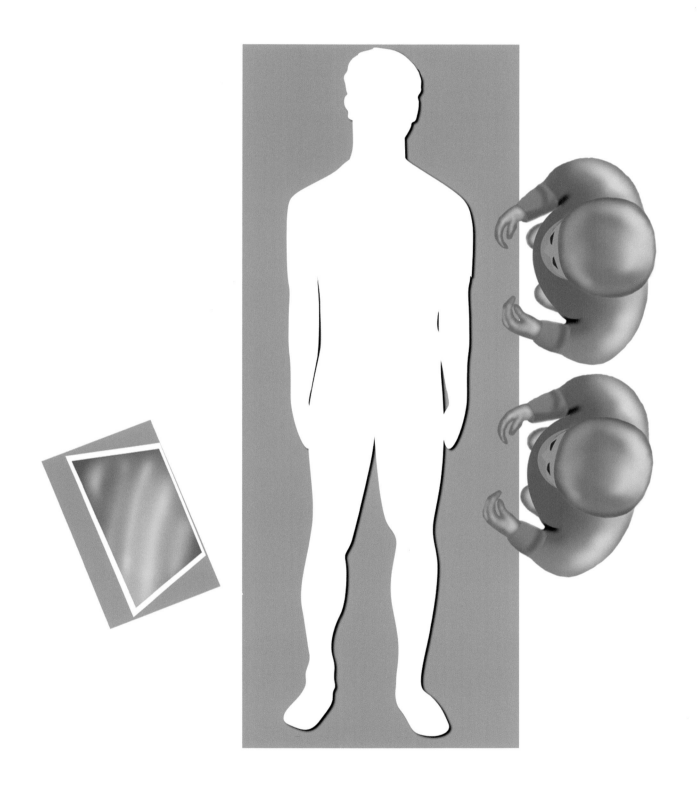

Access and Port Placement

5. Access is generally obtained via an open infraumbilical incision. A 10/12 mm Hasson port is placed under direct vision and pneumoperitoneum is established to a maximum pressure limit of 15 mm Hg. A closed-entry technique may be favored in obese patients.

6. A careful laparoscopic exploration is performed to ensure that no injury occurred during port insertion and that no other abnormalities are present. Although either a straight or 30° angled laparoscope may be used, the angled lens is preferred as it facilitates obtaining crucial images during the operation.

7. A 10/12 mm trocar is then placed under direct vision through an oblique incision in the left lower quadrant. Care is taken to avoid inadvertent injury to the inferior epigastric vessels.

8. Next, a 5 mm port is placed in the midline suprapubic area. Occasionally, another 5 mm port is necessary in either the right lower and/or right upper quadrant to better facilitate adequate dissection and exposure.

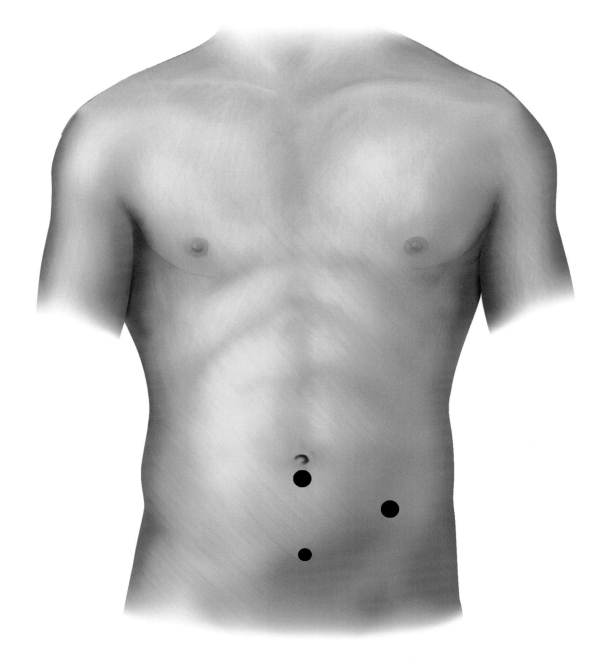

FIGURE C

Exposure and Dissection

9. After a thorough visual exploration of the abdomen, the patient is placed in Trendelenburg position and rotated left to enhance visualization of the right lower quadrant. The appendix is located by following the taeniae of the right colon/cecum to their convergence. Occasionally, the lateral peritoneal attachments to the cecum will need to be divided in order to expose a retrocecal appendix. Adhesions to the appendix are divided to facilitate full mobilization.

10. Atraumatic bowel clamps are used to manipulate the bowel. The appendix itself may also be directly manipulated, however, in the case of a severely inflamed and friable appendix, a loop ligature may be placed to facilitate gentle traction.

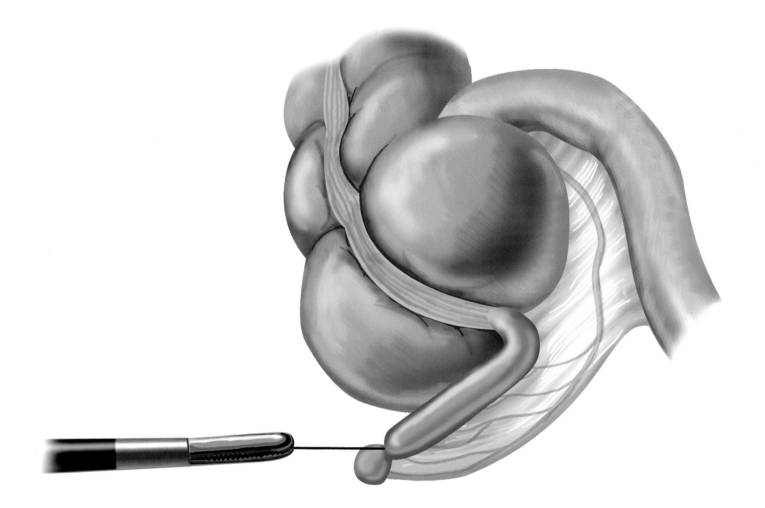

Dividing the Mesoappendix

11. With the mesoappendix under tension, a window is created bluntly near the appendiceal base (Figure D).

12. The mesoappendix, including the appendiceal artery and its branches, are then divided. This maneuver may be performed using bipolar cautery, ultrasonic coagulation, endoscopic clips (Figure E), or an endoscopic GIA stapling device loaded with 2.5 mm staples (Figure F). Multiple firings of the stapler may be required.

13. It is not recommended to staple and divide the mesoappendix and appendiceal base itself with one maneuver, unless the mesoappendix is severely inflamed and thickened, for which 3.5 mm staples may be preferred.

FIGURE D

FIGURE E

FIGURE F

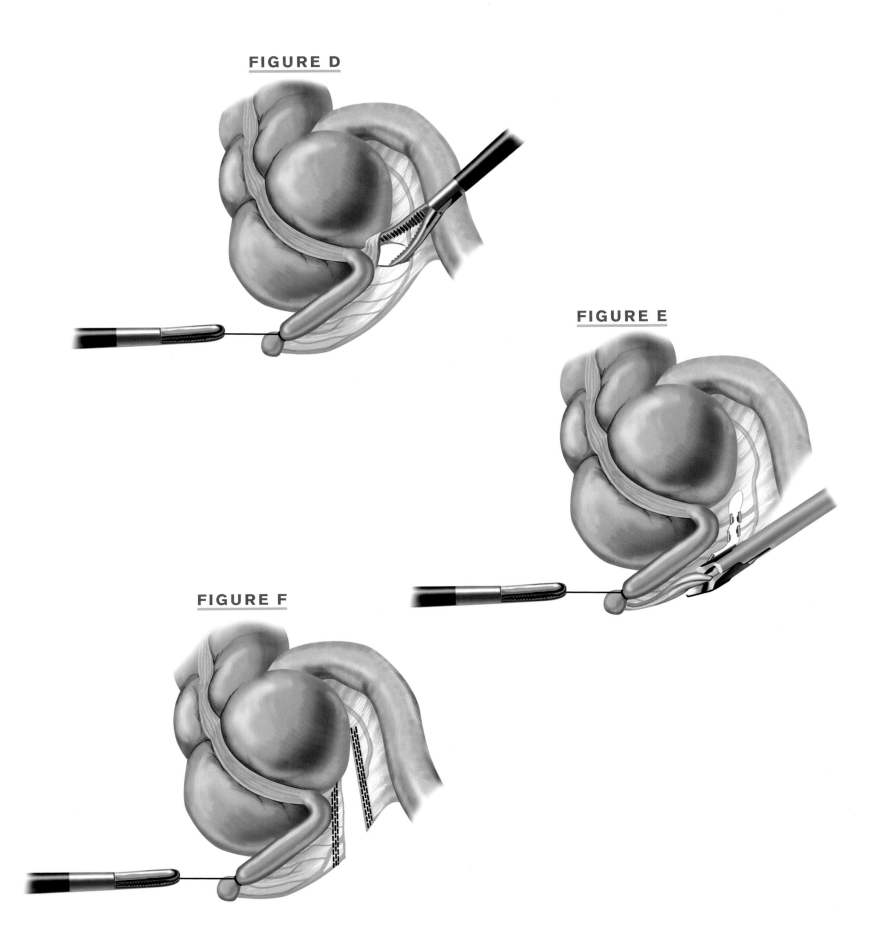

Dividing the Appendix

14. The appendix can be sharply divided in between two pretied loop ligatures placed at the appendiceal base (Figure G). For an inflamed base, two ties should be placed on the retained appendiceal stump.

15. Alternatively, a second firing of an endoscopic GIA stapling device (3.5–3.8 mm staples) can be used to divide the appendix at its base (Figure H). If the appendiceal base is necrotic, the stapler should be fired across the base of the appendix at the level of the cecum in order to incorporate healthy tissue in the staple line. Care must be taken to avoid narrowing the ileocecal junction.

16. If endoloops are used to divide the appendix, brief electrocautery may be applied to the appendiceal stump to prevent a mucocele, however, this practice introduces the risk of injury and is not necessary.

FIGURE G

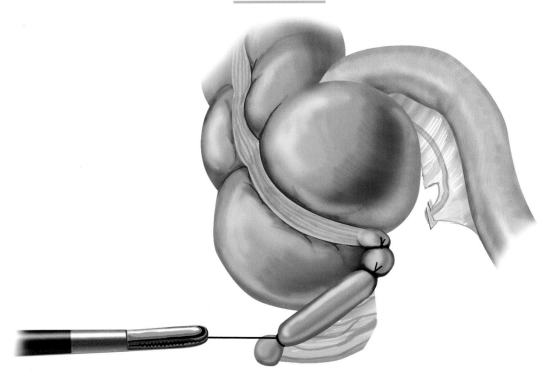

FIGURE H

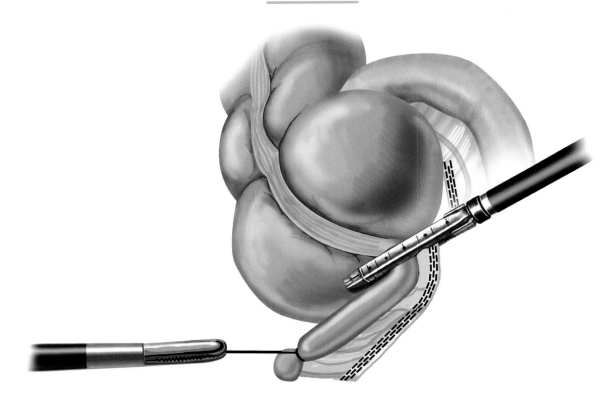

Removing the Appendix

17. The appendix can be removed through a 10/12 mm trocar directly (Figure I) or may be placed in a specimen retrieval bag (Figure J). A sac is recommended, especially if the appendix is purulent, fragmented, perforated, or suspected to harbor malignancy.

18. The patient is then placed in reverse Trendelenburg position and contaminated areas of the abdominal cavity are copiously irrigated. The cecum and ileum are carefully inspected for any inadvertent injury or bleeding. Trocars are removed under direct visualization.

19. The fascial incisions are closed in the usual manner and the skin incisions are closed with a subcuticular 4-0 absorbable suture.

FIGURE I

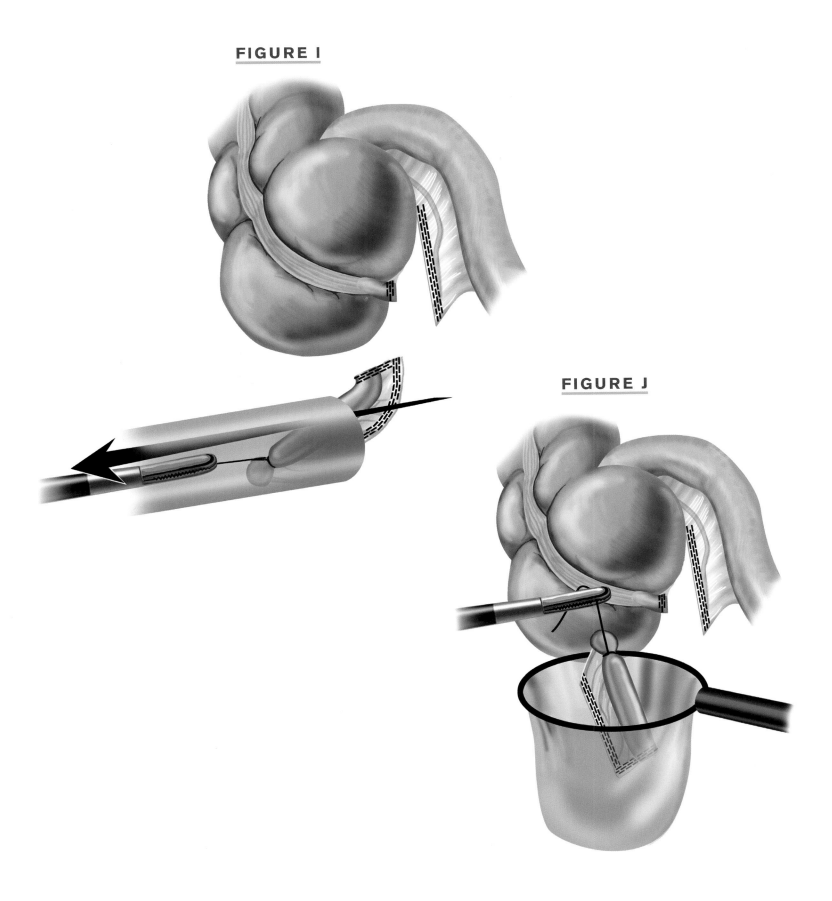

FIGURE J

Postoperative Care

Pneumatic compression devices and/or subcutaneous heparin are continued postoperatively. Continued use of antibiotics is at the discretion of the surgeon, depending on the status of the appendix at the time of operation. Patients are usually able to tolerate liquids and solid food within 24 hours after the operation.

Suggested Readings

1. Long KH, Bannon MP, Zietlow SP, et al. A prospective randomized comparison of laparoscopic appendectomy with open appendectomy: clinical and economic analyses. *Surgery*. 2001;129(4):390-400.

2. Martin LC, Puente I, Sosa JL, et al. Open versus laparoscopic appendectomy. A prospective randomized comparison. *Ann Surg*. 1995;222(3):256-262.

3. Laparoscopic versus open surgery for suspected appendicitis. *Cochrane Database of Syst Rev*. 2004;18(4):CD001546.

Commentary

Ronit Grinbaum, M.D., Beth Israel Deaconess Medical Center Harvard Medical School

Appendectomy has been the treatment of choice for acute appendicitis for more than 100 years since its introduction by McBurney in 1894. Semm was the first to describe laparoscopic appendectomy in 1983, inciting controversy that has since quieted but not disappeared. The laparoscopic approach slowly gained acceptance, because its advantages were not as obvious as laparoscopic cholecystectomy. However 22 years later, data accumulate as to the superiority of the laparoscopic approach in terms of a quicker and less painful recovery, less postoperative complications, and better cosmesis.

Laparoscopy per se may be used as a valuable diagnostic tool, reducing the frequency of unnecessary appendectomies, allowing superior visualization of the abdomen and pelvis. Studies over the last 20 years have shown laparoscopic appendectomy to be safe, successful, and recommended in the clinical setting of both simple and complicated appendicitis.

At the Hadassah University Medical Center in Jerusalem, we favor the use of endoscopic ligature, ultrasonic coagulation, or endoscopic clips for dividing the mesoappendix, allowing us to reduce costs. By sharply dividing the appendix in between pretied endoloops, we reserve the use of endoscopic GIA staplers for the more gangrenous appendicitis with severely inflamed appendiceal base or thickened inflamed mesoappendix.

Open appendectomy is sometimes advocated by some surgeons in the setting of young thin men, because of its simplicity, lower operative time, and lower operating room costs. We employ laparoscopy in young females, obese patients, or in cases of diagnostic uncertainty.

Fred Brody, M.D., M.B.A. George Washington University Medical Center

Appendectomy is one of the four most common procedures performed by general surgeons. Based on the ubiquitous nature of this procedure, there are multiple techniques to accomplish this task. The authors provide a concise assessment of the preoperative workup. We catheterize every woman due to the possibility of gynecological pathology. This is especially true of young females of child-bearing age. On the other hand, older men have the propensity for benign prostatic hypertrophy. Due to the presence of this pathology, each man should urinate before the procedure to avoid catheterization. We only catheterize men when the patient does not have a definitive diagnosis.

We utilize a Hasson at the umbilicus and two 5-mm ports in the lower abdomen. For women, the two 5-mm ports are placed along the bikini line. The first port does not have to be located in the suprapubic midline. But both ports can be placed along the bikini line within the left lower quadrant. Regardless of the definitive placement, the working ports and the appendiceal pathology should form an isosceles triangle to facilitate the dissection. Obviously, a 5-mm videoscope is necessary if staplers and this type of setup are used.

The authors discuss several techniques for dividing the mesoappendix. An alternative method includes stapling the mesoappendix without performing the window adjacent to the appendiceal lumen. Several surgeons at our institution apply a 2.5 mm endovascular stapler without dissecting a window. After the stapler is placed across the mesoappendix, the ileum should be inspected prior to deploying the stapler. Similarly, the cecum should be excluded from the gastrointestinal stapler. However, a portion of the cecum can be included in the specimen if the base of the appendix is perforated or severely inflamed. We currently do not oversew the appendiceal stump or cauterize the mucosa after using a stapler. The appendix can be brought into the port site and removed directly at the end of the procedure. If the specimen is removed without a bag, the port site should be irrigated copiously prior to closure. Alternatively, a specimen bag can be inserted through the Hasson trocar. We concur with perioperative antibiotics and the majority of patients are discharged within 28 to 48 hours.

In summary, this chapter reviews the prevailing techniques utilized by most surgeons for a laparoscopic appendectomy. Due to the incidence of this disease, several variants are available and this chapter manages to concisely review the prevailing techniques. These techniques will continue to change with the evolution of endoluminal therapies.

Craig G. Chang, M.D.
Citizens Medical Center

Although laparoscopic appendectomy is a commonly performed operation in private practice, there are several nuances that deserve mention. First, the clinical situation may make the laparoscopic approach more or less favorable. In the past, open appendectomy for perforated or gangrenous appendicitis (with or without abscess) was followed by a long recovery secondary to wound complications. Many wounds became infected or granulated over long periods. The laparoscopic approach is associated with significantly less wound morbidity. Wound infections are uncommon if the specimen is removed in a specimen bag and cosmesis is substantially better. However, laparoscopic appendectomy tends to be harder to perform in the face of active infection. Tissue planes are difficult to identify thus increasing the chance of injury to surrounding structures. Inflamed tissues are friable and handle less easily. Notwithstanding, the laparoscopic approach can be used in most cases of appendicitis.

Second, port size and placement may substantially affect the ease of the procedure. Alternative port configurations include using a dilating 10/12 mm port placed above the umbilicus and two 5 mm ports placed in the lower midline. This configuration avoids injury to the inferior epigastric vessels but requires a high-quality angled laparoscope. Since the supraumbilical port is further away from the appendix, this also allows easier insertion of the stapler (if used) into the abdomen. This configuration is not conducive for intracorporeal knot tying as the ports are too close. If suturing is anticipated, an additional 5 mm port in the right midclavicular line can be added. None of the fascial defects are closed unless they are enlarged to allow specimen removal.

Third, a necrotic appendiceal base is challenging even with an open approach. If there is significant inflammation around the cecum, closure of the stump may be difficult. Laparoscopically, the surgeon has a few choices. A portion of the cecum can be excised with a stapler. Alternately, large, full-thickness sutures can be placed across the stump defect. An omental patch closure ("Graham patch") provides yet another option. Suturing in this situation requires great care to avoid tearing inflamed tissues.